中医中文：文法与词汇 中医中文：文法与词汇 中
医中文：文法与词汇 中医中文：文法与词汇 中医
中文：文法与词汇 中医中文：文法与词汇 中医中
文：文法与词汇 中医中文：文法与词汇 中医中文
：文法与词汇 中医中文：文法与词汇 中医中文：
文法与词汇 中医中文：文法与词汇 中医中文：文

中医中文：文法与词汇

ZHŌNG-YĪ ZHŌNG-WÉN: WÉN-FǍ YǓ CÍ-HUÌ

Chinese Medical Chinese:
Grammar and Vocabulary

Nigel Wiseman (魏迺杰)

冯　晔 (Féng Yè)

中醫中文：文法與詞彙 中醫中文：文法與詞彙 中
醫中文：文法與詞彙 中醫中文：文法與詞彙 中醫
中文：文法與詞彙 中醫中文：文法與詞彙 中醫中
文：文法與詞彙 中醫中文：文法與詞彙 中醫中文
：文法與詞彙 中醫中文：文法與詞彙 中醫中文：
文法與詞彙 中醫中文：文法與詞彙 中醫中文：文
法與詞彙 中醫中文：文法與詞彙 中醫中文：文法
與詞彙 中醫中文：文法與詞彙 中醫中文：文法與

PARADIGM PUBLICATIONS　　2002　　BROOKLINE, MASSACHUSETTS

Chinese Medical Chinese: Grammar and Vocabulary

Zhōngyī Zhōngwén: Wénfǎ yǔ Cíhuì

中医中文：文法与词汇

Nigel Wiseman （魏迺杰） & 馮曄 (Féng Yè)

Copyright © 2002 Paradigm Publiations

44 Linden Street

Brookline, MA 02445 USA

www.paradigm-pubs.com

Library of Congress Cataloging-in-Publication Data

Wiseman, Nigel.
  Chinese Medical Chinese: grammar and vocabulary / Nigel Wiseman, Feng Ye
p.   cm.
Includes index.
Text in English and Chinese, with Pinyin.
ISBN 0-912111-65-8
1. Medicine, Chinese–Dictionaries. 2. Chinese Language–Dictionaries–English. I.
Feng, Ye, 1967-II. Title
[DNLM: Medicine, Chinese Traditional W 15 W814i 200]
R121 .W5347 2000
610'.951'03–dc21

                                                                    00-052436

Council of Oriental Medical Publishers (C.O.M.P.) Designation: Original document. English terminology from Wiseman N., 英汉汉英中医词典 *English-Chinese Chinese-Dictionary of Chinese Medicine*, Húnán Science and Technology Press, Chángshā, 1995.

Library of Congress Number: 00-52436
International Standard Book Number (ISBN): 0-912111-65-8
Printed in the United States of America

Contents

自序
Preface

Given the absence of a systematic approach to the westward transmission of Chinese medicine, and the paucity of texts translated from Chinese using a consistent terminology, the Western student unable to read primary Chinese literature has only limited access to Chinese medical knowledge, and therefore has much to gain by learning Chinese. This is not as daunting a task as is often thought. By narrowing the scope of study to Chinese medical texts, the task is made considerably easier. In the past, it took students over a year of intensive study of general and medical Chinese to approach Chinese medical texts. Since the terminology of Chinese medicine, especially in modern literature, rests largely on little more than a thousand characters, a focused approach to vocabulary learning should be able to reduce this even further.

This book assumes a knowledge of how Chinese characters are composed, how they are written by hand, and how they are pronounced. Anyone who has this basic knowledge of Chinese can tackle this book. Those lacking this basic knowledge can consult our *Chinese Medical Chinese: Characters*.

Part I describes the basic features of the literary language of Chinese medicine and its relationship to the language of the classical period and to the modern vernacular of northern China, Mandarin. It explains many grammatical constructions commonly encountered in Chinese medical texts and describes the buildup of Chinese medical terms in detail.

Part II breaks down the terminology of Chinese medicine into its component characters. The characters are introduced in lists according to subject matter, together with their Pīnyīn pronunciation and English equivalents (Kenyon and Knott transcription of English renderings is also given for the benefit of non-English-speaking learners). The lists are followed by examples of compound terms using only characters so far introduced. The examples are followed by drills that test the student on vocabulary items. The answers to questions are given at the end of the book.

Considerable space has been devoted to the explanation of terms. Until now, the English-language literature of Chinese medicine has been greatly marred by the absence of a standardized terminology that faithfully reflects the Chinese concepts. In the present text, we explain terms in relation to the concepts they denote, and in many cases explain the choice of the English terms used in this book. We hope that this will contribute to a greater awareness of terminological and translation issues, so that a well-chosen terminology may gradually be adopted by the English-speaking community of Chinese medicine as a whole.

Students wishing to find out more about Chinese medical terms and concepts can consult *A Practical Dictionary of Chinese Medicine*, by Wiseman N and Féng Y. Those who require a basic textbook of Chinese medicine applying the same terminology are recommended to use *Fundamentals of Chinese Medicine*, Wiseman N & Ellis A (Revised Edition 1994). Those interested in learning classical Chinese may appreciate the language study material contained in Appendix II of *Shāng Hán Lùn* (*On Cold Damage*): *Translation and Commentaries* by Mitchell, Féng, and Wiseman. All three titles are published by Paradigm Publications.

An English-Pīnyīn-Chinese and Pīnyīn-Chinese-English index of all single characters contained in the book provides access to the basic elements of the terminology.

It is hoped that the suitably prepared student, by working through the book systematically and doing each of the exercises, will gain the ability to approach a broad range of Chinese medical texts.

Thanks go to Thomas Dey and Frances Turner for proofreading and comments.

第一篇：文法
Part I: Grammar

1. Introduction

This part of the book aims to acquaint the English-speaking reader with the grammar of Chinese medical Chinese. It explains certain general features of the Chinese language and outlines basic patterns in the structure of Chinese medical terms. It is designed for students who have a basic knowledge of the construction of Chinese characters. However, the introductory material in particular should be of interest to any prospective learner of Chinese. Anyone wishing to learn 'Chinese medical Chinese' who is a complete newcomer to the Chinese language should study *Learn to Read Chinese* by Paul U. Unschuld.[1]

The following pages briefly sketch the main features of the language of Chinese medicine that concern students wishing to read modern texts. Even today, the language of Chinese medicine is essentially *literary Chinese* (文言文 *wén yán wén*), which has its roots in *classical Chinese* (古文 *gǔ wén*). Classical Chinese is the written language of antiquity and differs from the modern language in many ways, despite many similarities. Students wishing to know more about Chinese can consult the literature that provided an invaluable source in writing the present part of this book.[2]

---

[1]Unschuld, P.U., *Learn to Read Chinese*, Paradigm Publications, Brookline MA, 1994.

[2]For example, Norman, J., *Chinese*, Cambridge University Press, Cambridge UK, 1988; and Ramsey S.R., *The Languages of China*, Princeton University Press, Princeton NJ, 1987.

Classical Chinese was the written form of Old Chinese (古汉语 *gǔ hàn yǔ*), the modern linguistic term for the spoken language of China from the end of the Spring and Autumn Period to the end of the Hàn dynasty. This is the language of the early philosophers of China—Confucius, Mencius, and Laozi. Classical Chinese is believed to have reflected the spoken language of the times, though it probably differed from it just as written English differs from our spoken language. Classical Chinese was essentially monosyllabic; each word was a single syllable, written with a single character, and probably pronounced in a distinct tone.[3] It was virtually uninflected in the way European languages are, that is, words were not modified to indicate, say, the person or tense of verbs or plurality of nouns as in the English distinctions between 'want', 'wants', and 'wanted' or between 'dog' and 'dogs'.[4]

The spoken language underwent certain changes after the Hàn dynasty. It came to make increasing use of noun suffixes, noun compounds, and verb compounds—a development undoubtedly attributable to phonological attrition (reduction in the number of sounds) on the one hand, and to expanding vocabulary needs that were naturally met by compounding on the other. The spoken language also underwent changes in word-order, such as the shift of instrumental adverbials to before the verb. Furthermore, it developed measure words, resultative verbs, and verb aspects, and, of course, underwent changes in vocabulary. Since the classical language continued to be the standard for formal writing, these changes have been difficult to chart. Historical linguists tell us that when new features in the language started to occur frequently in written texts, they were probably already much more prevalent in the spoken language. For example, when the classical demonstrative 是 *shì* began to appear frequently as a copulative verb (like the English 'to be') as an optional alternative to classical construction that used no copulative verb, it is presumed that the Old Chinese construction had already been replaced by 是 in the spoken language and that its continuing appearance in written texts was merely a literary convention. Although classical Chinese ceased to reflect the spoken language two thousand years ago, it remained a standard for literary Chinese up to the beginning of this century, much as Latin remained the written language of Europe for centuries after it ceased to be anyone's mother tongue. But classical Chinese did not escape change; the ever-evolving ver-

---

[3] Norman, *Chinese*, page 54, discusses tentative propositions concerning the origin of tones in Chinese.

[4] In classical Chinese, the existence of two pronunciations of a single character is believed by some to represent the vestiges of inflections. Also, the distinctions between the nominative and genitive 吾 *wú* (I, my) and the accusative 我 *wǒ* (me) are considered to be vestiges of a case system.

nacular language left strong imprints on the writings of different eras that make literary Chinese different from classical Chinese.

Although literary Chinese partially reflected changes in the vernacular, it nevertheless remained close to its classical roots. Hence, by the Qīng dynasty, the spoken language had already drifted quite far from the written form. With the fall of the Qīng dynasty, literary Chinese was abandoned, and replaced with the written vernacular (白话文 *bái huà wén*), a style of writing that essentially reflected the spoken language of the north of China or Běijīng in particular, known as Mandarin, and called 普通话 *pǔ tōng huà* in the People's Republic of Chinese (PRC) and 国语 *guó yǔ* in Táiwān.[5] During the twentieth century, immense social, political, economic, and cultural changes due to the impact of Western civilization have influenced the Chinese language greatly. In particular, the terminological needs that came with the adoption of all branches of Western learning and technology have been met by a huge increase in compounds. Nevertheless, the literary language still lives on in various ways. It survives in the multitude of adages and stock phrases (成语 *chéng yǔ*) that especially mark the speech of the educated. It is still used in the generation of terminology, where, for example 足 *zú*, foot, is preferred to 脚 *jiǎo*, which has otherwise replaced it in the spoken language (e.g., 假足 *jiǎ zú*, pseudopodium). Furthermore, the literary form continues to provide models for concise and elegant writing that is free of the verbosity of the spoken language. Book titles, newspaper headlines, and political slogans often have a strong literary flavor. 'I love my city' expressed as 吾爱吾城 *wú ài wú chéng* is shorter and more expressive than 我爱我的城市 *wǒ ài wǒ de chéng shì*. The classical 吾 *wú* means 'my' as well as 'I', while in modern Chinese 'my' is expressed by two characters, 我的 *wǒ de*; 城 *chéng* means a '[walled] city' and its written form is not confused with the many homophones that make the compound with 市 *shì*, a market or market town, obligatory in the spoken language (城市 *chéng shì*). Not only are six characters reduced to four, but a pleasing four-character symmetry is also achieved.[6]

---

[5] 'Mandarin' is the language of mandarins (officials); in simple terms, it is the northern dialect of Chinese traditionally used in administrative circles, now promoted in the PRC and in Táiwān (and increasingly in Hong Kong) as the lingua franca of the Chinese people. Dialects in China are particularly pronounced. The Wú dialects of the Shànghǎi region, Mín dialects (notably dialects of Fúzhōu, Xiàmén, and Táiwān), and the Yuè dialects of Guǎngdōng (notably including Cantonese, the dialect of Guǎngzhōu), as well as the Kèjiā dialects (Hakka) north of the Mín-Yuè boundary, are for all intents and purposes different languages, but nevertheless share a common root with Mandarin.

[6] For a different view of the relationship between the classical and modern language, see DeFrancis *The Chinese Language: Fact and Fantasy*, University of Hawaii Press, Táiwān edition by Crane Publishing Company, Taipei, 1990.

Although Chinese script lies outside the scope of this book, its nature is inextricably related to other features of the Chinese language, and to this extent it concerns us. Like the cuneiform script of Sumer and the hieroglyphics of Egypt, the Chinese script is pictographic in origin. The sun, for example, was represented as a circle with a dot in the center (now written as 日 *rì*), while 'dog' was represented by an unequivocal representation of the animal (now stylized beyond recognition as 犬 *quǎn*). Certain concepts were not easily represented in picture form, and so more abstract ideographs were created: 'up' was represented in a form that has now become 上 *shàng* and 'down' as 下 *xià*. Other abstract ideas were expressed by combining pictographs: 'bright' was written as a combination of 'sun' and 'moon', now stylized as 明 *míng*. However, the earliest examples of Chinese writing on oracle bones and shells from the late Shāng dynasty (14th to 11th centuries B.C.) clearly show that the script had already developed from direct pictorial representation to a system of writing that reflected the spoken language of the time. The notion of 'come', for example, was expressed by the character that at the time was used for 'wheat', now written as 来. The borrowing of this character was based on a similarity in sound between the word 'wheat' and the word 'come'. As the borrowing of characters on the basis of sound introduced many potentially confusing homographs, derived meanings were differentiated by the addition of a *signific* that indicated the nature of the thing denoted. Thus the character now written as 工 *gōng*, originally meaning a 'carpenter's square' and later 'work', was used to mean river, 江 *jiāng*, by the addition of an element meaning 'water', which is written as three dots in the modern form of the character. The character 来 *lái*, to come, underwent no such modification, because it soon became obsolete in the sense of 'wheat'.

Combining significs with phonetic elements came to be the most productive method of character creation, and it is estimated that about 90% of characters now used were formed in this way.[7] However, the Chinese script never became fully phonetic as did other languages of the Old World. It did not follow the pattern of development observed in Egyptian from the hieroglyphic to the demotic script, in which a syllabic alphabet arose. In Chinese, the signific has never been discarded, and has remained as important as the phonetic. This conservatism would appear to be attributable to the monosyllabic and isolating nature of the language. Semantically, the Chinese script has nothing other than root meanings to account for. The Chinese verb 做 *zuò* is pronounced the same way whether it means 'do' or 'did'; and 牛 *niú* is pronounced the same way whether it means ox or oxen. Since Chinese words have no sound variations, they are adequately represented in writing by a single (phonetic or

---

[7]DeFrancis, *The Chinese Language: Fact and Fantasy*.

nonphonetic) sign, whereas the varying phonetic forms of words in languages such as English are logically best represented by a phonetic script. (The progressive movement toward phonetic representation in the Egyptian script, for example, is undoubtedly due to the phonetic variations of its words.) Furthermore, the relationship between sound and word is more robust in Chinese; because each morpheme is one of a limited set of single-syllable words, elisions are known but not numerous. In English, by comparison, the smallest sound units, phonemes (and in the writing system, letters representing them), are much freer to combine and separate, so that 'St. Audrey' in time could change into 'tawdry', the phonetic alphabetic script easily accommodating the change. Fusions of two words have occurred in Chinese, but they are far less numerous than in the polysyllabic Indo-European languages. The use of characters for their phonetic value has had a major place in the creation of new characters, but phonetic representation has never taken over completely. Characters were used for their phonetic value to create new characters, but once a character came into being, its structure was more or less permanently fixed, and even if its pronunciation changed so that it differed from that of the phonetic element, the written symbol was never revised. Thus, for example, 工, meaning 'work', was used as a phonetic element in the creation of 江 meaning 'river' (originally specifically the Yangtse). In modern Mandarin, the pronunciation of the two characters, which originally was identical or nearly identical, has diverged considerably (*gōng* and *jiāng*), although the written forms have not been changed. Sound changes that inevitably took place over the centuries have weakened the reliability of being able to guess the sound of characters by their phonetics. However, familiarity with the varying pronunciation of a phonetic element in different characters provides a rough indication of the range of sounds it can represent: 观 *guān*、 欢 *huān*、 权 *quán*、 劝 *quàn*.

After its initial development and refinement, the Chinese script reached maturity in the Hàn dynasty. Characters have changed little in their composition since that time, and the clerical script (隶书 *lì shū*) devised by Hàn scribes remains a commonly used font in the modern printshop and on the personal computer. The script has undergone a large systematic simplification under the PRC government. The new simplified characters, however, are largely based on simplifications developed in the 'running' and 'grass' calligraphic scripts (行书 *xíng shū* and 草书 *cǎo shū*) and on popular simplifications, that is, on existing variants of characters.[8] The pronunciation and

---

[8]The simplified characters have been adopted by the Chinese community of Singapore, but they have been hotly opposed by the Nationalist Government on Táiwān and resisted by laissez-faire Hong Kong. They are slowly being accepted by world sinologists together with the PRC's Pīnyīn system of transcription. However, the merging of multiple characters

syntax of Chinese has constantly changed, but the characters have remained essentially the same. With changes in vocabulary, each era created new and discarded old characters, but despite this, there is a common core of characters that runs through the writings of all eras. This situation is vastly different from that of English. While *Beowulf*, written during the 8th century in Old English, is unintelligible in its original form to modern English readers, *Zhū Bìng Yuán Hòu Lùn* (诸病源侯论 "The Origin and Manifestation of Disease"), which appeared in A.D. 610, is nearly as easy to read as Dickens.

The first major extant Chinese medical work, the *Huáng Dì Nèi Jīng* (黄帝内经 "The Yellow Emperor's Inner Canon"), is a product of the late classical period that underwent retranscription by later writers. Most subsequent works, that is, the bulk of Chinese medical literature before the modern era, were therefore essentially written in post-classical literary Chinese. The tradition of literary expression is sure to have been compounded by the attention paid to the writings of previous generations of physicians back to the *Huáng Dì Nèi Jīng*. Certainly, in the modern era, a continuing conservatism in Chinese medicine has prevented literary Chinese from being abandoned with the same decisiveness as in other activities. A large set of terms and a distinctive style of expression, which are clearly marked with the features of literary Chinese, still continue to form the core of Chinese medical discourse.

Despite the antiquity of Chinese medicine and the literary style of its expression, much of the basic vocabulary is formed with characters that are still used in the modern spoken language. Of the two thousand or so characters presented in this book, only a few are obsolete outside the realm of Chinese medicine. Of course, medical meanings and connotations have to be learned, but the Chinese student of Chinese medicine has nothing like the task of the English-speaking student of Western medicine in mastering unfamiliar words (derived from Latin and Greek word roots). Many texts that have been written over the ages contain obscure characters and phrases, but a mastery of the common core of terms and expressions used in modern texts and appearing recurrently over the centuries provides a firm basis for approaching any literature. Given the relative stability of the literary language over the centuries, the Western student who memorizes a basic set of commonly used characters and masters the grammatical constructions of literary Chinese is rewarded with the key to a body of medical literature that spans two millennia.

This book focuses on the terminology of Chinese medicine, that is, on the vocabulary of Chinese medical language rather than its grammar. However, given the nature of Chinese language and Chinese medical knowledge, the distinction is not so easily drawn. In modern disciplines, technical terms usually

---

into single forms affects the interpretation of historical texts. For this reason, even the PRC produces new editions of Chinese medical classics in complex, or unsimplified, script.

take the form of nouns or noun phrases and comparatively few are verbs (in a medical dictionary one generally finds 'evacuation' and 'lobotomy', but not 'evacuate' and 'lobotomize'). The analytical nature of modern science creates a tendency for any action that can be expressed by a verb to be considered as an event that can be analyzed into various components or as a complex procedure that is performed, and this is reflected in the tendency toward nominalization. In Chinese medicine, terminology is not so narrowly concentrated into particular parts of speech. The tendency towards nominalization, though it exists in Chinese medicine, is less pronounced, and verbs and verb phrases can serve as nouns without undergoing any morphological changes. In addition, the terminology includes many stock phrases from the classics expressing physiological and pathological laws and rules for treatment. For this reason, this book includes a concise grammar section covering the main constructions of literary Chinese used in Chinese medicine, and points out classical usages and correspondences in the modern language. Since the language of Chinese medicine is largely classical, the grammar section also serves the purpose of introducing the features of classical Chinese to students who have so far studied only the modern language. In learning Chinese, the hardest task is to learn the characters; the grammar, by contrast, is relatively simple. Students unfamiliar with the grammatical explanations need not be disheartened. Careful study of the 700 or more examples will lead to an intuitive understanding of the constructions.

2. Basic Sentences

Classical Chinese had two basic types of sentence, the nominal and the verbal. The nominal sentence is one in which one noun phrase identifies or explains the other without any verb linking the two. This was a feature of classical Chinese that has largely been replaced with a verbal sentence employing various verbs that correspond to the English verb 'to be'. All other complete Chinese sentences are verbal sentences as they are in English.

2.1 Nominal Sentences

The nominal sentence links a subject consisting of a noun, noun phrase, or pronoun to a predicate similarly consisting of a noun, noun phrase, or pronoun, for example, 脾者，脏也 *pí zhě, zàng yě,* 'the spleen is a viscus'.[9] Equivalent sentences in English require the interposition of the copulative

---

[9]'Viscus' is the singular form of the plural 'viscera'.

verb 'to be', but in early classical Chinese there was no such verb.[10] Nevertheless, the subject was often marked by 者 *zhě*, and the final particle 也 *yě* was usually added to mark the sentence as an explanation or judgment.

This construction could denote an equative relationship (A = B), where A is exactly equal to B.

1. 肝者，木脏也 *gān zhě, mù zàng yě*: the liver [is] the wood viscus
2. 六腑者，胆、胃、大肠、小肠、膀胱、三焦 *liù fǔ zhě, dǎn、wèi、dà cháng、xiǎo cháng、páng guāng、sān jiāo*: the six bowels [are] the gallbladder, stomach, large intestine, small intestine, bladder, and triple burner
3. 厥者，逆也 *jué zhě, nì yè*: reversal [is] counterflow

It can also denote an inclusive relationship (A ⊂ B), that is, one in which the subject is not the only item denoted by the noun of the predicate.

4. 耳聋者，肾经之病也 *ěr lóng zhě, shèn jīng zhī bìng yě*: deafness [is] a kidney channel disease
5. 目痛者，肝经之病也 *mù tòng zhě, gān jīng zhī bìng yě*: eye pain [is] a liver channel disease
6. 积聚者，脏腑之病也 *jī jù zhě, zàng fǔ zhī bìng yě*: accumulations and gatherings [are] diseases of the bowels and viscera
7. 补者，补其虚也 *bǔ zhě, bǔ qí xū yě*: supplementing [is] (means) supplementing vacuity

More loosely, B may be an explanation of A, where B is a whole verbal sentence.

8. 心痛者，风冷邪气乘于心也 *xīn tòng zhě, fēng lěng xié qì chéng yú xīn yě*: heart pain [is] wind-cold evil qì exploiting the heart

In the last example, the addition of 故 *gù*, 'therefore', before the final 也 would make the sentence more decidedly an explanation of cause ('heart pain is *due to* wind-cold evil qì exploiting the heart').

9. 风冷失音，风冷客于会厌故也 *fēng lěng shī yīn, fēng lěng kè yú huì yàn gù yě*: lit. 'wind-cold loss of voice: wind-cold settling

---

[10]Note that in formal definitions in English no copulative verb is used, for example, 'bladder: an organ in the lower abdomen that stores urine'. Note also that the copulative verb in Indo-European languages, as in Chinese, was a later development. The omission of the copula in the present tense is standard in modern Russian and was optional in Latin and ancient Greek. See *Introduction to Theoretical Linguistics*, Lyons, J., Cambridge University Press, London, 1968.

in the epiglottis, that's why', wind-cold loss of voice is due to wind-cold settling in the epiglottis

Sometimes the adverb 乃 *nǎi* is added between the subject and predicate.

10. 肛乃大肠之魄门 *gāng nǎi dà cháng zhī pò mén*: the anus corporeal [is] soul gate of the large intestine

11. 头痛乃风入太阳经也 *tóu tòng nǎi fēng rù tài yáng jīng yě*: headache [is due to] wind entering the greater yáng channel

The 乃 implies a reasonably precise equation between the subject and predicate. It is equivalent to the modern 就是 *jiù shì*.

12. 清者，乃治热之法也 *qīng zhě, nǎi zhì rè zhī fǎ yě*: clearing [is] the method of treating heat

Equational predicates in literary Chinese often take the more complex form of 'A 者 *zhě*, B 是也 *shì yě*', that is, 'A: B this'. Here, 'this' refers back to A.

13. 六气者，风、寒、暑、湿、燥、火是也 *liù qì zhě, fēng、hán、shǔ、shī、zào、huǒ shì yě*: the six qì [are] wind, cold, summerheat, dampness, dryness, and fire

14. 何为阴分？五脏之精气是也 *hé wéi yīn fèn? wǔ zàng zhī jīng qì shì yě*: What is the yīn aspect? It is the essential qì of the five viscera

15. 消者，去其壅也，经云'坚者消之'是也 *xiāo zhě, qù qí yōng ye, jīng yún 'jiān zhě xiāo zhī' shì yě*: dispersion is eliminating congestion; it is what the *Nèi Jīng* means by 'whittle away hardness'

Negative nominal sentences were expressed with the addition of the negative word 非 *fēi*, not normally used in verbal sentences: 是非疟疾 *shì fēi nuè jí*, 'this is not malaria'. Questions were expressed by the addition of other particles such as 乎 *hū*, which are discussed further ahead.

Toward the end of the classical period, 为 *wéi*, 'to act as', increasingly came to be a copula like the English verb 'to be'. Thus the nominal sentence was replaced by a verbal sentence. Both the nominal and verbal constructions are amply represented in the language of Chinese medicine.

16. 膀胱，津液之腑 *páng guāng, jīn yè zhī fǔ*: the bladder [is] the bowel of liquid and humor

17. 肺者，相傅之官也 *fèi zhě, xiāng fù zhī guān yě*: lung [is] assistant official

18. 疝者，气痛也 *shàn zhě, qì tòng yě*: mounting [is] qì pain

19. 厥者，逆也 *jué zhě, nì yě*: reversal [is] counterflow
20. 热病者，伤寒之类也 *rè bìng zhě, shāng hán zhī lèi yě*: heat diseases [are of] the cold-damage category
21. 肺为气之主，肾为气之根 *fèi wéi qì zhī zhǔ, shèn wéi qì zhī gēn*: lung is the governor of qì, kidney is the root of qì
22. 少阳为枢 *shào yáng wéi shū*: lesser yáng is the pivot
23. 阳明为阖 *yáng míng wéi hé*: yáng brightness is the closing
24. 肾为水脏 *shèn wéi shuǐ zàng*: the kidney is the water viscus

In modern spoken Chinese, 是 *shì*, which first came to be used as a copulative verb in the Hàn dynasty, is now standard.[11] It is often preceded by an adverb indicating precision such as 就 *jiù* in the spoken language or 便 *biàn* or 乃 *nǎi* in the written language. In modern writing, 是 *shì* is commonly replaced by 为 *wéi* and less commonly by 系 *xì*.

25. 气有余便是火 *qì yǒu yú biàn shì huǒ*: qì in superabundance is fire

The shift from the nominal to the verbal sentence was by no means definitive. Nominal sentences without a verb are not rare in the modern spoken language: 今天三号 *jīn tiān sān hào*, lit. 'today three number', that is, 'today is the third (of the month)'; 我山东人 *wǒ shān dōng rén*, 'I Shangdong person', that is, 'I'm from Shandong'. The copula is also often omitted announcing one's name as on the telephone. Furthermore, in the modern written language, the negative construction in which 非 *fēi* appears without a copula is still common.

The verb 属 *shǔ*, 'belong to' or 'to be classed as', can be used as 为 *wéi* and 是 *shì* when the noun in the predicate denotes a subset of the subject noun (A ⊂ B). It is usually followed by 于 *yú*, 'at', 'to' (A 属于 B).

26. 湿邪属于阴 *shī xié shǔ yú yīn*: damp evil is yīn
27. 气与水本属一家 *qì yǔ shuǐ běn shǔ yī jiā*: qì and water essentially belong to one [and the same] family

Both 属 and 为 are used to equate a set of symptoms with a diagnosis.

28. 白苔属于正常 *bái tāi shǔ yú zhèng cháng*: a white fur is normal
29. 发热恶风多属于外感热病 *fà rè wù fēng duō shǔ yú wài gǎn rè bìng*: heat effusion (fever) and aversion to wind are (constitute, indicate) an externally contracted heat disease

---

[11]The original meaning of 是 *shì* was 'this', and it is believed that it came to take on the function of a copula after serving as an emphatic marker of nominal predication. This development may have been reinforced by the fact that 是 was also used in the sense of 'right' as opposed to 非 *fēi*, 'wrong'. Since the *fēi* was the negative copula, it would have been natural to regard *shì* as filling the 'space' in the nominal sentence. See *Chinese*, Norman, J., 1988, page 125.

30. 鼻孔干燥为肺热 *bí kǒng gān zào wéi fèi rè*: dry nostrils are (constitute, indicate, are due to) lung heat

31. 舌质胖大多为阳气不足 *shé zhì pàng dà duō wéi yáng qì bù zú*: an enlarged tongue mostly is [due to] insufficiency of yáng qì

In the presentation of a diagnostic conclusion, the characters 属 and 为 are equivalent to the English 'indicate', and in fact 表示 *biǎo shì*, 'show' or 'indicate', now sometimes replaces them in modern texts, probably as an indirect result of English influence on the Chinese expression in Western medicine: 口唇干焦表示伤津 *kǒu chún gān jiāo biǎo shì shāng jīn*, 'dry, parched lips indicates damage to liquid'.

2.2 Verbal Sentences

Verbal sentences consist of a subject (noun, noun phrase, or pronoun) and a predicate consisting of a verb, sometimes with an object, and sometimes with adjuncts. Often, the subject is omitted if it is clear from the context. One of the simplest sentences is a subject with a verb, such as 腹痛 *fù tòng*, 'the abdomen hurts'. Verbal sentences notably include the subject + verb + object constructions that coincide with the English order.

32. 肺主气 *fèi zhǔ qì*: the lung governs qì

33. 目生粟疮 *mù shēng sù chuāng*: the eye grows a peppercorn sore

34. 白睛溢血 *bái jīng yì xuè*: white of the eye spills blood

35. 苦入心 *kǔ rù xīn*: bitterness enters the heart

36. 脾病及肝 *pí bìng jí gān*: spleen disease affects the liver

The existential verb was 有 *yǒu* in classical Chinese, as it still is in the modern vernacular. It corresponds to the English 'there is (are)', but while English adds the expletive ('dummy') subject 'there', no such subject exists in Chinese: 有热 *yǒu rè*, 'there is heat'. With a subject, 有 *yǒu* takes on the meaning of the English 'have', for example, 病人有痔疮 *bìng rén yǒu zhì chuāng*, 'the patient has hemorrhoids'.

In classical, literary, and modern Chinese, location is expressed with 在 *zài*. English has no such special verb, and the need is met by the verb 'to be'.[12] In English, the verb 'to be' functioning as the verb of location requires a preposition. In Chinese, 'location at' (or location in) does not normally require such addition.

37. 肝，其华在爪 *gān, qí huá zài zhǎo*: liver, its bloom is in the nails

38. 病在上 *bìng zài shàng*: the illness is in the upper body

---

[12]While English does not have a separate verb of location, Spanish, like Chinese, does have one (*estar*).

39. 伏热在里 *fú rè zài lǐ*: hidden heat is in the interior

All but a limited set of verbs are negated by 不 *bù*, placed before it.

40. 土不生金 *tǔ bù shēng jīn*: lit. 'earth not engender metal', earth is not engendering metal
41. 水不涵木 *shuǐ bù hán mù*: lit. 'water not moisten wood', water is not moistening wood

In the literary language, the negative 不 *bù* often carries connotations of unwillingness or (especially in the medical context) inability.

42. 不寐 *bú mèi*: does not sleep, cannot sleep
43. 不大便 *bú dà biàn*: does not defecate, cannot defecate

Another negative form, 未 *wèi*, is a factual assertion that something did not take place or has not taken place.

44. 恶露未尽 *è lù wèi jìn*: the lochia has not ceased (to flow)

The existential 有 *yǒu* has its own negative form: 无 *wú*, there is (are) not, has (have) not. In the modern language, this is expressed as 没 *méi* or 没有 *méi yǒu*.

45. 无力 *wú lì*: has no strength
46. 无形 *wú xíng*: has no form
47. 男子无月经 *nán zǐ wú yuè jīng*: men do not have menstrual periods

As already stated, the classical copulative sentence had its own negative 非 *fēi*. Classical Chinese had a variety of other negatives that are less common in the language of Chinese medicine.

2.3 Subjects and Topics

The Chinese language, through all its stages of its development, has been characterized by a loose relationship between 'subject' and predicate, and for this reason it is often more precise to speak of 'topic' rather than 'subject'.

As in English, the subject, or topic, can be the agent of the action denoted by the verb:

48. 心火上炎 *xīn huǒ shàng yán*: lit. 'heart fire upward flames', heart fire flames upward
49. 热邪伤阴 *rè xié shāng yīn*: heat evil damages yīn

Sometimes, the topic of the sentence is the object. The object of a transitive verb can be made its topic to express a passive sense. In the preceding example, 伤 *shāng*, 'to damage', is a transitive verb whose object is 阴 *yīn*,

'yīn'. By inverting the verb and its object as 阴伤 *yīn shāng*, the meaning is 'yīn is damaged'.[13] More will be said about this in the discussion of verbs.

50. 血夺 *xuè duó*: lit. 'blood: despoliate', the blood is despoliated;
51. 声不敢扬 *shēng bù gǎn yáng*: lit. 'voice: not dare to raise', not dare to raise one's voice
52. 手不可举 *shǒu bù kě jǔ*: lit. 'arm: cannot raise', cannot lift one's arm
53. 阳事不举 *yáng shì bù jǔ*: lit. 'male matter: (can)not raise', impotent
54. 发热多见于外感热病 *fā rè duō jiàn yú wài gǎn rè bìng*: lit. 'heat effusion: mostly see in externally contracted heat disease', heat effusion (fever) is mostly seen in externally contracted heat disease
55. 方剂可选用滋燥养营汤 *fāng jì kě xuǎn yòng zī zào yǎng yíng tāng*: as to formulas, [you] can choose Dryness-Enriching Construction-Nourishing Decoction
56. 症见发热、恶寒 *zhèng jiàn fā rè、wù hán*: lit. 'pathoconditions: [you] see heat effusion, aversion to cold', the pathoconditions observed include heat effusion (fever) and aversion to cold

Note in the preceding examples, English sometimes requires the addition of a subject (e.g., 'you', 'one') or transposition into the passive voice ('is seen in. . .'). In some cases, it requires a topic phrase introduced by a preposition such as 'in', 'for', or 'as to'.

A Chinese sentence may have two apparent subjects: 病人头痛 *bìng rén tóu tòng*, lit. 'patient: head hurts', that is, 'the patient has a headache'. In this case, *tóu tòng* appears so commonly with a human subject that we almost think of it as a verb that has 'absorbed' the original subject (*tóu*).

57. 妇人月经不调 *fù rén yuè jīng bù tiáo*: lit. 'women: menstruation irregular', women have irregular menstruation
58. 病人热胜阴伤 *bìng rén rè shèng yīn shāng*: lit. 'patient: heat exuberant, yīn damage', the patient suffers from exuberant heat and damage to yīn

Note in the preceding examples the tendency of English to express the intended notions in the form of subject + verb (have, suffer) + noun.

In the literary language, as we have already seen, a topic is often marked by 者 *zhě*.

59. 脾胃者，仓廪之官 *pí wèi zhě, cāng lǐn zhī guān*: the spleen and stomach is the official of the granaries

---

[13]Note that similar behavior is seen in a few English verbs, for example, to break: 'The man broke the vase' and 'the vase broke'.

60. 诸血者皆属于心 *zhū xuè zhě jiē shǔ yú xīn*: all blood belongs to the heart

61. 手少阴脉动甚者，孕子也 *shǒu shào yīn mài dòng shèn zhě, yùn zǐ yě*: lit. 'vessel of the hand lesser yīn markedly stirring PARTI-CLE: pregnancy PARTICLE', pronounced stirring of the vessel of the hand lesser yīn indicates pregnancy

3. Stative and Active Verbs

Verbs and adjectives are less clearly distinguished in Chinese than in English. In English, a predicative adjective requires the copula 'to be' (e.g., he is tall). In modern Chinese, the adjective is often marked by the 'dummy' adverb 很 *hěn*, very (as in 他很高 *tā hěn gāo*, he is tall), or with the copulative 是 *shì* (as in 啤酒是冰的 *pí jiǔ shì bīng de*, the beer is cold). In classical Chinese, adjectives required no extra wording: 脉浮 *mài fú*, 'the pulse is floating' (or 'the pulse floats'). Furthermore, all adjectives could act as verbs in the sense of becoming, a feature that is retained in the modern language: 他胖了 *tā pàng le*, lit. 'he's become fat', 'he's put on weight'. For these reasons, Chinese adjectives are now commonly referred to as 'stative verbs' and verbs as 'active verbs'.

A major feature of classical language was freedom from restraints of word-class. In addition to true verbs such as 走 *zǒu*, 'to run', 曰 *yuē*, 'to say', and 见 *jiàn*, 'to see', nouns could also function as verbs. For example, the names of professions, titles, and kinship terms were regularly used as intransitive verbs in the sense of 'to fulfill the duties of...'. Thus 君 *jūn*, 'sovereign', could be used as a verb: 君不君 *jūn bù jūn*, 'sovereign not sovereign', that is, 'the sovereign fails to act in a manner that befits a sovereign'. Similarly 父 *fù*, 'father' as a verb meant 'to fulfill one's paternal duties'. Nouns could also be used as transitive verbs. The names of tools and instruments could be used in the sense of 'to treat with (the given instrument)': 针 *zhēn*, 'a needle', could also be used to mean 'to needle'. Some nouns were used verbally in the sense of to 'treat as', that is, 人其人 *rén qí rén*, 'to treat him as a person'. The word 事 *shì*, 'matter', 'affair', 'duty', was commonly used as a verb in the sense of 'to serve' or 'to work': 事亲 *shì qīn*, 'to serve one's parents'. The word 医 *yī*, healer, was also used in the sense of 'to treat' or 'to heal'. In modern Chinese, this ability to use nouns as verbs has been reduced. In Chinese medicine, 'needle' and 'heal/er' retain their double usage.

62. 人皆宗之 *rén jiē zōng zhī*: lit. 'people all ancestor him', all look upon him as an ancestor

63. 杖犬，令血出 *zhàng quǎn, lìng xuè chū*: lit. 'stick dog, make blood come out', beat the dog with a stick to make it bleed

Furthermore, stative verbs could function as active verbs. In the following example, 明 *míng*, 'bright', means 'to penetrate with the brightness of intelligence', that is, 'to understand'. This, incidentally, has survived in the modern 明白 *míng bái*, 'to understand'.

64. 必明肝藏血之道 *bì míng gān cáng xuè zhī dào*: have to understand the logic (lit. Dao) of the liver storing blood

More importantly, intransitive verbs could be used in a causative sense. The terminology of Chinese medicine preserves some usages of this kind. The character 远 *yuǎn* meant 'distant' but read as *yuàn* could also mean 'to place at a distance,' 'to shun'[14]; 虚 *xū* means 'vacuity', but could be used to mean 'make (more) vacuous'; 为 *wéi*, 'to be', can be used to mean 'cause to be', i.e., 'make'; 去 *qù*, 'to go', 'to leave', can be used transitively in the sense of 'remove' or 'eliminate'. 下 *xià*, 'to go', is often used transitively in the sense of 'precipitate' (or 'purge').

65. 攻里不远寒 *gōng lǐ bù yuàn hán*: interior attack does not shun cold [medicinals]
66. 寒可去热 *hán kě qù rè*: cold can eliminate heat
67. 发表不远热 *fā biǎo bù yuàn rè*: exterior effusion does not shun hot [medicinals]
68. 虚虚实实 *xū xū shí shí*: to evacuate vacuity and replenish repletion (i.e., to exacerbate vacuity and repletion)
69. 为细末 *wéi xì mò*: lit. 'cause to be a powder', make into a fine powder
70. 为病 *wéi bìng*: cause disease
71. 复脉 *fù mài*: restore the pulse

In classical Chinese, transitive verbs could also be used in a causative meaning, but not without potential confusion: 饮之 *yǐn zhī* might mean to 'drink it', but (when 饮 *yǐn* is read as *yìn*), it could also mean to 'make him (her, them) drink'. Fortunately, such confusing usage is rarely seen in Chinese medical texts. A more general form of the causative is formed by means of the causative verbs 使 *shǐ* and 令 *lìng*.

---

[14]The difference in tone was originally a difference in the initial sound in old Chinese by which different functions of the same word were distinguished. These sound distinctions were mostly lost in subsequent sound changes. In some cases, the difference in pronunciation is preserved in the writing, for example, 见 *jiàn*, 'see', and 现 *xiàn*, 'cause to be seen' (to show). Among the classical pronouns, 吾 *wú*, 'I', 'my', and 我 *wǒ*, 'me'; 其 *qí*, 'he', 'his', and 之 *zhī*, 'it', are also sound variations corresponding to differences in function.

72. 使之吐 *shǐ zhī tù*: make him (her, them) vomit
73. 母能令子虚，子能令母实 *mǔ néng lìng zǐ xū, zǐ néng lìng mǔ shí*: the mother can make the child vacuous; the child can make the mother replete

Transitive verbs could (and still can) be used in a passive sense when they were not followed by their natural object:

74. 声不敢扬 *shēng bù gǎn yáng*: lit. 'voice: not dare to raise', not dare to raise one's voice
75. 头重不欲举 *tóu zhòng bú yù jǔ*: lit. 'head heavy, do not want to lift', to have a heavy head that one does not desire to lift

The agent could be expressed by 于 *yú*: 不伤于寒 *bù shāng yú hán*, 'not damaged by cold'. However, a true passive can be formed with 受 *shòu*, lit. 'to receive', or 被 *bèi*, lit. 'to be covered'.

76. 五脏之精分受伤 *wǔ zàng zhī jīng fēn shòu shāng*: the essence aspect of the five viscera is damaged
77. 胞脉受阻 *bāo mài shòu zǔ*: the uterine vessels are clouded
78. 心窍被蒙 *xīn qiào bèi méng*: the orifices of the heart are clouded

Another passive construction involves 为 *wéi* with 所 *suǒ* preceding the verb.

79. 血为肝所藏、为心所行 *xuè wéi gān suǒ cáng, wéi xīn suǒ xíng*: the blood is stored by the liver and is moved by the heart
80. 此皆心气不足所致 *cǐ jiē xīn qì bù zú suǒ zhì*: this is all caused by insufficiency of heart qi
81. 此为湿热所致 *cǐ wéi shī rè suǒ zhì*: this is caused by damp-heat

In certain set phrases, the 所, for reasons that will be explained later, is omitted.

82. 脾为湿困 *pí wéi shī kùn*: the spleen is encumbered by dampness

In classical Chinese, there were no verbal compounds. Two closely linked verbs could only be linked by 而 *ér*. Compounds started to appear in the Hàn dynasty. These included: a) compounds of synonyms or near synomyms such as 欢喜 *huān xǐ*, 'to be joyful', and 想念 *xiǎng niàn*, 'to think about'; b) resultative compounds such as 打杀 *dǎ shā*, 'to beat to death' (now 打死 *dǎ sǐ* in modern Chinese) and 学得 *xué dé*, 'to obtain by learning'; c) verbs with directional complements such as 流出 *liú chū*, 'to flow out'.

After the classical period, all three tendencies continued to develop. In resultative verb constructions, negation came to be expressed by placing the negative between the elements of the compound: 买未得 *mǎi wèi dé*, 'did not succeed in buying'. In this way, the 得 *dé* came to assume a potential function. Further development of this construction led to modern vernacular 买得到 *mǎi de dào*, 'can buy', negated as 买不到 *mǎi bu dào*, 'cannot buy'. Directional compounds developed in the same way: 流得出来 *liú de chū lái*, 'can flow out'; 流不出来 *liú bu chū lái*, 'cannot flow out'.

After the classical period, there were great changes in the function of verbs. In classsical Chinese, perfected action was signaled by the particle 既 *jì*. In the late classical period, this was replaced with the verb 已 *yǐ*, which originally meant 'to finish'. In the post-classical period 已 *yǐ* shifted to the end of the sentence. In the Táng dynasty, 了 *le* began to take over as the perfective marker. Subsequently, 了 *le* came to be suffixed to the verb, before rather than after any object that might follow the verb. With this last development, the format of the perfective aspect of verbs (V PERFECTIVE O) came in line with compound resultative verbs (V RESULTATIVE O).

Even today, in Chinese medical discourse, writers will use constructions that are obsolete in the spoken language.

83. 热势既退，冷气乃动 *rè shì jì tuì, lěng qì nài dòng*: when the heat has abated, cold qì then moves
84. 食已即吐 *shí yǐ jí tù*: lit. 'eat-finish immediately vomit', immediate vomiting after eating

The *perfective aspect*, which expresses completed action, is commonly associated with the English present perfect or past tense. This association is rather misleading because the correspondence is only partial. In the modern 我看到了一条狗 *wǒ kàn dào le yì tiáo gǒu*, 'I saw a dog', the perfective 了 *le* indeed corresponds to the past tense in English. However, in 累了就休息一下 *lèi le jiù xiū xī yí xià*, lit. 'tired PERFECTIVE then rest a moment', the perfective aspect merely sets 'becoming tired' in relation to 'resting'. This sentence could mean 'we would take a rest whenever we got tired' (past time), 'we will take a rest whenever we get tired' (future time), or even 'we would take a rest if we got tired' (conditional). The correct interpretation of the sentence would depend entirely on whether the context is a narrative about previous events or a discussion about future plans, and so forth.

It should be emphasized that Chinese has no tenses. An action in the past, present, or future is expressed by the same word. The presence of an adverb of time such as 'yesterday', 'today', and 'tomorrow' tells us when the action indicated by the verb in that same clause took place. Very often, an adverb of time sets the time context for a number of subsequent sentences in which the verbs, without any tense marking, are understood to have taken place. When no explicit time specification is given, the time of the action is understood through the extralinguistic situational context. In English, the difference in tense between 'I sit' and 'I sat' seems to imply a firm division between the present and past. Such a difference does not exist in Chinese.

Students who have difficulty getting used to the idea of verbs without tenses might reflect on the nature of the tenses in English. Although we speak of *present tense*, *past tense*, *future tense*, etc., it would be wrong to think of each tense as representing only the tense its name suggests. We often use the present tense for past, present, and future action (e.g., 'gravity causes unsupported objects to fall'); we use the present tense for future action (e.g., 'I leave for Paris tomorrow'); we use the past tense to represent possible future action (e.g., 'I would only help if he came too). Present, past, and future are not mapped onto our verb system with anything like the clarity we might imagine them to be.

Modern Chinese has a number of aspects that developed after the classical period. There is a continuative aspect marked before the verb by 在 *zài* or after it by 着 *zhe*: 我在想 *wǒ zài xiǎng*, 'I am thinking', and 坐着 *zuò zhě*, 'sitting'. There is a transitory aspect expressed by repetition of the verb: 试试看 *shì shì kàn*, 'have a try'. These, as with other aspects, are set against the common aspect, which is the unmarked verb. These aspects rarely appear in the technical discourse of Chinese medicine. The most common use of 着 *zhe* is seen in 有着 *yǒu zhe*, 'to have', where barely any continuative sense is implied.

In classical Chinese, instrumentality was expressed with 以 *yǐ*, 'with' or 'using' usually placed after the verb. In the late classical period, 用 *yòng*, 'to use', also started to appear in this usage, and is now standard in the modern vernacular. In the post-classical period, the instrumental phrase shifted to before the verb, and later, 将 *jiāng* and 把 *bǎ*, both verbs meaning 'to hold', began to be used in the same way: 把钱买药 *bǎ qián mǎi yào*, lit. 'hold money buy medicine', that is, 'buy medicine with money'. Later, these two verbs also came to be used to introduce the object of the main verb. In the modern language, they have lost their instrumental usage, and retain only their usage as pretransitive markers. In the spoken language, 把 *bǎ* is standard, but 将 *jiāng* is still common in the written language. The pretransitive construction is used in complex constructions where, for example, a directional or resultative element follows the main verb: 把药材放在锅里 *bǎ yào fāng zài guō lǐ*, lit. 'hold (take) drug materials put in wok', 'put the drug materials in the wok' (放药材在锅里 *fāng yào cái zài guō lǐ* would be incorrect Chinese).

3.1 Single-Character Verbs

In classical Chinese, most stative and active verbs were single characters. Many single-character active and stative verbs are among a core of basic terms that have been used ever since the time of the *Huáng Dì Nèi Jīng*.

85. 虚 *xū*, vacuous
86. 实 *shí*, replete
87. 胀 *zhàng*, distended
88. 满 *mǎn*, full
89. 滑 *huá*, slippery
90. 沉 *chén*, sunken, deep
91. 浮 *fú*, floating
92. 散 *sàn*, dissipated
93. 客 *kè*, visit, settle
94. 留 *liú*, stay, lodged
95. 遏 *è*, obstructed
96. 补 *bǔ*, supplement
97. 泻 *xiè*, drain
98. 阻 *zǔ*, obstruct
99. 养 *yǎng*, nourish
100. 清 *qīng*, clear
101. 结 *jié*, bind
102. 利 *lì*, disinhibit

3.2 Compound Verbs

In classical Chinese, two-character verbs were comparatively rare. However, reduplicates and semireduplicates were common. Examples include 濈濈 *jí jí*, 'stream-stream', 几几 *shū shū*, 'taut as the neck of a bird about to fly', 淅淅 *xī xī*, 'chilly', 翕翕 *xī xī*, 'warm', 逍遥 *xiāo yáo*, to wander freely, and 徘徊 *pái huái*, 'hesitate', 'pace back and forth', 'shilly-shally'. Most of these are descriptive or expressive. In the post-classical language of Chinese medicine, other compounds became more common. Active verbs combine in twos, either to represent the sum of the meaning of the component characters or the meaning of one qualified by the other. The English equivalent may be two verbs linked by the word 'and', but in some cases, one English verb covers the meanings of both characters (e.g., breathe).

103. 呼吸 *hū xī*: inhale and exhale; breathe
104. 发散 *fā sàn*: effuse and dissipate
105. 升发 *shēng fā*: upbear and effuse
106. 冲服 *chōng fú*: lit. 'drench and take', take drenched
107. 加减 *jiā jiǎn*: lit. 'add [and/or] subtract', vary [the ingredients in a formula]
108. 选用 *xuǎn yòng*: lit. 'select-use', select, use
109. 生用 *shēng yòng*: use raw

Stative verbs (adjectives) combine in the same way as active verbs.

110. 红绛 *hóng jiàng*: red or crimson
111. 青紫 *qīng zǐ*: purplish green-blue; green-blue or purple
112. 黄赤 *huáng chì*: reddish yellow; yellow or reddish
113. 灰白 *huī bái*: grayish white
114. 烦燥 *fán zào*: vexed and agitated
115. 错杂 *cuò zá*: complex

A stative or active verb may be qualified by a stative verb that precedes it. The modifier in such cases assumes an adverbial quality.

116. 淡红 *dàn hóng*: pale red
117. 萎黄 *wěi huáng*: withered-yellow
118. 微炒 *wéi chǎo*: stir-fry lightly
119. 频服 *pín fú*: lit. 'take frequently', taken in frequent, small doses
120. 妄行 *wàng xíng*: move frenetically
121. 复感外邪 *fù gǎn wài xié*: lit. 'repeat-contract external evil', contract external evil again
122. 过食 *guò shí*: eat excessively
123. 淡渗利水 *dàn shèn lì shuǐ*: lit. 'bland percolate disinhibit water', disinhibit water by bland percolation

Some verbal compounds are resultative.

124. 晒干 *shài gān*: sun-dry
125. 炒炭 *chǎo tàn*: lit. 'fry [till] charred', char-fry
126. 炒焦 *chǎo jiāo*: lit. 'fry [till] scorched', scorch-fry
127. 不易咯出 *bù yì kǎ chū*: lit. 'not easily coughed out', not easily expectorated

In combinations, a polarity action/state is sometimes expressed.

128. 升降 *shēng jiàng*: rise and fall
129. 老嫩 *lǎo nèn*: tough and tender

3.3 Auxiliary Verbs

The main auxiliary verbs used in literary Chinese are presented below.

130. 可 *kě*: can, may (expressing possibility, capability, permission)
131. 能 *néng*: can, may (expressing possibility or capability)
132. 得 *dé*: can (expressing capability)
133. 欲 *yù*: want to, desire to, about to
134. 宜 *yí*: ought to, is appropriate to
135. 必 *bì*: must, bound to (expressing obligation or necessity, or inevitability)

All these are still used in the modern vernacular writing style (*bái huà wén*). In the modern spoken language, 可 *kě* appears in the compound form 可以 *kě yǐ*; both 可 *kě* and 能 *néng* are used in the sense of capability; 能 *néng* is either used alone or in the compound 能够 *néng gòu* or 可能 *kě néng*; 堪 *kān* in the sense of 'can' is a nonclassical literary usage. In the vernacular, 要 *yào* or 想 *xiǎng* replaces 欲 *yù*; 应该 *yīng gāi*, 要 *yào*, and 必须 *bì xū*, expressing necessity, replace 必 *bì* and 宜 *yí*. The character 当 *dāng*, which came to be used in the sense of 'must' in the late classical period, survives in this sense in the compound 应当 *yīng dāng*.

The literary single-character forms commonly appear in Chinese medical terminology. Given that the medical context is dominated by illness, 可 *kě* and 能 *néng* are frequently used in the negative to describe the inability to perform functions.

136. 肩痛不可举 *jiān tòng bù kě jǔ*: lit. 'shoulder painful, cannot raise'
137. 不可忍 *bù kě rěn*: lit. 'cannot bear', insufferable, unbearable
138. 汗出不可止 *hàn chū bù kě zhǐ*: lit. 'sweat issues, cannot be stopped', sweat pours forth continuously
139. 寒可去热 *hán kě qù rè*: cold [medicinals] can eliminate heat
140. 肝受血而能视 *gān shòu xuè ér néng shì*: liver receives blood and [one] can see
141. 夜不能寐 *yè bù néng mèi*: cannot sleep at night

Inability to perform normal functions is often simply expressed by the negative 不 *bù*.

142. 不寐 *bú mèi*: does not sleep, cannot sleep
143. 不大便 *bú dà biàn*: does not defecate, cannot defecate
144. 不孕 *bú yùn*: does not get pregnant, cannot get pregnant

The verb 得 *dé* originally meant 'to get' or 'to obtain', and is still used in this sense to this day. Numerous examples are seen in Chinese medicine.

145. 腹痛，得热则缓 *fù tòng, dé rè zé huǎn*: lit. 'abdominal pain, [which when it] obtains heat, [is] then relieved', abdominal pain relieved by heat
146. 腹痛，得寒则甚 *fù tòng, dé hán zé shèn*: lit. 'abdominal pain, [which when it] obtains cold, [is] then exacerbated', abdominal pain exacerbated by cold
147. 重衣不得温 *chóng yī bù dé wēn*: lit. 'double clothing, cannot obtain warmth', cannot get warm despite extra clothing

The notion of 'obtaining' is very close to that of 'achieving', that is, ability. Examples of 得 *dé* used in the sense 'can' abound.[15]

148. 不得小便 *bù dé xiǎo biàn*: cannot urinate
149. 不得前后 *bù dé qián hòu*: lit. 'cannot obtain 'front' or 'back'', cannot urinate or defecate

---

[15]In 'I did not get to see the Eiffel tower' we see how the use of the English 'get' has developed a new sense of opportunity in addition to the meaning of 'obtain'.

150. 大小便不得 *dà xiǎo biàn bù dé*: cannot urinate or defecate
151. 不得卧 *bù dé wò*: cannot lie down (or cannot sleep)
152. 不得息 *bù dé xī*: cannot catch [one's] breath
153. 不得嚼 *bù dé jiáo*: cannot chew

The word 欲 *yù* means want or desire, but also means 'to be about to' or 'on the verge of'.

154. 口渴不欲饮 *kǒu kě bù yù yǐn*: thirst with no desire for fluids
155. 不欲言 *bù yù yán*: no desire to talk
156. 不欲饮食 *bù yù yǐn shí*: no desire for food and drink
157. 月经欲行不行 *yuè jīng yù xíng bù xíng*: menses about to come but not coming
158. 但欲寐 *dàn yù mèi*: desire only to sleep
159. 脉微欲绝 *mài wēi yù jué*: faint pulse verging on expiration

Examples of 宜 *yí* include:

160. 治疗宜清热泻火 *zhì liáo yí qīng rè xiè huǒ*: the treatment should be to clear heat and drain fire
161. 半夏不宜生用 *bàn xià bù yí shēng yòng*: pinellia should not be used raw

Examples of 必 *bì* include:

162. 治病必求于本 *zhì bìng bì qiú yú běn*: to treat disease, it is necessary to seek the root
163. 重阴必阳 *chóng yīn bì yáng*: double yīn must become yáng
164. 重阳必阴 *chóng yáng bì yīn*: double yáng must become yīn
165. 护处必痛 *hù chù bì tòng*: lit. 'protect(ed) spot must hurt', a protected spot indicates pain

4. Nouns

In classical Chinese, nouns were largely single characters. As with verbs, some noun compounds were reduplicates or semireduplicates: 猩猩 *xīng xīng*, an ape, 螳螂 *táng láng*, 'praying mantis', 螵蛸 *piāo xiāo*, 'mantis eggs', 蟋蟀 *xī shuài*, 'cricket' (pronounced *sjet sjuet* in Middle Chinese).[16]

---

[16] Note that reduplication abounds in the modern language. It appears notably in terms of affection such as 爸爸、妈妈 *bà ba, mā ma* 'mommy and daddy' (opposite order in Chinese), 弟弟 *dì di*, 'little brother', and 哥哥 *gē ge*, 'big brother', and in baby talk, 兔兔 *tù tu*, 'bunny' (rabbit) and 狗狗 *gǒu gou*, 'doggy'. In English, reduplication is seen commonly in baby talk ('wee-wee', 'caca', 'gee-gee'); semireduplicates also exist: 'helter-skelter', 'rumble-tumble', 'creepy-crawly', 'jiggery-pokery', 'hurdy-girdy', 'mish-mash', 'hocus-pocus', 'mumbo-jumbo'.

Other noun combinations were collocations such as 天子 *tiān zǐ*, Son of Heaven, whose meaning is essentially the sum of the meanings of the individual elements. However, some classical compounds represented more than the sum of the elements. The expression 水土 *shuǐ tǔ*, which literally means 'water [and] earth', represents the more abstract idea of 'geographical and climactic influences'; 山水 *shān shuǐ*, lit. 'mountains [and] water', means scenery; 风水 *fēng shuǐ*, lit. 'wind-water', means geomancy. Note this is rather like 'pots and pans' in English denoting kitchen utensils in general.

The basic resources of any language are limited, and compounding is a natural way of building vocabulary. Chinese has relied increasingly on compounding of characters just as English has increasingly relied on compounding of words and morphemes. In Chinese, the notion of 'telephone' is 电话 *diàn huà*, which literally means 'electric speech' (电 actually means 'lightening', and was coined to represent electricity). Though the elements of the compound are actually different in meaning from those of the English word (*tele,* distant; *phone,* sound) the principle of compounding is the same. While both 电 *diàn* and 话 *huà* are still used independently, this is not true of all characters. The character 军 *jūn* is now never used outside compounds such as 军队 *jūn duì*, 'army', 海军 *hǎi jūn*, 'navy', 空军 *kōng jūn*, 'air force', and 军事 *jūn shì*, 'military', except as an abbreviation. In the modern language, compounds are thus more cohesive than the collocations of the classical language.

Compounding was encouraged not only by the need to meet growing vocabulary needs, but also by a gradual reduction in sounds. For example, 25 characters now pronounced *jiàn* are known to have once represented eighteen distinct syllables.[17] When words once clearly distinguished in sound are no longer clearly distinguished, a combination of two words helped to restore the clarity. The classical word for the 'ear' was 耳 *ěr*, but in the modern spoken language, the same notion is expressed with a compound, 耳朵 *ěr duo*, lit. 'ear flower'. This process of compounding is often observed in names of body parts, as the list below shows. These compounds are used in the language of today, both spoken and written. They are, however, not inseparable. The additional elements disappear in compounds representing two or more parts of the body, for example, 耳鼻喉科 *ěr bí hóu kē*, 'ear, nose and throat department'. Even in Western medical texts, the colloquial compounds for single body parts are comparatively rare; and in Chinese medical literature, still to this day, single characters are the norm rather than the exception. Thus replacement of monosyllabic words with polysyllablic words is only partial.

166. 额 *é*, forehead, now 额头 *é tóu*, lit. 'forehead' with noun suffix

---

[17]This example comes from *Chinese*, Norman, J., page 133.

167. 目 *mù*, eye, now 眼睛 *yǎn jīng*, lit. 'eye eye'
168. 睑 *jiǎn*, eyelid, now 眼皮 *yǎn pí*, lit. 'eye skin'
169. 睫 *jié*, eyelash, now 睫毛 *jié máo*, lit. 'eyelash hair'
170. 耳 *ěr*, ear, now 耳朵 *ěr duo*, lit. 'ear flower'
171. 鼻 *bí*, nose, now 鼻子 *bí zi*, lit. 'nose', with noun suffix
172. 口 *kǒu*, mouth, now 嘴巴 *zuǐ bā*, lit. 'mouth' plus noun suffix
173. 齿 *chǐ*, tooth, now 牙齿 *yá chǐ*, lit. 'tooth tooth'
174. 舌 *shé*, tongue, is now 舌头 *shé tou*, lit. 'tongue' plus noun suffix
175. 喉 *hóu*, throat, now 喉咙 *hóu lóng*, lit. 'throat-throat'
176. 肩 *jiān*, shoulder, now 肩膀 *jiān bǎng*
177. 腹 *fù*, abdomen, now 肚子 *dù zi*
178. 脐 *qí*, umbilicus, now 肚脐 *dù qí*, lit. 'belly umbilicus'.
179. 膝 *xī*, knee, now 膝盖 *xī gài*, lit. 'knee cover' (probably originally referring to the kneecap)
180. 臀 *tún*, buttocks, now 臀部 *tún bù* or 屁股 *pì gǔ*
181. 骨 *gǔ*, bone, now 骨头 *gǔ tóu*
182. 发 *fà*, hair, now 头发 *tóu fà*

Note that modern vernacular names of body parts include all three of the noun suffixes, 子 *zi*, 头 *tou*, and 巴 *bā*, that are a feature of post-classical Chinese (鼻子 *bí zi*, 'nose', 骨头 *gǔ tóu*, 'bone', 下巴 *xià ba*, 'chin').

The tendency toward compounding is, of course, not limited to the names of body parts. We may presume that 痢 *lì*, 'dysentery' became 痢疾 *lì jí*, 'dysentery disease', by the need to distinguish 痢 *lì* from its many homophones. In compounds, however, the single character suffices to express the notion of dysentery: 赤痢 *chì lì*, 'red dysentery', 白痢 *bái lì*, 'white dysentery'.

Foreign borrowings constitute a major source of new vocabulary in most languages. Chinese has resisted borrowing from other languages, largely because the polysyllabic words and consonant clusters common in other languages are clumsy when assimilated to the sound patterns of Chinese. However, we do know that beyond a fundamental relationship with the Tibetan languages, Chinese appears to have affinities with other language groups. The ancient Chinese are known to have had contact with other peoples from the earliest times, and it would appear that the Chinese may have been strongly influenced by genetically unrelated languages. J. Norman posits, for example, that 狗 *gǒu*, 'dog', which has now largely replaced the competing synonym 犬 *quǎn*, is of Miáo-Yáo origin, that 虎 *hǔ*, 'tiger', is of an Austroasiatic origin, and that 犊 *dú*, 'calf', can be traced to an Altaic origin.

The foreign origins of the following plants and plant products would appear reasonably certain, attesting to contact with the distant civilizations of

India, the Middle East, and Southeast Asia. It is likely that further research could multiply these examples.

183. 荜拨梨 (荜茇) *bì bō lí, bì bá*, Sanskrit *pippali*, long pepper
184. 葡萄 *pú táo*, Iranian prototype **buddāwa*, grape[18]
185. 高良姜 *gāo liáng jiāng*, Arabic *khalanjān*, galangal
186. 诃黎勒 (诃子) *hē lì lì lè, hē zǐ*, Pashto *halīla-ī-kābulī*, myrobalan of Kabul, chebule
187. 茉莉 *mò li*, (Middle Chinese *m[u]ât li-*), Sanskrit *mallikā*, jasmine
188. 没药 *mò yào*, probably akin to Hebrew *mōr* and Arabic *murr*, myrrh
189. 槟榔 *bīn láng*, Malay *pinang*, areca (also called betel nut, pinang)
190. 苏枋 (木) *sū fāng, sū fāng mù*, Malay *sapang* of southern Indian origin, sappan
191. 栴檀 *zhān tán*, Sanskrit *candana*, sandal

The following sections discuss noun + noun, stative verb + noun, and possessive + noun, and noun phrases formed with numerals, measure words, quantifiers, and subordinative and nominalizing particles. In addition, proper nouns and pronouns are also discussed.

4.1 Single-Character Nouns

Many basic Chinese medical terms are single-word nouns. Some of these terms have been replaced by compounds in the modern spoken language (e.g., 肩膀 *jiān bǎng*, shoulder, 舌头 *shé tóu*, tongue), but even in modern Chinese medical texts, they continue to appear in their classical single-character form.

192. 肝 *gān*, liver	205. 目 *mù*, eye
193. 心 *xīn*, heart	206. 舌 *shé*, tongue
194. 脾 *pí*, spleen	207. 口 *kǒu*, mouth
195. 肺 *fèi*, lung	208. 齿 *chǐ*, tooth
196. 肾 *shèn*, kidney	209. 鼻 *bí*, nose
197. 胆 *dǎn*, gallbladder	210. 耳 *ěr*, ear
198. 胃 *wèi*, stomach	211. 发 *fà*, hair of the head
199. 肠 *cháng*, intestine	212. 头 *tóu*, head
200. 筋 *jīn*, sinew	213. 肩 *jiān*, shoulder
201. 肉 *ròu*, flesh	214. 手 *shǒu*, hand
202. 脉 *mài*, vessel	215. 足 *zú*, foot
203. 皮 *pí*, skin	216. 脐 *qí*, umbilicus
204. 骨 *gǔ*, bone	

---

[18]In linguistic convention, an asterisk before a word indicates a reconstructed pronunciation.

217. 肘 *zhǒu*, elbow
218. 膝 *xī*, knee
219. 血 *xuè*, blood
220. 精 *jīng*, essence
221. 气 *qì*, qi
222. 神 *shén*, spirit
223. 木 *mù*, wood
224. 火 *huǒ*, fire

225. 土 *tǔ*, earth
226. 金 *jīn*, metal
227. 水 *shuǐ*, water
228. 酸 *suān*, sour
229. 苦 *kǔ*, bitter
230. 甘 *gān*, sweet
231. 辛 *xīn*, acrid
232. 咸 *xián*, salty

It is interesting to note here most of the five viscera, 五脏 *wǔ zàng*, and six bowels, 六腑 *liù fǔ*, are represented by single-character names. All those that have single-character names are clearly identifiable as independent entities. The distinction between the large and the small intestine was made in Chinese, as in English, by the addition of adjectives (大、 小 *dà*、 *xiǎo*), and the pericardium was distinguished from the heart by the addition of 包络 *bāo luò*, 'envelope network', much as it is distinguished in English by the 'peri-', around, prefixed to 'card', heart. Being compounds, these terms may reflect the fact that they denoted technical distinctions not made in lay speech. The triple burner, 三焦 *sān jiāo*, another combination, was almost certainly not recognized by the lay since it was never even identified to the satisfaction of the whole of the medical community as anything more than a functional entity. Of the bowels and viscera, this leaves the bladder, 膀胱 *páng guāng*, a clearly identifiable organ represented by a noun compound that is most likely a semireduplication.

4.2 Noun + Noun Compounds

Nouns can be conjoined by 与 *yǔ* 'and', 'with' (e.g., 肝与胆 *gān yǔ dǎn*, 'the liver and gallbladder'). However, especially in fixed collocations and when the two (or more) items are considered to form a single entity, 与 is not used. Compare the following two examples.

233. 肝与胆相为表里 *gān yǔ dǎn xiāng wéi biǎo lǐ*: lit. 'the liver and gallbladder are exterior-interior to each other', they stand in interior-exterior relationship to each other
234. 肝胆有热 *gān dǎn yǒu rè*: lit. 'liver-gallbladder has heat', heat in the liver and gallbladder

Combinations of nouns display relationships similar to those existing between component characters of verb combinations. When they represent the sum of the components, the English equivalent takes the format of 'A and B', although combinations of evils and organ-phase appositions are hyphenated (e.g., wind-cold, spleen-earth).

235. 胸胁 *xiōng xié*: lit. 'chest/rib-side', chest and rib-side
236. 津液 *jīn yè*: liquid and humor; fluids
237. 崩漏 *bēng lòu*: flooding and spotting
238. 客主 *kè zhǔ*: Guest-Host (an acupuncture point name)
239. 心腹 *xīn fù*: heart [region] and abdomen
240. 心肺 *xīn fèi*: heart and lung
241. 癥瘕积聚 *zhēng jiǎ jī jù*: concretions, conglomerations, accumulations, and gatherings
242. 风寒 *fēng hán*: wind-cold
243. 湿热 *shī rè*: damp-heat
244. 脾土 *pí tǔ*: spleen-earth
245. 肺金 *fèi jīn*: lung-metal

Combinations may denote more than the sum of the individual meaning.

246. 水谷 *shuǐ gǔ*: grain and water, i.e., foodstuffs in general

The relationship between the components may involve a polarity.

247. 天地 *tiān dì*: heaven and earth
248. 寒热 *hán rè*: cold and/or heat
249. 标本 *biāo běn*: tip and root

Combinations may also take the form of premodification, that is, one noun qualified by a noun that preceeds it.

250. 精气 *jīng qì*: essential qì
251. 脾气 *pí qì*: spleen qì (splenic qì, the spleen's qì)
252. 心包 *xīn bāo*: lit. 'heart envelope', pericardium
253. 盗汗 *dào hàn*: lit. 'thief sweating', night sweating
254. 气淋 *qì lín*: qì strangury
255. 牛皮癣 *niú pí xiǎn*: ox-hide lichen
256. 梅核气 *méi hé qì*: plum-pit qì
257. 膀胱湿热 *páng guāng shī rè*: bladder damp-heat
258. 鹅爪风 *é zhǎo fēng*: goose-foot wind
259. 虾蟆瘟 *há má wēn*: toad-head scourge

4.3 Stative Verb + Noun Collocations

Noun phrases notably include stative verb (adjective) + noun constructions. A large number of Chinese medical terms are formed by this kind of premodification.

260. 浮脉 *fú mài*: floating pulse
261. 白苔 *bái tāi*: white [tongue] fur

262. 迟脉 *chí mài*: slow pulse
263. 白秃疮 *bái tū chuāng*: bald white scalp sore
264. 小便 *xiǎo biàn*: lit. 'lesser convenience', urine
265. 少阳 *shào yáng*: lesser yáng

4.4 Numerals, Measures, and Quantifiers

In classical Chinese, a number could also be placed directly before the noun. Numerous Chinese medical terms are numeral + noun combinations.

266. 二阴 *èr yīn*: the two yīn, that is, the anus and genitals
267. 三因 *sān yīn*: the three causes
268. 四关 *sì guān*: the four gates
269. 五痹 *wǔ bì*: five impediments
270. 六腑 *liù fǔ*: six bowels
271. 七冲门 *qī chōng mén*: seven gates
272. 八法 *bā fǎ*: the eight methods
273. 九窍 *jiǔ qiào*: the nine orifices
274. 十剂 *shí jì*: ten formulas
275. 十一科 *shí yī kē*: the eleven branches of medicine
276. 十二经筋 *shí èr jīng jīn*: the twelve channel sinews
277. 十三鬼穴 *shí sān guǐ xuè*: the thirteen ghost points
278. 十四经 *shí sì jīng*: the fourteen channels
279. 十五络 *shí wǔ luò*: the fifteen network vessels
280. 十六郄穴 *shí liù xī xuè*: the sixteen cleft points
281. 十七椎穴 *shí qī zhuī xué*: the seventeenth vertebral point
282. 十八反 *shí bā fǎn*: the eighteen clashes
283. 二十椎穴 *èr shí zhuī xué*: the twentieth vertebral point
284. 二十三蒸 *èr shí sān zhēng*: the twenty-three steamings
285. 二十八脉 *èr shí bā mài*: the twenty-eight pulses

'Number one', 'number two', 'number three', and so on, are expressed as numeral + 号 *hào*.

286. 驱蛔汤二号 *qū huí tāng èr hào*: Roundworm-Expelling Decoction No. 2

The ordinals 'first', 'second', 'third', etc., are expressed in Chinese by 第 *dì* + numeral.

287. 第二章 *dì èr zhāng*: lit. 'second chapter', chapter two
288. 第二十八页 *dì èr shí bā yè*: lit. '28th page', page 28

Note that sometimes the ordinal marker 第 is dropped, for example, 二十八页 *èr shí bā yè*, 28th page, page 28. Two examples of this are also to be seen in the list of examples of numerals above.

Points in a discussion are frequently labelled with the character 则 *zé*.

289. 一则无热象，二则有明显的气虚、阳虚之象 *yī zé wú rè xiàng; èr zé yǒu míng xiǎn de qì xū、yáng xū zhī xiàng*: First, there are no heat signs; second, there are marked signs of qì vacuity and yáng vacuity.

A distinctive characteristic of modern Chinese is the use of measure words with nouns. English, too, has measure words, but they only apply to things or substances that are not naturally differentiated into distinct units, represented in English by what are known as noncount nouns (nouns that normally have no plural form): 'a cup of milk', 'a bucket of water', 'a bag of flour', and so forth. In modern Chinese, there are not only measures for noncount nouns like flour and water, but also for classes of objects: 一支笔 *yì zhī bǐ*, 'a stick of pen'; 一篇文张 *yì piān wén zhāng*, 'a piece of article' (an essay or article); 一个人 *yì ge rén*, 'a unit of person'; 一层楼 *yì céng lóu*, 'a layer of building' (a story). Abstract notions appearing with a number are often preceded by 种 *zhǒng*, 'kind', for example, 两种治法 *liǎng zhǒng zhì fǎ*, 'two methods of treatment'.

The obligatory use of measure words is a fairly late development. Classical Chinese, like English, did not have measure words for things naturally taking the form of differentiated units. When the measure words started to be used, they were generally placed after the noun.

290. 病机十九条 *jī bìng shí jiǔ tiáo*: the 19 pathomechanisms
291. 大枣三枚 *dà zǎo sān méi*: three jujubes
292. 生姜五片 *shēng jiāng wǔ piàn*: five slices of fresh ginger

A number of single- or two-character quantifiers expressing relative quantity precede the noun they qualify. The most commonly used in Chinese medicine are:

293. 诸 *zhū*, all, various
294. 各 *gè*, each, various
295. 每 *měi*, each
296. 数 *shù*, several
297. 整 *zhěng*, whole
298. 全 *quán*, whole
299. 多 *duō*, much, many
300. 少 *shǎo*, little, few
301. 一切 *yí qiè*, all

Examples include:

302. 诸虫 *zhū chóng*: all worms; the various worms

303. 一切疾病 *yí qiè jí bìng*: all diseases
304. 多气少血 *duō qì shǎo xuè*: much qì and little blood
305. 全蝎 *quán xiē*: whole scorpion
306. 桂枝、白芍各五钱 *guì zhī、bái sháo gè wǔ qián*: cinnamon twig and white peony, five qián of each

Two of the above quantifiers, 多 *duō* and 少 *shǎo*, also act as predicative stative verbs, as the following examples show.

307. 痰多 *tán duō*: phlegm is copious.
308. 病种众多 *bìng zhǒng zhòng duō*: the kinds of illness are numerous

4.5 Noun Phrases Formed with Particles

The particle 之 *zhī*, equivalent to the 的 *de* of the modern spoken language, expresses a possessive or subordinative relationship similar, in some of its uses, to the English *'s* or 'of'. It can be placed between a premodifier and the noun it modifies, though usually only when the premodifier is more than one character.

309. 经络之气 *jīng luò zhī qì*: lit. 'channel-network's qì', qì of the channels and network vessels
310. 仓廪之官 *cāng lǐn zhī guān*: lit. 'granaries' official', official of the granaries
311. 五藏之精气 *wǔ zàng zhī jīng qì*: lit. 'five viscera's essential qì', the essential qì of the five viscera
312. 经脉之海 *jīng mài zhī hǎi*: the sea of the channels and vessels
313. 一身之表 *yī shēn zhī biǎo*: lit. 'one body's exterior', the exterior of the entire body
314. 人之一身 *rén zhī yì shēn*: the whole of the human body
315. 春夏之令 *chūn xià zhī lìng*: the seasons of spring and summer

The premodifier may be a stative verb or stative verb phrase.

316. 苦寒之剂 *kǔ hán zhī jì*: cold bitter formulas
317. 辛热之剂 *xīn rè zhī jì*: hot acrid formulas
318. 新旧之疾 *xīn jiù zhī jí*: new and old diseases

Note that if the modifier is comprised of a single character, the 之 is unnecessary: 寒剂 *hán jì*, 'cold formulas'.

Verb + object phrases are commonly turned into modifiers with the addition of the subordinative 之. Notice that similar premodification in English sometimes requires the verb and object to switch positions.

319. 受盛之官 *shòu shèng zhī guān*: lit. 'receive-plenitude PARTICLE official', official receiving plenitude

320. 清热泻火之剂 *qīng rè xiè huǒ zhī jì*: lit. 'clear-heat drain-fire PARTICLE formulas', heat-clearing fire-draining formulas; formulas that clear heat and drain fire

321. 肺为贮痰之器，脾为生痰之原 *fèi wéi zhǔ tán zhī qì, pí wèi shēng tán zhī yuán*: lit. 'lung is hold-phlegm PARTICLE receptacle; spleen is engender-phlegm PARTICLE source', the lung is the receptacle that holds phlegm; the spleen is the source of phlegm formation

The particle 者 *zhě*, which we have already seen as a topic marker, can be added to adjectives, verbs, and verb + object phrases to make them into nouns. It corresponds to 'thing(s) which,' 'person(s) who', 'situation in which', or 'where'.

322. 患者 *huàn zhě*: lit. 'a person who is sick', a patient, patients

323. 医者 *yī zhě*: healer

324. 失音有虚有实，虚者属于肺虚，实者属于肺闭 *shī yīn yǒu xū yǒu shí, xū zhě shǔ yú fèi xū, shí zhě shǔ yú fèi bì*: As to loss of voice, there is vacuity and there is repletion. The vacuity situations (or cases) are due to lung vacuity; the repletion situations (or cases) are due to lung block.

325. 前者 *qián zhě*: the former

326. 后者 *hòu zhě*: the latter

327. 附子之大者 *fù zǐ zhī dà zhě*: lit. 'aconite's large ones', the large forms of aconite

Verb phrases may also be nominalized by 者 (the thing/person that, situation in which).

328. 克我者 *kè wǒ zhě*: lit. 'the one that restrains me', the phase that restrains this one

329. 热毒甚者 *rè dú shèn zhě*: lit. 'heat toxin pronounced person/situation', a patient with pronounced heat toxin, or when (wherever) heat toxin is pronounced

The word 凡 *fán* can be added at the beginning of the phrase to emphasize all-inclusiveness (*any* person who, *any* situation in which, when*ever*, where*ever*).

330. 凡皮肤热者 *fán pí fū rè zhě*: lit. 'any skin hot person', anyone with hot skin, or wherever the skin is hot

Another important particle is 所 *suǒ*, previously discussed in the context of passive constructions. The original meaning of 所 was 'place' or 'location', and it is still used in that sense today. It is also used in the phrase 所在 *suǒ zài*, 'place [where something or someone] is', or 所向 *suǒ xiàng*, 'place [where something or someone] is heading'.

331. 足太阴所出 *zú tài yīn suǒ chū*: lit. 'the place where the greater yīn issues', an epithet of the acupuncture point SP-1
332. 足太阴所入 *zú tài yīn suǒ rù*: lit. 'the place where the greater yīn enters', an epithet of SP-9

Further, 所 is used in the sense not only of 'place where', but more loosely as 'thing which' or 'what'.

333. 五脏所藏 *wǔ zàng suǒ cáng*: lit. 'what the five viscera store'
334. 五味所入 *wǔ wèi suǒ rù*: lit. 'what [organs] the five flavors enter'

Thus while 者 *zhě* marks the agent of the verb, 所 *suǒ* marks the object of the action of transitive verbs: 所胜 *suǒ shèng*, 'the one (i.e., phase) that is overcome'. It is also used in a more abstract sense, as the following examples show:

335. 邪之所凑，其气必虚 *xié zhī suǒ còu, qí qì bì xū*: where evil encroaches, qì must be vacuous
336. 筋失所养 *jīn shī suǒ yǎng*: lit. 'sinews lose what nourishes [them]', the sinews are deprived of nourishment

From this it is quite easy to show how 所 is used with 之 *zhī* to form relative adjective phrases corresponding to English relative clauses: 其所用之方 *qí suǒ yòng zhī fāng*, lit. 'he uses PARTICLE formula', that is, 'the formula that he uses'.

4.6 Proper Nouns

Proper nouns in Chinese medicine include the names of medicinals, formulas, and acupuncture points (and other elements of channel system nomenclature). Since the names of formulas are complex terms made up of medicinal names, terms describing therapeutic effect, and preparation form, they are not discussed here.

Because Chinese medicinals are raw or simply processed vegetable, animal, and mineral products, their names mostly derive from the plant, animal, or mineral from which they are derived. The simplest plants, animal, and mineral names are formed by combining significs such as grass (⁺⁺ *cǎo*), wood (木 *mù*), stone (石 *shí*), insect (虫 *chóng*), and fish (鱼 *yú*) with a phonetic. Examples include 葱 *cōng*, scallion, 柏 *bǎi*, arborvitae, 硫 *liú*, sulfur, 虻

méng, tabanus (or gadfly), and 鳖 *biē*, turtle. These names are primary morphemes in Chinese, that is, we cannot break the name down into semantic components or trace their origin to metaphors in Chinese. Usually these occur in combinations that ensure they will be distinguished from homophones. The additional element is usually a generic category (tree, insect) or other distinguishing feature 松树 *sōng shù*, 'pine tree', 柏树 *bǎi shù*, 'arborvitae tree', 虻虫 *méng chóng*, 'tabanus insect', and 乌龟 *wū guī*, 'black tortoise' (no two-character form exists for 葱 *cōng*, scallion). Sometimes a compound is a semireduplicative or reduplicative such as 桑螵蛸 *sāng piāo xiāo*, 'mantis egg-case', 海螵蛸 *hǎi piāo xiāo*, 'cuttlefish bone', and 蟋蟀 *xī shuài*, 'cricket'. Sometimes the origin of compounds is unclear 薏苡 *yì yǐ*, coix (Job's-tears) or 枸杞 *gǒu qǐ*, lycium. As has been shown, a number of such terms are known to be loans from other languages, e.g., 槟榔 *bīn láng*, which has also given 'pinang', an uncommon equivalent of 'areca' or 'betel nut' in English (from Penang, the port on the west coast of the Malaysian Pininsula).

Names of medicinals are derived from the names of the original entity by the addition, if necessary, of a part name or other distinguishing feature.

337. 松脂 *sōng zhī*: lit. 'pine resin', rosin
338. 龟板 *guī bǎn*: lit. 'tortoise board', tortoise plastron
339. 柏子仁 *bó zǐ rén*: lit. 'arborvitae seed kernel', arborvitae seed
340. 鳖甲 *biē jiǎ*: turtle shell
341. 生姜 *shēng jiāng*: raw ginger

Some names are not primal, but are meaningful word compounds, and are constructed in the same way as other noun terms. Of these, noun + noun combinations are among the most common.

342. 人参 *rén shēn*: lit. 'man wort', ginseng
343. 丹砂 *dān shā*: lit. 'cinnabar sand', cinnabar
344. 牛膝 *niú xī*: lit. 'ox knees', achyranthes
345. 云母 *yún mǔ*: lit. 'cloud mother', muscovite
346. 地黄 *dì huáng*: lit. 'earth yellow', rehmannia
347. 木香 *mù xiāng*: lit. 'wood fragrance', saussurea
348. 沙参 *shā shēn*: lit. 'sand wort', adenophora/glehnia
349. 蛇床子 *shé chuáng zǐ*: lit. 'snake bed seed', cnidium seed
350. 龙眼肉 *lóng yǎn ròu*: lit. 'dragon's-eye flesh', longan
351. 石膏 *shí gāo*: lit. 'stone paste', gypsum
352. 地骨皮 *dì gǔ pí*: lit. 'earth bone skin', lycium root bark
353. 丁香 *dīng xiāng*: lit. 'nail fragrance', clove

Some are premodified nouns:

354. 甘草 *gān cǎo*: lit. 'sweet grass', licorice

355. 紫草 *zǐ cǎo*: lit. 'purple grass', arnebia/lithospermum (Arnebiae/Litho-spermi Radix

356. 远志 *yuǎn zhì*: lit. 'far-ranging mind/will', polygala

357. 沉香 *chén xiāng*: lit. 'sinking fragrance', aquilaria

358. 陈皮 *chén pí*: lit. 'old skin', tangerine peel (matured until it turns black)

359. 滑石 *huá shí*: lit. 'slippery stone', talcum

360. 红花 *hóng huā*: lit. 'red flower', carthamus (safflower)

Some names involve active verbs:

361. 独活 *dú huó*: lit. 'alone moving', pubescent angelica (Angelicae Pubscentis Radix)

362. 续断 *xù duàn*: lit. 'join breaks', dipsacus

363. 当归 *dāng guī*: lit. 'must return', Chinese angelica

364. 淫羊藿 *yín yáng huò*: lit. '[cause]-lust [in]-sheep grass', epimedium (a medicinal used to invigorate the sexual function)

365. 益母草 *yì mǔ cǎo*: lit. 'boost-mother herb', leonurus, motherwort

366. 防风 *fáng fēng*: lit. 'protect [against] wind', saposhnikovia

367. 升麻 *shēng má*: lit. 'raising hemp', cimicifuga

Some names include numbers:

368. 半夏 *bàn xià*: lit. 'half summer', pinellia

369. 一支箭 *yī zhī jiàn*: lit. 'one arrow', ophioglossum

370. 三七 *sān qī*: lit. 'three-seven', notoginseng

371. 五味子 *wǔ wèi zǐ*: lit. 'five-flavor seed', schisandra

372. 六麴 *liù qū*: lit. 'six leaven', medicated leaven

373. 八角 *bā jiǎo*: lit. 'eight corners', star anise

374. 九节菖蒲 *jiǔ jiè chāng pú*: lit. 'nine-node acorus', Altai anemone

375. 十大功劳叶 *shí dà gōng láo yè*: lit. 'ten-great-achievements leaf', mahonia

376. 百合 *bǎi hé*: lit. 'hundredfold union', lily bulb

377. 千日红 *qiān rì hóng*: lit. 'thousand days red', globe amaranth

378. 万年青根 *wàn nián qīng gēn*: lit. '10 thousand years green root', rohdea root

Interestingly, three drug items have Chinese names that are constructed in a manner logically similar to that of their English names: 丁香 *dīng xiāng*, lit. 'nail fragrance' to the English 'clove', which derives from the Latin *clavus*, a nail; 益母草 *yì mǔ cǎo*, lit. 'mother-boosting herb' to 'motherwort'; 甘草 *gān cǎo*, lit. 'sweet herb', to 'licorice', which derives from the Greek *glucur-rhiza*, *glukus*, sweet, + *rhiza*, root. Many others, though dissimilar from the

English, are nevertheless logical: 五味子 *wǔ wèi zǐ* is so named because it is considered to have all five flavors (sour, bitter, sweet, acrid, and salty); 沉香 *chén xiāng*, lit. 'sinking fragrance', because it sinks in water and has a scent; 人参 *rén shēn*, lit. 'man wort', because the root is shaped like the legs of man; 龙眼肉 *lóng yǎn ròu*, lit. 'dragon's-eye flesh', because it is the dried flesh of the longan fruit, which, when fresh, has a black kernel (pupil) surrounded by white flesh (sclera); 百合 *bǎi hé*, lit. 'hundredfold union', because of the multiple fleshy leaves forming the single bulb (this is identical to the origin of the English 'onion', from the Latin *unio*, 'union', which denotes a bulb of similar architecture).

Channel and acupuncture point nomenclature differs in nature from the names of medicinals in that none of the terms is primal. Virtually all terms are compounds of two or more characters and most are clearly metaphorical even if the origin of the metaphor is not always clear.

379. 经 *jīng*: lit. 'warp, major line', channel
380. 络 *luò*: lit. 'network, connecting', network
381. 井、荥、输、经、合 *jīng, yíng, shū, jīng, hé*: lit. 'well, brook, stream, channel, uniting', i.e., the five transport points
382. 云门 *yún mén*: lit. 'Cloud Gate', LU-2
383. 水道 *shuǐ dào*: lit. 'ST-28', Waterway
384. 犊鼻 *dú bí*: lit. 'Calf's Nose', ST-35
385. 丰隆 *fēng lóng*: lit. 'Bountiful Bulge', ST-40
386. 风市 *fēng shì*: lit. 'Wind Market', GB-31
387. 少海 *shào hǎi*: lit. 'Lesser Sea', HT-3
388. 曲泽 *qū zé*: lit. 'Marsh at the Bend', PC-3
389. 阳池 *yáng chí*: lit. 'Yáng Pool', TB-4
390. 天井 *tiān jǐng*: lit. 'Celestial Well', TB-10
391. 中渎 *zhōng dú*: lit. 'Central River', GB-32
392. 四渎 *sì dú*: lit. 'Four Rivers', TB-9
393. 三间 *sān jiān*: lit. 'Third Space', LI-3
394. 悬钟 *xuán zhōng*: lit. 'Suspended Bell', GB-39
395. 三阴交 *sān yīn jiāo*: lit. 'Three Yīn Intersection', SP-6
396. 迎香 *yíng xiāng*: lit. 'Welcome Fragrance', LI-20
397. 养老 *yǎng lǎo*: lit. 'Nursing the Aged', SI-6

4.7 Pronouns

The discourse of Chinese medicine is characterized by a predominance of the third person. As in the discourse of the modern sciences, 'I', 'my', 'you', and 'your' are not commonly seen. The various first-person pronouns are seen in prefaces and case histories, but second-person pronouns are rare.

Pronouns abounded in classical Chinese; the list below is not complete. Those used in modern Mandarin constitute a minimal set.

First-person pronouns (I, me)

398. 吾 *wú* (classical)

399. 我 *wǒ* (in classical Chinese, mainly object 'me'; in modern Chinese, object and subject)

400. 余 *yú* (classical)

401. 予 *yú* (classical)

Second-person pronouns (you)

402. 汝 *rǔ* (classical)

403. 尔 *ěr* (classical)

404. 你 *nǐ* (general form)

405. 您 *nín* (polite form)

Third-person pronouns (he, she, it)

406. 其 *qí* (classical subject and possessive form, he, she, it, they; his, her, its, their)

407. 之 *zhī* (classical object form corresponding to 其)

408. 他 *tā* (modern he)

409. 她 *tā* (modern she)

410. 它 *tā* (modern it)

Demonstrative pronouns

411. 此 *cǐ* (classical)

412. 彼 *bǐ* (classical)

413. 是 *shì* (classical)

414. 斯 *sī* (classical)

415. 这 *zhèi, zhè* (modern)

416. 那 *nèi, nà* (modern)

In the classical language, all the personal pronouns are both singular and plural. Additional words could be tacked on to make the notion of plurality explicit, for example, 吾等 *wǔ děng* or 吾辈 *wǔ bèi*, 'we'. The modern pronouns are made plural by the addition of the character 们 *men*.[19]

Of the first-person pronouns, 吾 *wú* was used in classical Chinese as the subject or possessive, while 我 *wǒ* tended to be used only as the object pronoun. In modern spoken Mandarin, the latter is the only first-person pronoun and is used as subject and object. In classical Chinese, first-person pronouns were often replaced by deferential forms, such as 臣 *chén*, 'vassal'.

In classical Chinese, second-person pronouns were used between family members and intimate friends. When talking to superiors, they were replaced by honorifics such as 君 *jūn*, 'master', and 子 *zǐ*, 'lord'. The avoidance of second-person pronouns has continued into the present. In polite speech, one addresses one's superiors by title, for example, 老师 *lǎo shī*, 'teacher'.

Of the third-person pronouns, 其 *qí* can be used in the sense of 'he, she, it, or they', but is most commonly used in the sense of 'his, her, its, their', while 之 *zhī*, which we have already encountered in its use as a subordinative particle, is usually an object pronoun.

---

[19] 们 is believed to be a contraction of 每人 *měi rén*, 'each person'.

As we have already explained, the subject is not obligatory in a Chinese sentence. In general, a third-person subject is either a noun or nothing. Hence neither the classical 其 *qí*, nor the modern 他 *tā*, 'he', 她 *tā*, 'she', 它 *tā*, 'they', which became established in the 7th or 8th century, are so commonly seen as their English counterparts in subject position, for example, 脾胃俱旺，则能食而肥 *pí wèi jù wàng, zé néng shí ér féi*, 'when the spleen and stomach are effulgent, [he, one] can eat and become fat'. However, the classical 其 *qí* is commonly encountered in premodern texts since, in addition to its possessive usage, it is often used in the personally less specific sense somewhat like the English definite article. Thus, 察其色，诊其脉 *chá qí sè, zhěn qí mài*, 'examine his (or her, i.e., the patient's) complexion, and take his (or her) pulse' would be more naturally rendered in English as 'examine the complexion and take the pulse'. In 知其常而通其变 *zhī qí cháng ér tōng qí biàn*, 'understand the norm and be fully conversant with the transmutations (deviations from the norm)', 其 cannot possibly refer to any human subject and serves only to nominalize the verbs 常 *cháng*, 'normal', and 变 *biàn*, 'transmute'.

417. 虚者补其母 *xū zhě bǔ qí mǔ*: lit. 'vacuity: supplement its mother', in vacuity, supplement the mother (i.e., the organ engendering the affected one in five-phase theory)

418. 实者泻之 *shí zhě xiè zhī*: lit. 'repletion: drain it', drain repletion

419. 衰者补之 *shuāi zhě bǔ zhī*: lit. 'debility: supplement it', supplement debility

We should note that classical Chinese possesses an indeterminate personal pronoun, 或 *huò*, 'someone': 或曰 *huò yuē*, 'someone has said', 'it has been said'.

The work done by English reflexive and reciprocal pronouns is performed in Chinese by 自 *zì*, 'self', 'subjectively', and 相 *xiāng*, 'each other', 'mutually'.

420. 脾与胃相为表里 *pí yǔ wèi xiāng wéi biǎo lǐ*: lit. 'the spleen and stomach are exterior-interior to each other', they stand in interior-exterior relationship to each other

421. 自觉冷 *zì jué lěng*: lit. 'self feel cold', experience a subjective feeling of cold

The word 自 originally meant 'self',[20] and is used as a reflexive or disjunctive pronoun (e.g., 自欺欺人 *zì qī qī rén*, 'to fool oneself and others') or adverbially in the sense of 'by oneself', 'by itself', or 'spontaneously' (for

---

[20] The character 自 was a pictographic representation of a nose, the organ to which the Chinese point when indicating 'self' ('me') by gesture.

example, 自汗 *zì hàn*, 'to sweat spontaneously'), but is also used prepositionally in the sense of 'from' (as will be explained later).

The word 相 would appear to be a verb or adverb meaning 'to face (another)' or 'in relationship to another'. In the seven relationships between drugs, 相畏 *xiāng wèi* describes a relationship in which one drug 'fears' another, that is, its toxicity is counteracted by another drug. In the five phases, 相生 *xiāng shēng* and 相克 *xiāng kè*, for example, denote one-way engendering and restraining relationships between each phase and another. In both these cases, the relationship is not one of mutuality. A similar usage is observed in 相信 *xiāng xìn*, 'to believe' (to have trust in another).

The demonstrative pronouns of classical and literary Chinese are 彼 *bǐ*, 'that' and 此 *cǐ*, 'this'. However, in literature, where demonstratives have antecedents in the linguistic context rather than the physical context, 彼 *bǐ*, 'that', is rare. The word 此 *cǐ*, 'this', is often seen even in modern literature in the conjunction 因此 *yīn cǐ*, 'because of this', 'therefore'. In older literature, 是 *shì* (which, as we have seen, has long been the copulative verb of spoken Chinese) is commonly used in the sense of 'this', as is 斯 *sī*.

422. 彼痛风者 *bǐ tòng fēng zhě*: those people suffering from pain wind
423. 并无是字，焉有是病 *bìng wú shì zì, yān yǒu shì bìng*: if no such word exists, how can this disease exist?
424. 斯可以言虚劳之嗽矣 *sī kě yǐ yán xū láo zhī sòu yǐ*: this can be called vacuity-taxation cough

One other demonstrative that should be mentioned is 本 *běn*, which means 'this' in the sense of 'the captioned item'. Under the heading of Cinnamon Twig Decoction (*guì-zhī tāng*), the formula would be consistently referred to as 本方 *běn fāng*, 'this formula', whereas 此方 *cǐ fāng* would refer to the last-mentioned formula (one other than Cinnamon-Twig Decoction). Similarly, 本书 *běn shū* means 'this book' in the sense of 'the present work', whereas 此书 *cǐ shū* refers to a book (by another author) just mentioned. The word 本 *běn* in this sense also appears in some technical terms:

425. 本经自发 *běn jīng zì fā*: to originate in this channel
426. 本经选穴 *běn jīng xuǎn xué*: selection of same-channel points

Classical Chinese has no indefinite pronouns corresponding to 'something' and 'nothing'. These notions are expressed with 所 adding yet another dimension to the complex use of this particle.

427. 目无所见 *mù wú suǒ jiàn*: lit. 'eyes don't have what they see', loss of vision
428. 妄有所见 *wàng yǒu suǒ jiàn*: lit. 'recklessly having what is seen', hallucination

5. Adverbials

Adverbials express manner, time, place, and instrumentality. They include a small class of single-character adverbs that modify the verbs they precede. They also include noun, verb, and prepositional phrases.

5.1 Single-Character Adverbs

The following adverbs, all placed before the verb, commonly appear in Chinese medical texts.

429. 皆 *jiē*, 俱 *jù*, 均 *jūn* (modern 都 *dōu*), 'all'. Discussed below.

430. 独 *dú* and 惟 *wéi* were the classical adverbs corresponding to the English 'only'. The character 但 *dàn* started to be used in this sense in the late Hàn. In the modern language, 'only' is expressed as 只 *zhǐ*, and 但 *dàn* survives in 不但... 而且 *bú dàn... ér qiě*, 'not only... but also, and in 但是 *dàn shì*, 'however'.

431. 乃 *nǎi*, 便 *biàn*, 则 *zé*, and 就 *jiù*, all have a common usage in expressing promptness of action, immediacy of logic, and preciseness of equation. Discussed below.

432. 即 *jí*, 'immediately'; also used in the sense of 乃 *nǎi*, etc., above.

433. 方 *fāng*, just, not until (modern 才 *cái*).

434. 将 *jiāng*, future marker

435. 尤 *yóu*, 'especially'

436. 反 *fǎn*, 'on the contrary', 'contrary to expectation', 'instead'

437. 再 *zài*, 'again'

438. 尚 *shàng*, 仍 *réng*, and 犹 *yóu*, 'still', 'yet'. Of these, only 尚 can be used with the negative: 尚未 *shàng wèi*, 'not yet'. In the modern written language, both 尚 and 仍 continue to be used; and 还 *hái*, which has taken their place in the modern spoken language, is also seen.

439. 亦 *yì* (modern 也 *yě*), 'also' in the sense of a further subject (different subject but same action)

440. 又 *yòu*, 'also' in the sense of a further action (same subject but different action); furthermore

441. 素 *sù*, 'ordinarily', in the medical context emphasizes the patient's constitution or his normal state before the onset of illness: 素有内热 *sù yǒu nèi rè*, 'ordinarily has (suffers from) internal heat'.

442. 鲜 *xiǎn* and 罕 *hǎn*, 'rarely'

443. 多 *duō*, 'mostly', 'usually'

444. 少 *shǎo*, 'less', 'rarely'

445. 或 *huò* (或许 *huò xǔ*, 也许 *yě xǔ* in the modern vernacular), 'perhaps', 'maybe'

The adverb 皆 *jiē* means 'all'. It is often not emphatic and merely serves to mark the subject as plural. It also frequently means 'in all instances' or 'always'. Close synonyms of 皆 *jiē* are 均 *jūn*, and 俱 *jù*. The character 全 *quán* is more emphatic. When the subject is dual, 两 *liǎng*, 'both' (lit. 'two') can be used instead.

446. 疫者，民皆疾也 *yì zhě, mín jiē jí yě*: an epidemic is when all the people are sick

447. 风、火、暑皆属于阳 *fēng, huǒ, shǔ jiē shǔ yú yáng*: wind, fire, and summerheat are yáng

448. 天有暴寒者，皆为时行寒疫也 *tiān yǒu bào hán zhě, jié wéi shí xíng hán yì yě*: sudden cold weather always causes seasonally current cold epidemics

449. 气阴两虚 *qì yīn liǎng xū*: qì and yīn both vacuous

450. 心脾俱虚 *xīn pí jù xū*: heart and spleen both vacuous

451. 胃气全无者，危矣 *wèi qì quán wú zhě, wéi yǐ*: cases where stomach qì is completely absent are critical!

The adverbs 乃 *nǎi*, 则 *zé*, 便 *biàn*, and 就 *jiù* have no exact counterparts in English. The first of these, 乃, which has already been introduced, is classical, while the other three were later developments. Accordingly, in copulative sentences, 乃 and 则 can be used without a copulative verb, whereas 便 and 就 require a copulative verb.

452. 此乃不幸致生灾变 *cǐ nǎi bú xìng zhì shēng zāi biàn*: lit. 'this [is] just unfortunately meeting life catastrophic turn', this is an unfortunate catastrophic turn in life

453. 气有余便是火 *qì yǒu yú biàn shì huǒ*: qì in superabundance is fire

454. 此则时行之气也 *cǐ zé shí xíng zhī qì yě*: this, then, [is] seasonally current qì

In two-clause verbal sentences, these adverbs mark the event of the second clause as a temporal or logical sequel to that of the first. Very often, this is expressed in English with 'when' or 'if'.

455. 阴阳离决，精气乃绝 *yīn yáng lí jué, jīng qì nǎi jué*: lit. 'yīn and yáng separate, then essential qì expires', when yīn and yáng separate, essential qì expires

456. 阳强不能密，阴气乃绝 *yáng qiáng bù néng mì, yīn qì nǎi jué*: lit. 'yáng is [over]strong [and] cannot [keep] tight, yīn qì then expires', when yáng is overstrong and does not constrain itself, yīn qì expires

Of the above adverbs, 即 *jí*, 'immediately', is the only one that commonly appears in terms. The same idea is sometimes expressed with 辄 *zhé*.

457. 见食即吐 *jiàn shí jí tù*: lit. 'see food, immediately vomit', vomiting at the sight of food
458. 睡即惊觉 *shuì jí jīng jué*: lit. 'sleep, immediately fright awake', waking with a sudden fright or start after falling asleep
459. 疹出即收 *zhěn chū jí shōu*: lit. 'papules come out, immediately disappear', disappearance of papules immediately after eruption
460. 食入即吐 *shí rù jí tù*: lit. 'eat, immediately vomit', immediate vomiting of ingested food
461. 水入则吐 *shuǐ rù zé tù*: lit. 'water enters, [patient] immediately vomits', immediate vomiting of ingested fluids
462. 动辄气急 *dòng zhé qì jí*: lit. '[patient] moves, immediately qì urgent', rapid breathing at the slightest exertion

The adverb 反 *fǎn* implies an event or state that is contrary to expectation.

463. 不恶寒反恶热 *bú wù hán fǎn wù rè*: not averse to cold, but averse to heat instead
464. 冬时应寒而反大温者，此非其时而有其气 *dōng shí yìng hán ér fǎn dà wēn zhě, cǐ fēi qí shí ér yǒu qí qì*: lit. 'winter time, should be cold, but [if] on the contrary is greatly warm, this is not the time but there is the qì (weather type)', in winter, when it is greatly warm when it should be cold, this is an untimely presence of a qì

As previously discussed, descriptive verbs placed before an active verb have an adverbial function: 微炒 *wéi chǎo*, 'stir-fry lightly'; 清炒 *qīng chǎo*, 'stir-fry plainly' (i.e., without additives). Nouns are also occasionally used.

465. 目连札 *mù lián zhá*: eyes blinking continually

Finally, nouns could also function as adverbs. Two used very commonly in this way are:

466. 原 *yuán* (modern 原来 *yuán lái*), 'originally', 'actually'
467. 本 *běn* (modern 本来 *běn lái*), 'at root', 'essentially', 'originally'

Certain time nouns are also used adverbially. These will be discussed further ahead.

5.2 Adverbials of Manner

Some of the simple adverbs that have been introduced are adverbs of manner. In literary Chinese, many descriptive adverbs of manner take the form of verbs or phrases added after the verb. These appear to have the nature of separate clauses.

468. 汗出濈濈 *hàn chū jí jí*: sweat flows forth streamingly
469. 歌笑不休 *gē xiào bù xiū*: sing and laugh incessantly
470. 连绵不绝 *lián mián bù jué*: continuous
471. 咳嗽连声不已 *ké sòu lián shēng bù yǐ*: bouts of continuous coughing

Adverbs of manner in literary Chinese could also precede the verb. The following examples are formed with 然 *rán*, 'like this', '-like'.

472. 豁豁然空 *huò huò rán kōng*: gapingly empty
473. 濈然汗出 *jí rán hán chū*: sweat flows drizzlingly

In modern Chinese, adverbs of manner may similarly precede or follow the verb. Those that precede the verb are sometimes marked with 地 *de*, and that follow it are sometimes marked by 得 *de*. Adverbs that precede the verb describe the attitude of the agent or the manner in which the action starts: 他慢慢地开了门 *tā màn màn de kāi le mén*, 'he slowly opened the door'. Adverbs that follow the verb describe the action itself: 他开门开得很慢 *tā kāi mén kāi de hěn màn*, 'he opened the door slowly'. As these examples show, a similar distinction operates in English. The manner adverbials of literary Chinese can also precede or follow the verb, but they do not reveal a clear distinction between attitude and manifestation.

5.3 Prepositions

Many adverbials, especially ones specifying place and cause, take the form of a phrase introduced by a preposition. Prepositions in literary Chinese, as in the modern language, are mostly said to be verbs in origin, and many can be used as main verbs. The main prepositions in the literary discourse of Chinese medicine are listed below. Their usage will be discussed in the following sections.

Locatives (where?)
474. 于 *yú*, at, to
475. 在 *zài*, at
476. 当 *dāng*, at

Ablatives (from where, what?)

477. 自 *zì*, from
478. 由 *yóu*, from
479. 从 *cóng*, from

Instrumentals (by what?)
480. 以 *yǐ*, with, using

481. 用 *yòng*, with, using
Benefactive (for whom, what?)
482. 为 *wèi*, for
Causal (because of what?)

483. 因 *yīn*, because of, in response to

Comparative (in relation to what?)
484. 于 *yú*, than, in relation to

All these are used in the modern spoken language, although 从 *cóng* has largely replaced 自 *zì* and 由 *yóu*.

5.4 Adverbials of Comparison

Analogies, which are rather plentiful in the language of Chinese medicine, are expressed with 如 *rú*, which in origin is a verb similar to the English 'resemble'. A simple analogy is expressed as 'X 如 Y', 'X resembles (is like) Y'.

485. 下焦如渎 *xià jiāo rú dú*: the lower burner is like a sluice
486. 大便如鸭溏 *dà biàn rú yā táng*: stool resembling duck's slop
487. 声如拽锯 *shēng rú zhuài jù*: sound resembling the rasping of a saw

When 如 follows an active or stative verb, it introduces an adverbial phrase. In this usage, it can be thought of as a preposition similar to the English 'like'.

488. 腹胀如鼓 *fù zhàng rú gǔ*: abdomen distended like a drum
489. 牙齿干燥如枯骨 *yá chǐ gān zào rú kū gǔ*: teeth dry as desiccated bones
490. 视赤如白 *shì chì rú bái*: seeing red as white
491. 汗出如油 *hàn chū rú yóu*: lit. 'sweat comes out like oil', put forth oily sweat
492. 血出如注 *xuè chū rú zhù*: blood issuing as if pouring

If the object of comparison is a stative or active verb, 如 thus corresponds to the English 'as if'.

493. 目如脱 *mù rú tuō*: lit. 'eyes are as if [about to] pop out', eyes fit to burst from their sockets
494. 头痛如破 *tóu tòng rú pò*: lit. 'head hurt, as if split', have a splitting headache

Less commonly, the 如 phrase may precede the verb (as the modern vernacular construction 象 *xiàng*... 一样 *yí yàng* in the case of stative verbs), e.g., 如麻子大 *rú má zǐ dà*, 'as big as (the size of) a sesame seed'. In such cases, the word 如 can disappear: 梧桐子大 *wú tóng zǐ dà*, 'make into pills the size of firmiana seeds'. Notice that a similar disappearance of a preposition is observed in adverbials of instrumentality discussed ahead.

In classical Chinese, comparative constructions were expressed in the form 'noun + stative verb + 于 *yú* (than) + noun': 热重于寒 *rè zhōng yú hán*, 'the heat is more pronounced than the cold'.[21] This construction is still used on occasion in the modern written and spoken language, but is limited to one-word verbs (e.g., 高于 *gāo yú*, higher than). It has largely been replaced by 'noun + 比 *bǐ* (compared with) + noun 比较 *bǐ jiào* (comparatively) + stative verb'. In the modern written language, the formula 'noun + 较 *jiào* (compared with) + noun + stative verb' is also common. Note that 比, like 如, is a verb in origin.

495. 热证较寒证少见 *rè zhèng jiào hán zhèng shǎo jiàn*: heat patterns are rarer than cold patterns

5.5 Adverbials of Place and Movement

In classical Chinese, the preposition of location was 于 *yú*. In modern spoken Chinese, it has been completely replaced by 在 *zài*, the verb of location, except in set phrases. It is nevertheless still used in the written language, and is common in modern Chinese medical texts. Notice in the following examples that the 于 can sometimes be omitted.

496. 肺主输精于皮毛 *fèi zhǔ shū jīng yú pí máo*: lung governs transportation of essence to the skin and [body] hair
497. 寒邪客于肺 *hán xié kè yú fèi*: cold evil settles in the lung
498. 热结 (于) 大肠 *rè jié (yú) dà cháng*: heat binds in the large intestine
499. 邪留 (于) 三焦 *xié liú (yú) sān jiāo*: evil lodges in the triple burner

In the language of Chinese medicine, 在 appears occasionally as a preposition. In the example below, it has a specific sense.

500. 脾，在华为爪，在志为思 *pí, zài huá wéi zhǎo, zài zhì wéi sī*: lit. 'the spleen in [the context of] bloom is the nails, in [the context of] minds, it is thought'

Adverbial phrases of place can take the form of a place noun followed by a localizer such as 上 *shàng*, above, 下 *xià*, below, 内 *nèi* (also 里 *lǐ* and 中 *zhōng*), inside, 外 *wài*, outside, 后 *hòu*, behind, and 前 *qián*, in front of. Localizers are thus 'postpositions' by comparison with their English counterparts, which are all prepositions. Thus the postposition 中 *zhōng* corresponds to the English preposition 'in': 喉中 *hòu zhōng* means 'in the throat'. Notice that adverbials of place at the beginning of the sentence have no 于.

501. 喉中有水鸡声 *hóu zhōng yǒu shuǐ jī shēng*: there is a frog rale in the throat

---

[21] The English 'than' differs from 于 in being classed as a conjunction.

502. 梦中呓语 *mèng zhōng yì yǔ*: talk in [one's] sleep
503. 胸中烦热 *xiōng zhōng fán rè*: vexed and hot in the chest
504. 胃中有热 *wèi zhōng yǒu rè*: there is heat in the stomach
505. 耳内长肉 *ěr nèi zhǎng ròu*: flesh growing in the ear
506. 目下卧蚕 *mù xià wò cán*: sleeping silkworms beneath the eyes
507. 渗湿于热下 *shèn shī yú rè xià*: percolate dampness down [and out of] the heat
508. 透风于热外 *tòu fēng yú rè wài*: outthrust wind out of the heat
509. 内服 *nèi fú*: take internally
510. 邪留皮肉之间 *xié liú pí ròu zhī jiān*: evil lodges in the skin and flesh

Beginners of Chinese are often confused by the notion of postpositions. However, they might find it easier to grasp when they realize that there are vestiges of this in English in words like 'hereafter' (which means 'after this'), 'thereby' (which means 'by this'), 'herein' ('in this'), etc. Also, postpositions make more sense when they are regarded as nouns. Thus if 膝下 *xī xià*, 'under the knee', is thought of as the 'knee's under side', the logic of the Chinese order becomes apparent. In some cases, this logic is borne out by the fact that the localizer is attached to the noun with the subordinative particle 之 *zhī*, 's: 下极之下 *xià jí zhī xià*, 'below the lower extreme'.

In Chinese medicine, 上 *shàng*, 下 *xià*, 内 *nèi*, and 外 *wài* may denote the upper part of the body, the lower part, the inside, and the outside, respectively, and as such stand independently as adverbials of place, just before the verb.

511. 肝风内动 *gān fēng nèi dòng*: liver wind stirs internally
512. 心火内焚 *xīn huǒ nèi fén*: heart fire deflagrates internally
513. 水饮内停 *shuǐ yǐn nèi tíng*: water-rheum collects internally
514. 内有热，外有寒 *nèi yǒu rè, wài yǒu hán*: there is heat in the inner body and cold in the outer body

So far we have seen that location is expressed largely by a preposition, or by localizing phrase, or—much more rarely—by both. The prepositions 于 *yú* and 在 *zài*, indicate the general idea of 'at' or 'in'. Localizers are used where a more specific position in relation to the location noun needs to be marked. In the literary language, the preposition does not usually appear when the location noun starts the sentence: 胃中有热 *wèi zhōng yǒu rè*, there is heat in the stomach. It tends to disappear when it follows the main verb: 热结（于）大肠 *rè jié (yú) dà cháng*, 'heat binds in the large intestine'. However, it cannot disappear when it follows a verb + object phrase because it would bring two nouns into a confusing contiguity. For example, if 于 *yú* were removed from the sentence 渗湿于热下 *shèn shī yú rè xià*, 'percolate dampness down [and out of] the heat', 湿 *shī* and 热 *rè* would be contiguous and might be understood as the compound 'damp-heat'. The same is true of 输精于皮毛 *shū jīng yú pí máo* given above.

If the preposition indicates a rough location expressed in English as 'at' or 'in', it might be contended that the localizer 中 *zhōng* in 胸中烦热 *xiōng zhōng fán rè*, 'vexed and hot in the chest', and 胃中有热 *wèi zhōng yǒu rè*, 'there is heat in the stomach', is superfluous. Indeed, the localizer often disappears in the latter term, but in both cases its presence is upheld by a tendency toward symmetry generally observed in the literary language. A four-character expression would seem to have an esthetic value. More will be said later about the esthetic value of four-character expressions.

Although 于 does not normally appear at the beginning of a sentence, 当 *dāng*, 'at', 'right at', can.

515. 当心痛 *dāng xīn tòng*: pain [right] in the heart
516. 卧当风 *wò dāng fēng*: sleeping in a draft (lit. wind)

Before leaving the discussion of the preposition 于, we should note that it occurs in a fused form, 焉 *yān*, 'therein', 'thereat', 'therefrom', etc., which is explained in Chinese as meaning 于此 *yú cǐ*, 'at/from it' (herein, therein, therefrom, etc.).[22]

517. 气之所至，水亦无不至焉 *qì zhī suǒ zhì, shuǐ yì wú bú zhì yān*: lit. 'the places qì reaches, there is no water that cannot reach there too', wherever qì reaches, water always reaches too
518. 脾胃者，仓廪之官也，五味出焉 *pí wèi zhě, cāng lǐn zhī guān yě, wǔ wèi chū yān*: the spleen and stomach hold the office of the granaries; the five flavors emanate therefrom

In the literary language, adverbs of direction are usually undistinguished from adverbs of location. Thus 外 *wài* can mean 往外 *wǎng wài*, toward the outside (outward), or 在外 *zài wài*, on the outside.

519. 痰火上扰 *tán huǒ shàng rǎo*: lit. 'phlegm-fire upwardly harassing', phlegm-fire harassing the upper body
520. 宗气外泄 *zōng qì wài xiè*: discharge of ancestral qì
521. 内陷 *nèi xiàn*: inward fall
522. 肝火上炎 *gān huǒ shàng yán*: liver fire flaming upward
523. 舌出口外 *shé chū kǒu wài*: tongue (hanging) out of the mouth

Examples of the ablatives 自 *zì* and 由 *yóu* include:

524. 自表入里 *zì biǎo rù lǐ*: pass from the exterior into the interior

---

[22]It is considered by historical linguists to be a fusion of 于 *yú*, at, not with 此 *cǐ*, this, but with a now unknown demonstrative or pronoun with the initial sound [*n].

525. 气由脏发 *qì yóu zàng fā*: qì effuses from the viscera

5.6 Adverbials of Instrumentality

In classical Chinese, adverbial phrases indicating instrumentality are mostly formed with the preposition 以 *yǐ*, and placed after the verb. However, an early development in the post-classical period was the shifting of such phrases to before the verb. Chinese medicine presents examples of both constructions.

526. 形不足者，温之以气 *xíng bù zú zhě, wēn zhī yǐ qì*: insufficiency of the [physical] body is warmed with qi
527. 精不足者，补之以味 *jīng bù zú zhě, bǔ zhī yǐ wèi*: insufficiency of essence is supplemented with flavor
528. 以毒攻毒 *yǐ dú gōng dú*: treat poison with poison

The verb 用 *yòng*, 'to use', was only a main verb in classical Chinese. In the modern vernacular, it has largely replaced 以 as the instrumental preposition 'using': 用苦寒药清热 *yòng kǔ hán yào qīng rè*, 'use cold bitter medicinals to clear heat' or 'clear heat with cold bitter medicinals'.

In certain conventional expressions the 以 disappears, and its noun becomes an enclitic to the verb:

529. 水煎服 *shuǐ jiān fú*: take decocted in water

5.7 Adverbials of Time

As has been explained, adverbial phrases are mostly nouns or verbs. Adverbial phrases of time are mostly nouns or include nouns.

The time at which an action or event occurs is often expressed by a single noun. The word 日 *rì*, day, also means 'in the day'; The word 夜 *yè*, night, also means 'at night'. These are placed before the verb.

530. 夜间多尿 *yè jiān duō niào*: lit. 'night-period much urinate', urinate frequently during the night
531. 夜多尿 *yè duō niào*: lit. 'night much urinate', urinate frequently during the night
532. 朝食暮吐 *zhāo shí mù tù*: lit. 'morning eat, evening vomit', vomiting in the evening of food ingested in the morning

Note that in the above example 间 *jiān*, 'period' or 'interval', is not indispensable for 夜 *yè*, 'night', to perform the adverbial function of 'at night'.

Adverbial phrases indicating time of occurrence may be composed of a noun with a postposition. Again, phrases of this kind are placed before the verb.

533. 饭前服 *fàn qián fú*: lit. 'food-before take', take before meals

534. 伤寒病後 *shāng hán bìng hòu*: after a cold-damage disease

535. 食远服 *shí yuǎn fú*: lit. 'food-far-away take', take between meals, not close to mealtimes

In the above examples, 前 *qián*, 'before', is a postposition like 上 *shàng*, 'above', and 下 *xià*, 'below'. As its opposite, 后 *hòu*, it can be used in time (before, after) and place expressions (in front of, behind).

Adverbial phrases of time may take the form of noun phrases made with 时 *shí*, time. In modern Mandarin, 时 is usually replaced by the noun compound 时候 *shí hou*, and is linked to a verb phrase by the subordinative particle 的 *de*: 他睡觉的时候流涎 *tā shuì jiào de shí hou liú xián*, lit. 'he sleeps PARTICLE time, flow saliva', that is, 'he drools when he is asleep'. In a more literary style, 睡觉的时候 is reduced to 睡时.

536. 睡时口角流涎 *shuì shí kǒu jiǎo liú xián*: lit. 'sleep time mouth corner flow drool', drooling from the corner of the mouth during sleep

In the modern vernacular, 有时候 *yǒu shí hou*, 'there are times', expresses the notion of 'sometimes'. In the literary language, this is expressed as 有时 *yǒu shí* or, more commonly, simply as 时 *shí* in the literary language.

537. 语言时断时续 *yǔ yán shí duàn shí xù*: lit. 'speech sometimes halts, sometimes continues', speak haltingly

538. 时轻时重 *shí qīng shí zhòng*: sometimes mild, sometimes severe

The word 时 *shí* is doubled to express repetitiveness.

539. 时时发热 *shí shí fā rè*: intermittent heat effusion

540. 时时惊醒 *shí shí jīng xǐng*: frequent awakening from fright

The word 间 *jiān*, 'interval', is used in the adverbial sense of 'at intervals', for example, 寒热间作 *hán rè jiān zuò*, 'heat [effusion] and [aversion to] cold occurring intermittently'.

The repetition of 日 *rì*, 'sun' or 'day', is not necessary to convey the meaning of 'every day' or 'daily' (modern 天天 *tiān tiān*).

Adverbs of duration are placed after the verb when the verb is in the affirmative, and before the verb when the verb is in the negative.

541. 服用一年 *fú yòng yī nián*: take for one year

542. 三日不食 *sān rì bù shí*: not eat for three days

Phrases expressing the number of times an action occurs are placed after the verb.

543. 蒸八次 *zhēng bā cì*: steam eight times

An additional adverbial phrase indicating the period in which the occurrences of the action take place may be placed before the verb.

544. 日服一次 *rì fú yī cì*: take once a day

The word 久 *jiǔ* expresses the idea of 'a long time'.

545. 日久 *rì jiǔ*: after a long time
546. 久咳 *jiǔ ké*: to have had a cough for a long time

5.8 Adverbials of Cause

Causal constructions are made with 因 *yīn* or 由 *yóu*.

547. 因热为病 *yīn rè wéi bìng*: sick owing to heat
548. 气由脏发 *qì yóu zàng fā*: qì is effused by the viscera

5.9 Sentence Modifiers

Some adverbial phrases modify the whole sentence. Sentence modifiers commonly seen in modern texts include the following:

549. 实际上 *shí jì shàng*: in fact
550. 当然 *dāng rán*: of course
551. 此外 *cǐ wài*: furthermore
552. 另外 *lìng wài*: furthermore
553. 同时 *tóng shí*: at the same time, used (as in English) not only in the temporal sense, but also in the sense of 'furthermore'

5.10 Other Adverbials

Many adverbial phrases are formed with prepositions, which are nearly all derived from other parts of speech and barely distinguishable from them. Verbs that can be used 'prepositionally' are not a closed class.

The verbs 去 *qù*, 'go', 'leave' (equivalent to 离 *lí*, 'leave', in the modern vernacular) and 隔 *gé*, 'separate', are commonly used to express location away from a given point.

554. 去爪甲如韭叶 *qù zhǎo jiǎ rú jiǔ yè*: lit. 'go from nail like a Chinese leek leaf', the breadth of a Chinese leek leaf from the nail
555. 隔水炖 *gé shuǐ dùn*: lit. 'separate-by-water boil', to double-boil.
556. 隔姜灸 *gé jiāng jiǔ*: lit. 'separated-by-ginger moxa', moxa on ginger

The word 随 *suí*, 'to follow', is commonly used 'prepositionally' in the sense of 'according to', 'depending on'.

557. 随证取穴 *suí zhèng qǔ xué*: select points according to signs
558. 随证加减 *suí zhèng jiā jiǎn*: vary the formula in accordance with signs

Other verbs may have an adverbial sense in certain contexts. The following example sentences can be interpreted to have equal emphasis on both phrases, or to be a main verb phrase qualified by an adverbial phrase made up of a verb functioning as a preposition.

559. 辨证论治 *biàn zhèng lùn zhì*: identify patterns and determine treatment, to determine treatment according to pattern
560. 审因施治 *shěn yīn shī zhì*: assess the cause and administer treatment, administer treatment according to cause

6. Conjunctions

Conjunctions are words that act as connectors between words, phrases, clauses, and sentences. The commonly used conjunctions in Chinese medical texts are as listed below.

561. 而 *ér*, 'and' and 'but', is classical and modern.
562. 且 *qiě*, 而且 *ér qiě*, 'and', 'moreover', 'besides', is classical and modern.
563. 则 *zé*, 'so', 'then' is classical, and is widely used in modern formal writing.
564. 然 *rán* and 然而 *rán ér* were the classical adversative conjunctions corresponding to the English 'but' or 'however'; 但 *dàn*, 但是 *dàn shì*, 可是 *kě shì* are modern usage.
565. 虽 *suī* (now 虽然 *suī rán* in the spoken language), 'although'.
566. 因 *yīn*, 'because', is classical, while 因为 *yīn wei*, 'because', is standard in the modern language.
567. 故 *gù*, 所以 *suǒ yǐ*, 是以 *shì yǐ*, 因而 *yīn ér*, and 因此 *yīn cǐ* are classical expressions 'so', 'therefore', 'hence'. All are still commonly used in modern writing with the sole exception of 是以 *shì yǐ*. In the modern spoken language, 所以 *suǒ yǐ* is the standard, and 因此 *yīn cǐ* is heard in formal speech.
568. 若 *ruò*, 如 *rú*, and 苟 *gǒu* were the classical words for 'if'. The first two are still used in modern writing, 如果 *rú guǒ* is standard in speech and writing, and 要是 *yào shi* is colloquial.

569. 以 *yǐ* is the classical 'in order to'. It is still used in modern writing, but is replaced by 来 *lái* in modern Mandarin.

570. 或 *huò* (或者 *huò zhě*), 'or'

Of the above conjunctions, the one most commonly appearing in classical Chinese and in medical terminology is 而 *ér*, which is used both in the additive sense of 'and' and in the adversative sense of 'but'. However, note in the examples below that sentences formed with 而 *ér* often correspond to English sentences formed with 'when'; sentences formed with 而不 *ér bù* often correspond to English phrases formed using 'without'.

Examples of additive meaning include:

571. 痰少而黏 *tán shǎo ér nián*: the phlegm is scant and sticky

572. 脉迟而紧 *mài chí ér jǐn*: the pulse is tight and slow

573. 按之窅而不起 *àn zhī yǎo ér bù qǐ*: lit. 'press it, [it] pits and does not rise', pits when pressure is applied

Examples of adversative usage are given below.

574. 欲便而不得便 *yù biàn ér bù dé biàn*: desires to defecate but cannot defecate

575. 坐而不得卧 *zuò ér bù dé wò*: lit. 'sit but not lie', ability to sit but not to lie down

576. 不梦而遗 *bú mèng ér yí*: lit. 'not dream but emit', seminal emission without dreaming

The conjunction 而 *ér* also appears within adverbial phrases and can be used to join adverbial phrases (in the examples, below 当心 *dāng xīn* and 环脐 *huán qí*) to the main verb.

577. 自上而下 *zì shàng ér xià*: from top to bottom

578. 自叔和而下 *zì shú hé ér xià*: down from (since the time of) [Wáng] Shú-Hé

579. 当心而痛 *dāng xīn ér tòng*: pain in the heart

580. 因霍乱而死 *yīn huò luàn ér sǐ*: died of cholera

581. 环脐而痛 *huán qí ér tòng*: pain around the navel

The word 则 *zé*, 'then', expresses a logical outcome such as 'if. . ., then. . .' or 'when. . ., then. . .'.

582. 燥在中焦则宜养胃 *zào zài zhōng jiāo zé yí yǎng wèi*: lit. 'dryness is in the middle burner, then [one] should nourish the stomach', when the dryness is in the middle burner, it should be treated by nourishing the stomach

583. 阴胜则阳病 *yīn shèng zé yáng bìng*: lit. 'when yīn prevails, then yáng ails', when yīn prevails, yáng ails

584. 阴虚则内热 *yīn xū zé nèi rè*: when yīn is vacuous, there is internal heat

585. 风胜则动 *fēng shèng zé dòng*: lit. 'wind prevails, then stir', prevalence of wind gives rise to stirring

Clauses can be joined together without conjunctions. In such cases, the relationship between the two clauses is indicated only by the meaning content. The absence of conjunctions is called parataxis, which will be discussed ahead.

586. 重衣不得温 *chóng yī bù dé wēn*: lit. '[even if he] doubles [his] clothing, [he] does not get warm', inability to get warm despite extra clothing

7. Empty Words

In classical Chinese a distinction is made between 'empty words' (虚字 *xū zì*) and 'full words' (实字 *shí zì*). Empty words are function words with no concrete meaning, used to express grammatical relationships and personal attitudes; this category includes pronouns, demonstratives, prepositions, and particles. Full words have a concrete meaning; they include mainly nouns and stative and active verbs. Empty words include the negatives 非 *fēi* and 无 *wú*, and particles such as 之 *zhī* and 者 *zhě*, which have already been mentioned.

In Chinese, some empty words perform the function of signaling grammatical structure. Others, importantly, serve to express personal attitude, such as doubt, surprise, confidence. In English, personal attitude is largely expressed by intonation. In Chinese, fixed tonality of words limits the variability of intonation, and so empty words are added to help out. This major difference between English and Chinese explains why many particles cannot be translated lexically.

In modern Chinese, a grammatical pause can be indicated by the empty words 呢 *ne* and 啊 *a*. Personal attitude is expressed through a variety of empty words: 了 *le* (also 啦 *la* and 罗 *luo*) indicates affirmation; 吧 *ba* marks advice, conjecture, or resignation; 嘛 *ma* highlights what the speaker feels to be an obvious fact. 啊 *a*, indicates surprise. Question particles such as 吗 *ma* and 呢 *ne* offer nuanced alternatives to the standard interrogatives of the verb + negative + verb type.

The empty words of classical Chinese were roughly the same in number as the modern ones. They included initials as well as finals. They have no exact correspondences to the modern ones and notably perform more grammatical functions.

7.1 Initial and Final Particles

Chinese has a limited set of particles that begin and end clauses, modifying the clause or sentence. Final and initial particles mostly express feelings such as doubt, certainty, surprise.

Initials

587. 夫 *fú* is a sentence-initial particle that expresses certainty or obviousness.

588. 盖 *gài* is a sentence-initial particle that expresses supposition or uncertainty.

Finals

589. 也 *yě*, particle indicating explanation or judgment

590. 矣 *yǐ* indicates positive affirmation, or exclamation.

591. 哉 *zāi* indicates an exclamation or a rhetorical question.

592. 耳 *ěr* only, just, that's all

The initials 夫 *fú* and 盖 *gài* both introduce a sentence, but whereas the former indicates certainty on the part of the writer, the latter implies that the writer is offering his ideas tentatively.

593. 夫酒者大热有毒 *fú jiǔ zhě dà rè yǒu dú*: [Now] liquor is greatly hot and toxic

594. 少食而肥，虽肥而四肢不举，盖脾实而邪气盛也 *shào shí ér féi, suī féi ér sì zhī bù jǔ, gài pí shí ér xié qì shèng yě*: [if the patient] eats little yet is fat, and although fat, he cannot lift his limbs, it is likely that the spleen is replete and evil qì is exuberant

The final particle 也 *yě*, already mentioned, indicates judgment or explanation, and is often used in the classical nominal sentence. It is also used in the middle of sentences to indicate a pause. The second example below illustrates both usages.

595. 肝者，脏也 *gān zhě, zàng yě*: the liver is a viscus

596. 血之行也，气运之而行也 *xuè zhī xíng yě, qì yùn zhī ér xíng yě*: as to the movement of blood, it is moved by qi

The particle 矣 *yǐ* shows that the writer is emphasizing a point. As a perfective marker, it can also indicate the emergence of a new situation. In both its meanings it is equivalent to the modern 了 *le* when used as a final particle.[23]

597. 肺肾俱病，则他脏不免矣 *fèi shèn jù bìng zé tā zàng bù miǎn yǐ*: when the lung and kidney are both ill, then other viscera are not spared!

598. 只此不同而已矣 *zhǐ cǐ bù tóng ér yǐ yǐ*: only this is different, that's all!

599. 汗出则愈矣 *hàn chū zé yù yǐ*: when sweat flows, it is cured

The final 哉 *zāi* marks an exclamation. It is also often in sentences containing question words such as 何以 *hé yǐ*, meaning 'how' or 'why'.

600. 呜呼，哀哉 *wū hū, āi zāi*: Alas!

601. 何以女子有月信，而男子无月信哉？ *hé yǐ nü zi yǒu yuè xìn, ér nán zi wú yuè xìn zāi?*: Why is it that women have menstrual periods and men do not?

602. 何以言水即化气哉？ *hé yǐ yán shuǐ jí huà qì zāi?*: Why [do we] say that water transforms into qì?

The particle 耳 *ěr* indicates limitation and finality, somewhat as the English 'only', 'just', 'that's all', and equivalent to the 而已 *ér yǐ* (lit. 'and stop') used in both classical and modern Chinese.

603. 此六气中之一气耳 *cǐ liù qì zhōng zhī yī qì ěr*: this is one of the six qi only

604. 余继先人志耳 *yú jì xiān rén zhì ěr*: I am carrying forward the aspirations of previous people, that's all

The initial and final particles are a major feature of literary Chinese that distinguishes it from other forms of written Chinese, notably the modern vernacular form (*bái huà wén*). They abounded in traditional academic discourse, but are almost never seen in modern writing of any kind. In the modern spoken language, the final particles of classical Chinese have been replaced by a new array of particles expressing speaker attitude (了、罗、吧 *le, luo, ba*, etc). These, however, are normally considered inappropriate for modern academic discourse, which is now very much modeled on the sober, unrhetorical patterns of Western languages. The two classical initial particles discussed above have no counterparts in the spoken language, and are therefore, for all intents and purposes, obsolete. It must be borne in mind that Chinese texts were traditionally never punctuated, and that final and initial particles to some extent

---

[23]Note 了 *le, h*as previously been mentioned as a perfective aspect marker following the verb. At the end of a sentence, it has the wide function of expressing affirmation, surprise, insistence, etc.

served the function of marking sentence beginnings and endings. The modern adoption of Western punctuation (slightly modified for Chinese needs) has undoubtedly decreased the need for these particles in the modern written language.

In Chinese medical discourse, even highly literary styles of writing that freely tap literary Chinese rarely use any classical initial and final particles. Nevertheless, it should be noted that certain adverbial phrases, such as 基本上 *jī běn shàng*, 'basically', 实际上 *shí jì shàng*, 'in actual practice', and 事实上 *shì shí shàng*, 'in fact', which are often heard in modern speech, are often seen in modern writing and in modern Chinese medical texts. These are readily translated into English, and they most probably arose under foreign influence. Although the language of Chinese medicine is still very much classical in its terminology, it is distinctly modernized in its discourse.

7.2 Interrogatives

Interrogatives are rarely seen in modern Chinese medical texts. Nevertheless, medical discourse of the past was often highly rhetorical and hence in premodern texts interrogatives abound.

Classical interrogatives are of two kinds: yes/no questions and questions eliciting specific information.

Interogatives

605. 乎 *hū* is a final particle indicating a question of the yes/no type, roughly equivalent to the modern 吗 *ma*

606. 耶 *yé* carries a mild tone of surprise

607. 何 *hé* 'what', 'why', 'how', 'where'

608. 岂 *qǐ*, a question particle

609. 孰 *shú*, 'who', 'which', 'what'

610. 谁 *shuí*, (*shéi*), 'who'

611. 焉 *yān*, 'how'

The particle 乎 *hū* usually indicates a yes/no question. It may also be used with other question words. 耶 *yé* carries a mild tone of surprise.

612. 能有子乎？ *néng yǒu zǐ hū?*: Can he have children?

613. 病在根本，尚堪治不求本乎？ *bìng zài gēn běn, shàng kān zhì bù qiú běn hū?*: The disease is in the root. Could one still treat it without seeking the root?

614. 天下之病，孰有多于温病者乎？ *tiān xià zhī bìng, shú yǒu duō yú wēn bìng zhě hū?*: Of all the diseases under heaven, which is there more of than warm diseases?

In modern Chinese, 吗 *mā* is the equivalent of 乎, but yes/no questions may also be expressed as 'V NEGATIVE V', for example, 他是不是医生？ *tā shì bú shì yī shēng*, 'Is he a doctor?' The latter format is slightly more blunt.

The particle 何 *hé* is a general question marker equivalent to 'what', 'why', 'how', 'where'. It is combined with other characters for greater precision: 何以 *hé yǐ*, 'why' or 'how'; 何人 *hé rén*, 'what person' (who); 何时 *hé shí*, 'what time' (when); and 何处 *hé chù*, 'what place' (where).

> 615. 何为阴分？五脏之精气是也 *hé wèi yīn fēn? wǔ zàng zhī jīng qì shì yě*: What is the yīn aspect? It is the essential qì of the five viscera.
>
> 616. 男子何以不行经？ *nán zǐ hé yǐ bù xíng jīng?*: Why do men not menstruate (lit. perform menstruation)?

In the modern vernacular, these classical forms are not used: 'why' is expressed as 为什么 *wèi shén me*; 'how' as 怎么 *zěn me*; 'who' as 什么人 *shén me rén* or 谁 *shuí, shéi*; 'when' as 什么时候 *shén me shí hou*; and 'where' as 什么地方 *shén me dì fāng*, 哪里 *nǎ lǐ*, or 哪儿 *nǎr*.

The interrogative 孰 *shú* is narrower in meaning than 何, 'who', 'which', 'what'.

> 617. 天下之病，孰有多于温病者乎？ *tiān xià zhī bìng, shú yǒu duō yú wēn bìng zhě hū?*: Of all the diseases under heaven, which is there more of than warm diseases?

As previously indicated, when 何以 is used rhetorically, the final particle 哉 *zāi* often appears at the end of the sentence.

The word 岂 *qǐ* means 'how' or 'how is it possible' and expresses disbelief. For example, 岂能不辞而别？ *qǐ néng bù cí ér bié?*: 'How could you possibly leave without saying good-bye?' When directly followed by a negative, it marks a rhetorical question: 岂不善乎？ *qǐ bù shàn hū?*: 'How can that possibly not be good?' (would not that be good?)

8. Distinctive Features

Chinese probably has no feature that it does not share with some other language. Its nonalphabetic script is unique among modern languages, but even our own writing system preserves ideographs in the Roman numerals I, II, and III and (less conspicuously) in the Arabic numerals 1, 2, and 3 that are very similar to the Chinese 一、二、三. Nevertheless, Chinese has a number of features that are more marked than in other languages. Three features of the literary language, all clearly illustrated in the language of Chinese medicine, have been isolated for discussion here. The first is the ability of words to function as different parts of speech (multifunctionality). The second is a strong tendency to express ideas through juxtaposition without explicit marking of logical relationships (parataxis), and the related tendency towards ellipsis and chronologically ordered description. The third is a tendency to manipulate the variability of single- and double-character expressions to achieve a rhythmic symmetry of expression (elasticity and symmetry). Interestingly, all three of these features are intimately related to the noninflexional and originally monosyllabic nature of the Chinese language.

8.1 Multifunctionality

We have already seen how intransitive verbs could be used in a causative sense, and how nouns and verb phrases are used as premodifiers. We have also seen that some Chinese words are used in so many ways that any classification of them by word-class is difficult. A feature of classical Chinese is its failure to mark word-classes and its great freedom for multifunctional usage. For example, 人 *rén*, 'person', 'human being', can be used as a verb or an adverb. Thus in 人其人 *rén qí rén*, the first 人 is a verb meaning 'to treat humanly'. In 豕人立而啼 *shǐ rén lì ér tí*, 人 *rén* is an adverb meaning 'like a human being', so that the meaning of the whole sentence is 'the pig stood up like a human and wept'. The modern slang expression 鬼叫 *guǐ jiào*, 'scream like a ghost', follows the same pattern.

The technical vocabulary of Chinese medicine contains examples of nouns being used as verbs.

618. 不药而愈 *bú yào ér yù*: lit. 'not medicine (verb), and (yet) cure', to cure without using drugs
619. 不月 *bú yuè*: lit. 'not month', to not have menstrual periods
620. 冬石 *dōng shí*: lit. '[in] winter [it is] stone', in winter it (the pulse) is stonelike
621. 小便 *xiǎo biàn*: lit. 'smaller convenience (urine)', used as 'to urinate'
622. 大便 *dà biàn*: lit. 'greater convenience (stool)', used as 'to defecate'

Stative and active verbs can be used as nouns when used in the position normally occupied by a noun.

623. 太阳为开 *tài yáng wéi kāi*: greater yáng is the opening
624. 哭为肺之声 *kū wéi fèi zhī shēng*: crying is the sound of the lung

625. 赤为热 *chì wéi rè*: red is (i.e., indicates) heat

626. 肾主开阖 *shèn zhǔ kāi hé*: the kidney governs opening and closing

Verb + object phrases are commonly used as nouns. The phrase 清热 *qīng rè*, 'to clear heat', is also used as a noun phrase denoting the name of the method, 'clearing heat'. It also functions as an adjective, for example, 清热剂 *qīng rè jì*, 'heat-clearing' formula. Despite different functions, Chinese terms undergo no change in form, although a change of syntax or morphology is seen in English. All terms describing therapeutic action have this triple function.

627. 解表 *jiě biǎo*: resolve the exterior; resolving the exterior (or exterior resolution); exterior-resolving

628. 理气 *lǐ qì*: rectify qì; rectifying qì; qì-rectifying

629. 利水 *lì shuǐ*: disinhibit water; disinhibiting water; water-disinhibiting

630. 温中祛寒 *wēn zhōng qū hán*: warm the center and dispel cold; warming the center and dispelling cold; center-warming cold-dispelling

Verb phrases and subject + verb phrases are also used as nouns. The term 腹痛 *fù tòng*, means 'the abdomen is painful'; as a predicate with a subject, it means 'to have abdominal pain'; and used as a noun phrase, it means 'abdominal pain'. The fact that the Chinese literally means 'abdomen painful' should not lead the learner to believe that attributive adjectives follow the nouns they qualify as in French and Spanish. The order here derives from the predicative construction 'abdomen is painful'. In general, most symptom terms evince this kind of multifunctionality. Generally, English expresses symptoms in noun phrases, which are often quite different from the verb phrases.

631. 不寐 *bú mèi*: not sleeping, sleeplessness

632. 阳痿 *yáng wěi*: 'yáng wilt', impotence

633. 伤寒 *shāng hán*: to be damaged by cold, cold damage

634. 易伤于风邪 *yì shāng yú fēng xié*: easily damaged by wind evil, tendency to be damaged by wind evil

635. 交接出血 *jiāo jiē chū xuè*: lit. 'have intercourse, bleed', coital bleeding

636. 不梦而遗 *bú mèng ér yí*: lit. 'not dream but emit', seminal emission without dreaming

637. 夜不能寐 *yè bù néng mèi*: lit. 'cannot sleep at night', inability to sleep at night

638. 不得小便 *bù dé xiǎo biàn*: cannot urinate, inability to urinate

In some cases, there would appear to be a difference between subject + verb collocations and verb + noun collocations. Pulse terms follow the pattern of 脉浮 *mài fú*, 'pulse (is) floating' in diagnostic descriptions, but are expressed as 浮脉 *fú mài*, 'floating pulse' in a noun phrase. Multiple-quality pulses are always expressed in the descriptive noun + verb format 脉浮滑而数 *mài fú huá ér shuò*, 'pulse (is) floating, slippery, and rapid'. One single quality may be expressed in the verb + noun format.[24]

Terms describing physiological and pathological conditions also evince the dual function of noun phrase and verb phrase. The term 木生火 *mù shēng huǒ*, is both a description of a universal law, 'wood engenders fire', and an instance of its operation, 'wood engendering fire'. Similarly, 肝火上炎 *gān huǒ shàng yán*, 'liver fire flames upward', describes an action of the liver in terms of a verb phrase, but can also represent the condition or an instance of the pathology as a noun phrase 'liver fire flaming upward'.

In the medical context, what appears a topic + predicate in Chinese, often most naturally translates into English as a noun + relative clause or qualifying phrase.

639. 妇人月经不调、胁痛、乳房胀痛、经血夹块等证，宜疏肝解郁、活血化瘀 *fù rén yuè jīng bù tiáo、xié tòng、rǔ fáng zhàng tòng、jīng xuè jiā kuài děng zhèng, yí shū gān jiě yù、huó xuè huà yū*: for women who have (or with) menstrual irregularities, rib-side pain, distention and pain of the breasts, and clots in the menstrual discharge, the treatment should be to course the liver and resolve depression, and to quicken the blood and transform stasis

It is interesting to note that in the above example the closest formal equivalent to the English relative clause would be 'symptoms a, b, c + 的 + 妇人'. Such constructions abound in modern Chinese, probably due to the influence of Western languages, but they tend not to be used when there are numerous qualifiers (as the four symptoms here). The simpler subject + predicate construction is still preferred. The above example could also be rendered into English as an 'if' clause: 'if a woman has...'. (We have already seen how the notion of 'if' or 'when' does not often appear in Chinese.) Of course, relative or conditional clauses can also be avoided in English too, provided all the symptoms appear in noun form: 'In women, menstrual irregularities, etc., should be treated by...'. However, whichever option is chosen by the translator, English requires decisions about parts of speech, and the addition of markers indicating relationships ('in women', 'women with', 'women who have'), whereas Chinese prefers the simplest construction in which the re-

---

[24]See Wiseman N and Féng Y (1999) "Translation of Chinese Medical Pulse Terms: Taking Account of the Historical Dimension." In *Clinical Acupuncture and Oriental Medicine*. 1.1.

lationships between the elements of the sentence are deduced from context created by the sentence as whole.

This example sentence is an illustration of grammatical multifunctionality. It is also an example of parataxis, the juxtaposition of phrases without explicit marking of the relationships between them. The abundance of paratactical constructions is a striking feature of Chinese, and accounts largely for the fabled tersity of the classical and literary languages. More must be said about it.

8.2 Parataxis, Ellipsis, and Chronological Description

Parataxis is the juxtaposition of words or phrases without any explicit connections. The sense of a paratactical expression is implicit in the context. In English an oft-quoted example of literary parataxis is 'I came; I saw; I conquered', in which the relationship between the actions is not explicitly expressed. This type of construction is common in everyday English: 'prices have dropped; there's a mad rush to buy'. It also occurs with a certain degree of ellipsis in stock phrases: 'in for a penny, in for a pound'; 'nothing ventured, nothing gained'; 'out of sight, out of mind'. Here the main semantic components of the sentence are stripped of the normal grammatical necessities of English ('if one is confident enough to invest a penny, one might as well invest a pound').

In Chinese, parataxis is more prevalent and more developed. The dropping of conjunctions is more common in Chinese speech than in English: 房子盖好了，买不出去 *fáng zi gài hǎo le, mài bu chū qu*, 'house finish building, cannot sell' (the house is finished; [but] we can't sell it). Furthermore, other features of Chinese grammar show marked paratactical tendencies. As we have seen, nouns are regularly not conjoined as they have to be in English: 阴阳 *yīn yáng*, 'yīn and yáng', 天地 *tiān dì*, 'heaven and earth', 兄弟姊妹 *xiōng dì jiě mèi*, lit. 'big brothers, little brothers, big sisters, little sisters' (brothers and sisters), 癥瘕积聚 *zhēng jiǎ jī jù*, 'concretions, conglomerations, accumulations, and gatherings'. The loose relationship of certain topics to their predicates are also paratactical: 病人头痛 *bìng rén tóu tòng*, lit. 'patient: headache'. In the common language, paratactical stock phrases also abound: 南腔北调 *nán qiāng běi diào*, lit. 'southern lilt, northern twang', to speak with mixed local accents. While such phrases in English often represent platitudes, many in Chinese have their origin in the literary language where parataxis has been strongly cultivated. While English attains elegance through refined manipulation of its more complex grammar (as, for example, through the use of relative clauses), Chinese seeks esthetic expression in the succinct paratactical juxtaposition of images, the logical relationships between which, outside stock phrases, the readers must supply for themselves.

The absence of conjunctions between nouns and between verbs is a commonly occurring form of parataxis. Examples abound in Chinese medicine.

640. 水谷 *shuǐ gǔ*: grain and water

641. 天地 *tiān dì*: heaven and earth

642. 加减 *jiā jiǎn*: lit. 'add and/or subtract', vary [the ingredients in a formula]

643. 真虚假实 *zhēn xū jiǎ shí*: true vacuity and false repletion

644. 半表半里 *bàn biǎo bàn lǐ*: half interior and half exterior

645. 重衣不得温 *chóng yī bù dé wēn*: lit. 'double clothing, cannot obtain warmth', cannot get warm despite extra clothing

646. 癥瘕积聚 *zhēng jiǎ jī jù*: concretions, conglomerations, accumulations, and gatherings

Parataxis is commonly used to express comparisons:

647. 多寒少热 *duō hán shǎo rè*: lit. 'much [aversion to] cold, little heat [effusion]', [aversion to] cold more pronounced than heat [effusion]

648. 热重寒轻 *rè zhòng hán qīng*: lit. 'pronounced heat, mild cold', heat more pronounced than cold

649. 太阳多血少气 *tài yáng duō xuè shǎo qì*: greater yáng has copious blood and scant qì

In the conjoining of verb phrases, parataxis can express addition or purpose.

650. 活血化瘀 *huó xuè huà yū*: quicken the blood and transform stasis

651. 益气解表 *yì qì jiě biǎo*: boost qì and resolve the exterior

652. 泄卫透热 *xiè wèi tòu rè*: discharge defense and outthrust heat

653. 导滞通腑 *dǎo zhì tōng fǔ*: abduct stagnation and free the bowels

654. 提壶揭盖 *tí hú jiē gài*: lift the pot and remove the lid

655. 急下存阴 *jí xià cún yīn*: to precipitate urgently in order to preserve yīn

656. 回阳救逆 *huí yáng jiù nì*: return yáng in order to stem counterflow

657. 增液行舟 *zēng yè xíng zhōu*: increase humor in order to move the grounded ship

658. 辨证论治 *biàn zhèng lùn zhì*: identifying patterns as a basis for determining treatment

In the above examples, we see that English conjoins nouns and verbs with conjunctions that are absent in the original Chinese expression. This is not to say that there is a conjunction missing in Chinese; there is simply no need for one. For this reason, it has been said that while parataxis in English is now the exception rather than the rule, in Chinese it is the rule rather than the exception.[25]

Parataxis is distinct from, but nevertheless related to, ellipsis insofar as in literary Chinese both are used together to achieve the terse elegance the Chinese traditionally cultivated.

659. 朝食暮吐 *zhāo shí mù tù*: lit. 'morning eat, evening vomit', vomiting in the evening of food ingested in the morning
660. 饮一溲二 *yǐn yī sōu èr*: lit. 'drink one, urinate two', passing twice as much fluid as is drunk
661. 夜梦鬼交 *yè méng guǐ jiāo*: lit. 'night dream ghost intercourse', dreaming of intercourse with ghosts
662. 迎风流泪 *yíng fēng liú lèi*: tearing on exposure to wind
663. 重按无力 *zhòng àn wú lì*: lit. 'pressing heavily, there is no force', forceless under heavy pressure

In all these examples, substantial parts of the meaning are not explicit. The first sentence, on the surface, would appear to be a description of morning and evening activities, but in fact, tells us when food eaten at a certain time of the day is vomited. The second sentence omits the measures to which 'one' and 'two' refer. The third sentence is ambiguous since it could mean dreaming of a) having intercourse with ghosts, b) ghosts having intercourse, or c) having intercourse like a ghost. The fourth example omits the relationship between being exposed to wind and tearing, although the order of the elements ('being exposed to wind' before 'tearing') reflects a chronological order.

Note that the literal English translations are not always fully intelligible. Even after adjustment to natural English syntax (e.g., 'eating in the morning and vomiting in the evening'), an English speaker still might ask if the patient only eats in the morning.

Parataxis is closely related to a natural chronology embedded in Chinese discourse. A description of a development of events in time and causally related events tends to follow their sequence in time. Most of the preceding examples follow a chronological or causal sequence. If 'drinking one and urinating two' were reversed as 'urinating two and drinking one', the implication would be that patients suffering from dispersion-thirst (diabetes) gauged their fluid intake in proportion to the amount urinated, which is of course not the case. In such contexts, clear descriptive English pinpoints the logical relationship between the observed phenomena. What is described in Chinese as

---

[25]Wáng Lì, "Zhōng Guó Yǔ Fǎ Lǐ Lùn" (中国语法理论 "The Theory of Chinese Grammar") in *Wáng Lì Wén Jí* (王力文集 "Wáng Lì's Collected Writings") Shāndōng Jiàoyù Chūbǎnshè, 1984, vol. 1, p. 90. Original version, Shāngwù Yìnshūguǎn, 1947.

'drinking one and urinating two' is more naturally expressed in English as 'passing twice as much fluid as is drunk', that is to say, through a comparison between the amount of fluid drunk and the amount discharged through urination. Such a comparison does not reflect the chronological aspect of the events.

The natural chronological order is reflected in Chinese grammar. As we have seen, a chronological sequence can be expressed in either of two ways. One is by two clauses, for example, 至冬其病即发 *zhì dōng qí bìng jí fā*, 'come winter, his disease recurs'; the other by turning the first clause into an adverbial phrase 冬时其病即发 *dōng shí qí bìng jí fā*, 'when winter comes, his disease recurs'. In both cases, the Chinese sequence cannot be changed. While 'his disease recurs when winter comes' is equally acceptable English, it is impossible in Chinese. The latter of the two Chinese constructions (the one using 时 *shí*) was rare in classical Chinese, and has only become more common in modern times. It is derived from the former by the process of turning a clause into a nominal adverb of time. The derivation is more clearly apparent in another chronological sequence. The phrase 未红即痛 *wèi hóng jí tòng*, lit. 'not yet red, hurts', that is, 'it hurts before it reddens', could also be expressed as 未红前即痛 *wèi hóng qián jí tòng*, lit. 'before [it] is not yet red, [it] hurts'. Here, the presence of the negative indicates that the verb phrase is, as it were, not completely nominalized and reflects the original construction of two distinct verbal clauses. Compare also:

664. 未发病前服 *wèi fā bìng qián fú*: take before [having] an attack
665. 临睡前服 *lín shuì qián fú*: lit. 'close to sleep before take', take just before bedtime

The chronological pattern of discourse is widely seen in Chinese medical texts. Let us take for example a literal rendering of a Chinese sentence describing an etiology: 'Liver wind is a form of internal wind, caused mostly by liver and kidney yīn humor being excessively depleted, the liver's yáng qì not receiving the nourishment and counterbalancing of liver-kidney yīn-humor, and liver yáng's upbearing and stirring not being restrained'. This description follows the pattern: 'X is brought about by (the sequence) a), b), and c)'. An English speaker describing the same events may well choose this order, but may equally prefer to highlight the importance of one of the elements, for example, 'X is a direct result of c), which stems from a) followed by b)'. English expression tends to give more detail of the causal relations between the individual elements of the sequence, whereas the natural Chinese expression follows the chronology of events. By simply stating all the events as they occur in time, the necessity to mark relationships between events is lessened.

8.3 Elasticity and Symmetry

In most of the examples of Chinese medical terms we have seen so far, each character within the term is used with its own distinct meanings, and in translation it is rendered with a separate English word, for example, 心肺 *xīn fèi*, heart and lung. This reflects the fact that the basic terminology of Chinese medicine was formed at a time when combinations were much less frequent. However, we have also seen that in the modern vernacular many ideas expressed by a single character in classical Chinese are expressed in compounds. This tendency toward disyllabic expression is to some extent reflected in premodern as well as modern Chinese medical texts.

666. 身体 *shén tǐ*: body
667. 形体 *xíng tǐ*: body
668. 眼睛 *yǎn jīng*: eye
669. 目睛 *mù jīng*: eye
670. 胞睑 *bāo jiǎn*: eyelid
671. 口唇 *kǒu chún*: lit. 'mouth lip', lip

In most of the above examples, the combination is comprised of near-synonyms; in 口唇 *kǒu chún*, 'lips', 口 *kǒu*, mouth, is a logical addition.

The same process of doubling is seen in verbs, both stative and active.

672. 肥胖 *féi pàng*: fat; obese
673. 消瘦 *xiāo shòu*: emaciated
674. 宣通 *xuān sàn*: diffuse and free
675. 宣散 *xuān tōng*: diffuse and dissipate
676. 调和 *tiáo hé*: regulate and harmonize

Chinese combinations tend to be of two or four characters, and characters are often supplied or removed to fit this format. Thus 唇 *chún* can be used singly or combined with 口 *kǒu* depending on whether the postmodifier is a single or multiple stative verb.

677. 唇焦 *chún jiāo*: parched lips
678. 唇裂 *chún liè*: cracked lips
679. 唇肿 *chún zhǒng*: swollen lips
680. 唇紫 *chún zǐ*: purple lips
681. 口唇干焦 *kǒu chún gān jiāo*: dry parched lips
682. 口唇紧缩 *kǒu chún jǐn suō*: tightly contracted lips
683. 口唇淡白 *kǒu chún dàn bái*: pale lips
684. 口唇青紫 *kǒu chún qīng zǐ*: green-blue or purple (purplish green-blue) lips

Combinations of three characters are possible, but they tend to be less frequent.

685. 唇燥裂 *chún zào liè*: dry cracked lips
686. 唇口聚 *chún kǒu jù*: pursed lips and mouth
687. 唇青紫 *chún qīng zǐ*: green-blue or purple (purplish green-blue) lips

In the following example, 面 *miàn*, face, and 面色 *miàn sè*, facial complexion, are interchanged in the same way.

688. 面白 *miàn bái*: white face
689. 面青 *miàn qīng*: green-blue face
690. 面色㿠白 *miàn sè huǎng bái*: bright white facial complexion
691. 面色青紫 *miàn sè qīng zǐ*: green-blue or purple (purplish green-blue) facial complexion
692. 面色黄 *miàn sè huáng*: yellow facial complexion

From the point of view of technical meaning, the apparent elasticity of compounds causes one to wonder to what degree the components of a combination are dictated by meaning or esthetics. In other words, the clinical significance of the difference between 面青 *miàn qīng*, green-blue face, and 面色青紫 *miàn sè qīng zǐ*, green-blue or purple (purplish green-blue) facial complexion, may be less than one might expect.

The above examples follow the pattern of noun + verb or noun-noun + verb-verb. Other patterns also exist: noun-verb + noun-verb and verb-noun + verb-noun. All these phrase patterns are seen in diagnostic terms.

693. 四肢拘急 *sì zhī jū jí*: hypertonicity of the limbs
694. 手舞足蹈 *shǒu wǔ zú dào*: flailing of the limbs
695. 扬手踯足 *yáng shǒu zhí zú*: flailing of the limbs
696. 筋惕肉瞤 *jīn tì ròu rùn*: jerking sinews and twitching flesh
697. 囟门下陷 *xìn mén xià xiàn*: depressed fontanels
698. 囟填 *xìn tián*: bulging fontanels
699. 撮空理线 *cuō kōng lǐ xiàn*: lit. 'grope space, order threads', groping in the air and pulling at [invisible] threads
700. 循衣摸床 *xún yī mō chuáng*: lit. 'fumble clothes, stroke bed', picking at bedclothes; carphology
701. 头晕目眩 *tóu yūn mù xuàn*: dizzy head and vision

Symmetry is sometimes achieved by the addition of 'dummy' verbs such as 作 *zuò* and 发 *fā*.

702. 寒热大作 *hán rè dà zuò*: lit. 'cold heat greatly doing', great heat [effusion] and [aversion to] cold

703. 喉中作声 *hóu zhōng zuò shēng*: lit. 'in throat doing noise', throat rale

704. 蛔虫作嘈 *huí chóng zuò cáo*: lit. 'roundworm doing noise', round-worm clamor

705. 两腿交替作痛 *liǎng tuǐ jiāo tì zuò tòng*: lit. 'two legs alternatingly doing hurt', pain alternating between the legs

706. 乳房作胀 *rǔ fáng zuò zhàng*: lit. 'breasts doing distend', distention of the breasts

707. 嗓子发干作痒 *sǎng zǐ fā gān zuò yǎng*: lit. 'larynx becoming dry doing itch', dry itchy larynx

708. 食入作胀 *shí rù zuò zhàng*: lit. 'food enters and does distend', distention after eating

709. 隐隐作痛 *yǐn yǐn zuò tòng*: lit. 'dully dully doing hurt', dull pain

710. 发黄 *fā huáng*: yellowing

711. 发痉 *fā jìng*: tetany

712. 经来发狂 *jīng lái fā kuáng*: lit. 'menses come, become manic', menstrual mania

The tendency towards symmetry is observed in terms denoting methods of treatment. Here, verb-verb + noun-noun and noun-verb + noun-verb patterns are seen. Symmetry is usually achieved by doubling the verb. In the first example, however, the character 血 *xuè* is repeated. Note that three-character combinations do appear, but much less frequently.

713. 凉血散血 *liáng xuè sàn xuè*: cool the blood and dissipate the blood; cool and dissipate the blood

714. 宣通水道 *xuān tōng shuǐ dào*: free the waterways

715. 滑利关节 *huá lì guān jié*: disinhibit the joints

716. 调和肝胃 *tiáo hé gān wèi*: [regulate and] harmonize the liver and stomach

717. 祛风散寒 *qū fēng sàn hán*: dispel wind and dissipate cold

718. 祛风寒 *qū fēng hán*: dispel wind and cold

719. 强筋壮骨 *qiáng jīn zhuàng gǔ*: strengthen sinew and [strengthen] bone

720. 强筋骨 *qiáng jīn gǔ*: strengthen sinew and bone

721. 泻水逐饮 *xiè shuǐ zhú yǐn*: drain water and expel rheum

722. 逐水饮 *zhú shuǐ yǐn*: expel water-rheum

It is often difficult to determine whether the esthetics of symmetry have taken precedence over meaning content. However, when an otherwise indispensable grammatical word is missing from a symmetrical expression, there can be little doubt about it. In 水火不济 *shuǐ huǒ bú jì*, lit. 'water and fire not helping', a negative statement derived from 水火相济 *shuǐ huǒ xiāng jì*, 'water and fire helping each other', it is fairly conclusive that 相 *xiāng* has been dropped to maintain symmetry. The same applies to 脾为湿困 *pí wéi shī kùn*, 'spleen is encumbered by dampness'.

The literary language in which Chinese medicine is traditionally expressed is a development of the largely monosyllabic classical language, but also reflects the increasing disyllablic and polysyllabic tendencies of the vernacular. It reserves the freedom to choose between changing states of the language.

9. Translation

The translation of terms into English in this book follows definite principles.[26] An important distinction is made between terms used more or less as they are in the everyday language of the lay, and terms that have been purposefully created to represent technical concepts. Terms of the first category, which include organ names, body parts, and environmental phenomena, have been translated with their natural English equivalents (nose, eye; spleen, heart, kidney; cold, heat, dampness, and so on). Terms of the second category have mostly been rendered with English terms of equivalent literal meaning (heart fire flaming upward, triple burner, life gate).

The use of modern Western medical terms that do not reflect the Chinese medical understanding of the concept and that introduce alien Western medical notions into Chinese medicine has been systematically avoided. Thus 风火眼 *fēng huǒ yǎn* is rendered as 'wind-fire eye' rather than 'acute conjunctivitis' since the literal rendering preserves the Chinese frame of reference. The only modern medical terms that have been adopted are those whose literal meanings do not imply any modern technical knowledge that is alien to the Chinese frame of reference. 'Diphtheria' has been adopted as the equivalent of 白喉 *bái hóu*, lit. 'white throat', because its literal connotation of 'leatheriness' of the throat does not clash with the Chinese understanding.

Transliteration has been used for Chinese terms such as qì and yīn-yáng that have already been adopted in the English language, but it has been used beyond this very little since it conveys no meaning to the English speaker. Transliteration has been used for 癞 *lài* and 疳 *gān*, where the literal meaning of the Chinese words is questionable. Many terms are commonly transliterated where there is no need to do so. The term 卫 *wèi* conveys no meaning when transliterated as 'wei' and potentially deprives the Western reader of insight into the concept.

In general, a literal approach to translation has been adopted to preserve a faithful representation of Chinese medicine. In particular, attention has been paid to preserving metaphor that enlightens us to the original understanding of concepts. A few exceptions have been made in deference to dubiously established conventions (e.g., point for 穴 *xuè*, bowels and viscera for 脏腑 *zàng fǔ*).

A major aim of the terminology presented in this book is that it should achieve as close a one-to-one relationship with the Chinese as possible. Many

---

[26]For a fuller discussion, see *English-Chinese Chinese-English Dictionary of Chinese Medicine*, Wiseman, N., Húnán Science and Technology Press, Chángshā, 1995, and *Approaches to Traditional Chinese Medical Literature*, Unschuld, Paul U. (ed.), Kluwer Academic Publishers, Dordrecht, Netherlands, 1989.

Chinese words have multiple equivalents, and the best English equivalent may depend on the context. When a word is given multiple renderings, translators wishing to use a systematic English terminology find the burden of remembering equivalents very difficult. Ideally, therefore, the number of renderings should be kept to a minimum. For example, the word 生 *shēng* has a variety of meanings including 'to engender', 'to be born' (or be engendered), 'life', 'raw', etc. In the context of the five phases and therapeutic action, we have chosen to translate *shēng* as 'engender'; in the realm of therapeutic actions, we systematically render it as 'engender', whatever object it applies to: 生肌 *shēng jī*, 'engender flesh', 生津 *shēng jīn*, 'engender liquid', etc. Although more idiomatic English verbs could might be found for each context, we have placed a priority on parity because, in the end, it is the only way to ensure consistency of English terminology. In the pharmaceutical context, 生 *shēng* means having undergone no processing. The word 'raw' is used for plants and 'crude' is used for minerals, in keeping with English usage. Three different words thus economically cover the senses of 生 *shēng* that commonly appear in medical terminology.

The question of whether the 'word' in a Chinese medical text is a character or a compound is very important to the method of translation adopted. A meticulous method of translation, which allows the target-language reader to gain all the information and hints that the original text offers, must take account of the fact that traditional Chinese medicine tends to base its reasoning on the statements of early texts such as the *Nèi Jīng, Nàn Jīng, Shāng Hán Lùn*, etc., which were written in the early post-classical period. In these texts, a 'word' was still essentially a 'character'.

723. 惊悸 *jīng jì*: fright palpitation
724. 怔忡 *zhēng chōng*: fearful throbbing
725. 烦燥 *fán zào*: vexation and agitation
726. 烦闷 *fán mèn*: vexation and oppression
727. 痞满 *pǐ mǎn*: glomus and fullness
728. 胀满 *zhàng mǎn*: distention and fullness
729. 肿胀 *zhǒng zhàng*: swelling and distention
730. 瘰疬 *luǒ lì*: scrofula (large and small)
731. 癃闭 *lóng bì*: dribbling urinary stoppage
732. 呕吐 *ǒu tù*: vomiting (and retching)
733. 咳嗽 *ké sòu*: cough (sonorous and productive)

In all but the last three of the above examples each character originally had a distinct meaning, and a definite reason to be included in the compound term. Although many of these terms could conceivably each be translated with single English words, the compounds can be reproduced in English without difficulty. Even though the translated term may be unwieldy, it nevertheless brings the reader closer to the original meaning.

It should be pointed out that in this part of the book, renderings have been chosen to reflect the original parts of speech as in the Chinese in order to help the student understand the grammar of Chinese medical terminology. The actual renderings used in the body of the text in many cases are formulated to come closer to natural English usage. Thus, the term 腹痛 *fù tòng*, which means 'abdomen painful', is given the standard rendering of 'abdominal pain'.

Finally, in Part II of this book, explanations of English term choices have been included with the explanations of Chinese terms and their meanings.

第二篇：词汇
Part II: Vocabulary

In Part II, Chinese characters are presented in sets according to subject matter. Each set of characters is followed by examples made of compound terms composed of previously introduced characters and by drills.

In each character set, each character is given in both its new simplified form and its old complex form, in each case with the signific in brackets in smaller print. This is followed by the Pīnyīn. On the right hand side of the page is the English rendering (or renderings) with pronunciation given in Kenyon and Knott (KK) phonetic transcription, and, where pertinent, an indication of its part of speech. This information has been included for the benefit of native Chinese students and teachers. The renderings of key characters (defined in the introduction) are given in regular type, while those of non-key characters are given in italics.

Each character in the lists of single characters is numbered for easy communication in the classroom. Each new key character that is introduced is given a unique serial number (e.g., n-245).

The English terminology presented in this volume has largely been created by literal translation, and Chinese compound terms have mostly been translated on a component-by-component basis. In the lists of single characters, each character with a corresponding English word that appears in translations of compound terms is marked with an asterisk. The asterisked characters are thus the basic building blocks of Chinese medical terminology. Some asterisked characters are used in distinct senses that call for different equivalents in English (e.g., 滑 *huá* is translated as 'slippery' in the context of the pulse, but as 'glossy' in the context of the tongue). The single characters not marked with an asterisk are characters appearing in terms that are translated by existing English equivalents For example, 落枕 *lào zhěn*, which literally means "fall [off the] pillow," is translated as 'crick in the neck', which is an existing English term not a loan-translation. The English equivalents of characters not literally translated are given in italics to draw attention to the fact that they merely explain the Chinese term and do not appear in English compound terms.

The index at the end of the book allows any individual character to be accessed by Pīnyīn or any of its English equivalents.

Finally, located before the index are appendices containing the names of medicinals, formulas, and acupuncture points.

第一节：基础理论
Section 1: Basic Theories

第一节　第一组	SECTION 1: SET 1

阴阳   **Yīn & Yáng**

1-n1	* 阴 阝	陰 阜	*yīn*	yīn /jɪn/ *n., adj.*
2-n2	* 阳 阝	陽 阜	*yáng*	yáng /jɑŋ, jæŋ/ *n., adj.*

注 Note:

Yīn and yáng are categories for classifying paired phenomena according to their nature and mutual relationship. By the ideographic composition of the characters, 阴 *yīn* is the north side of the mountain that does not receive sunlight, and 阳 *yáng* is the south side of the mountain that receives sunlight. Both terms are therefore natural metaphors.

复合词 Compounds:

1. 阴阳 *yīn yáng*, yīn and yáng; yīn-yáng
2. 二阴 *èr yīn*, the two yīn
3. 三阳 *sān yáng*, the three yáng (channels)
4. 二阴 *èr yīn*, the two yīn (i.e., the anus and genitals)

第一节　第二组	SECTION 1: SET 2

五行   **Five Phases**

3-n3	* 五 二	五 二	*wǔ*	five /faɪv/
4-n4	* 行 彳	行 彳	*xíng*	phase /fez/
5-n5	* 木 木	木 木	*mù*	wood /wʊd/ *n.*
6-n6	* 火 火	火 火	*huǒ*	fire /faɪr/ *n.*
7-n7	* 土 土	土 土	*tǔ*	earth /ɚθ/ *n.*
8-n8	* 金 金	金 金	*jīn*	metal /ˈmɛtl̩/ *n.*
9-n9	* 水 水	水 水	*shuǐ*	water /ˈwɔtɚ/ *n.*
10-n10	* 生 丿	生 生	*shēng*	engender /ɪnˈdʒɛndɚ/ *vt.*
				engendering /ɪnˈdʒɛndərɪŋ/ *n.*

11-n11	相 木	相 目	*xiāng*	inter-, mutual, reciprocal
12-n12	* 克 十	剋 刀	*kè*	restrain /rɪˈstren/ *vt.* restraining /rɪˈstrenɪŋ/ *n.*
13-n13	* 乘 禾	乘 丿	*chéng*	overwhelm /ovɚˈwɛlm, -ˈhwɛlm/ *vt.* overwhelming /ovɚˈwɛlmɪŋ, -ˈhwɛlm-/ *n.*
14-n14	* 侮 亻	侮 人	*wǔ*	rebel /rɪˈbɛl/ *vi.* rebellion /rɪˈbɛljən/ *n.*
15-n15	反 厂	反 又	*fǎn*	revolt, oppose, counter

注 Notes:

1. The five phases are five classes by which a vast array of different phenomena are classified and related. The names of the phases are words denoting natural phenomena. The five same symbols are also known under the name 五才 *wǔ cái*, the 'five materials'.

2. The word 'phase' has been widely adopted as the translation of 行 *xíng*. The Chinese term literally means to 'go', 'move', and by extension, 'act'. The ancient Chinese regarded wood, fire, earth, metal, and water as physical things that had systematic correspondences with other phenomena including not only physical things but also states occurring in cycles (e.g., days, seasons). The word 行 *xíng* denotes five movements that form the complete cycle. The word 'phase' is a segment of the entire cycle. Since the word 行 *xíng* also means action, another well-chosen equivalent that has been proposed is *agent*.[27]

Some writers still refer to the 五行 *wǔ xíng* as 'five elements', suggestive of elements that the Greeks considered to constitute essential stuff of the universe.

3. As to the names of the phases, only one is problematic. Chinese has two words, 土 *tǔ* and 地 *dì*, that can be translated as earth. *Tǔ* is the earth that is tilled, and *dì* is the counterpart of heaven. Paul Unschuld has proposed that *tǔ*, the word used in the context of the five phases, should be rendered as 'soil' rather than 'earth'. Although 'soil' is narrower in meaning than 'earth', the suggestion is valid if confusion arises when two distinct Chinese terms are conflated into one equivalent.

4. The orders of engendering and restraining are as follows:

相生: 木→ 火→ 土→ 金→ 火→

[27]Harper D (1998) *Early Chinese Medical Literature: The Mawangdui Medical Manuscripts*. London, Kegan Paul.

相克: 木→ 土→ 水→ 火→ 金→

Overwhelming is the same as restraining (except that it is due to abnormal weakness of the restrained phase). Rebellion is restraining in opposite order.

5. The relationships between the phases are described in metaphor. The character 侮 *wǔ*, rendered here as 'rebellion', literally means to 'insult', 'humiliate', 'cheat', 'encroach upon'. In the five phases, it is used alone or in the combination 反侮 *fǎn wǔ* to denote one of the four interrelationships. The character 反 *fǎn*, turn over, return, opposite, is used in the political context to mean 'revolt' and in the military context to mean 'counterattack'. The five-phase relationship of rebellion is the reverse of the normal restraining relationship.

6. The character 相 means 'inter', 'reciprocal', or 'mutual'. The compound 相生 *xiāng shēng* literally means 'inter-engendering'. In practice, the meaning is sufficiently clear if the 相 is left untranslated.

复合词 Compounds:

5. 相生 *xiāng shēng*, engendering
6. 相克 *xiāng kè*, restraining
7. 相乘 *xiāng chéng*, overwhelming
8. 相侮 *xiāng wǔ*, rebellion
9. 木生火 *mù shēng huǒ*, wood engenders fire
10. 火生土 *huǒ shēng tǔ*, fire engenders earth
11. 土生金 *tǔ shēng jīn*, earth engenders metal
12. 金生水 *jīn shēng shuǐ*, metal engenders water
13. 水生木 *shuǐ shēng mù*, water engenders wood
14. 木克土 *mù kè tǔ*, wood restrains earth
15. 土克水 *tǔ kè shuǐ*, earth restrains water
16. 水克火 *shuǐ kè huǒ*, water restrains fire
17. 火克金 *huǒ kè jīn*, fire restrains metal
18. 金克木 *jīn kè mù*, metal restrains wood
19. 木乘土 *mù chéng tǔ*, wood overwhelms earth
20. 水乘火 *shuǐ chéng huǒ*, water overwhelms fire
21. 土侮木 *tǔ wǔ mù*, earth rebels against wood
22. 木侮金 *mù wǔ jīn*, wood rebels against metal
23. 金反侮火 *jīn fǎn wǔ huǒ*, metal rebels against fire
24. 火反侮水 *huǒ fǎn wǔ shuǐ*, fire rebels against water

习题 Exercise:

1.   木生火   ....

2. *mù kè tǔ* ....

3. earth restrains water ....

4. 水克火 ....

5. *jīn kè mù* ....

6. earth engenders metal ....

7. 金乘木 ....

8. *tǔ kè shuǐ* ....

9. fire restrains metal ....

10. 金乘木 ....

11. *huǒ fǎn wǔ shuǐ* ....

12. water rebels against earth ....

13. 土反侮木 ....

第一节　第三组	**SECTION 1: SET 3**

方位			**Positions**	
16-n16	方 方	方 方	*fāng*	place; square; method
17-n17	* 位 亻	位 人	*wèi*	position /pəˈzɪʃən/
18-n18	* 东 一	東 木	*dōng*	east /ist/
19-n19	* 南 十	南 十	*nán*	south /sɑʊθ/
20-n20	* 西 覀	西 襾	*xī*	west /wɛst/
21-n21	* 北 匕	北 匕	*běi*	north /nɔrθ, norθ/
22-n22	* 中 中	中 丨	*zhōng*	center /ˈsɛntɚ/
23-n23	* 属 尸	屬 尸	*shǔ*	belong to /bɪlˈɔŋ tu/

复合词 Compounds:

25. 东南 *dōng nán*, southeast
26. 西北 *xī běi*, northwest
27. 西南 *xī nán*, southwest
28. 东属木 *dōng shǔ mù*, east belongs to wood
29. 南属火 *nán shǔ huǒ*, south belongs to fire
30. 西属金 *xī shǔ jīn*, west belongs to metal
31. 北属水 *běi shǔ shuǐ*, winter belongs to water
32. 中属土 *zhōng shǔ tǔ*, center belongs to earth

习题 Exercise:

14. *dōng běi* ....
15. southeast ....
16. 南属火 ....
17. *xī shǔ jīn* ....

第一节 第四组 | **SECTION 1: SET 4**

时令 | **Seasons**

24-n24	* 时 日	時 日	*shí*	season	/ˈsizən/
25-n25	* 令 人	令 人	*lìng*	season	/ˈsizən/
26-n26	* 季 禾	季 子	*jì*	season	/ˈsizən/
27-n27	天 天	天 大	*tiān*	*heaven*	
28-n28	* 春	春 日	*chūn*	spring	/sprɪŋ/
29-n29	* 夏 夂	夏 夂	*xià*	summer	/ˈsʌmɚ/
30-n30	* 秋 禾	秋 禾	*qiū*	autumn	/ˈɔtəm/
31-n31	* 冬 夂	冬 冬	*dōng*	winter	/ˈwɪntɚ/
32-n32	* 长 丿	長 長	*cháng*	long	/lɔŋ/

注 Notes:

1. The Chinese 天 *tiān* has the primary meaning of sky (or the heavens) and a wide range of other meanings, including 'heaven', 'season', 'weather', and 'nature'. Its use in the present context as 'season' is chiefly a vernacular usage.

2. The Chinese 长夏 *cháng xià*, long summer, is the third month of summer in the Chinese calendar, i.e., the sixth month in the lunar calendar (roughly the last half of July and first half of August). This term is sometimes misleadingly translated as Indian summer, which refers to "a period of mild, warm, hazy weather following the first frosts of late autumn" (*Websters New World College Dictionary*).

复合词 Compounds:

33. 春天 *chūn tiān*, spring
34. 夏天 *xià tiān*, summer
35. 春令 *chūn lìng*, spring
36. 秋天 *qiū tiān*, autumn

37. 冬天 *dōng tiān*, winter
38. 四时 *sì shí*, four seasons
39. 四季 *sì jì*, four seasons
40. 长夏 *cháng xià*, long summer
41. 春属木 *chūn shǔ mù*, spring belongs to wood
42. 夏属火 *xià shǔ huǒ*, summer belongs to fire
43. 秋属金 *qiū shǔ jīn*, autumn belongs to metal
44. 冬属水 *dōng shǔ shuǐ*, winter belongs to water
45. 长夏属土 *cháng xià shǔ tǔ*, long summer belongs to earth

习题 Exercise:

18. four seasons ....

19. 冬天 ....

20. *chūn shǔ mù* ....

21. autumn belongs to metal ....

22. 冬属水 ....

第一节　第五组				**SECTION 1: SET 5**

脏腑   Bowels & Viscera

33-n33	* 脏 月	臟 肉	*zàng*	viscus /ˈvɪskəs/
				viscera /ˈvɪsərə/ *pl.*
34-n34	* 腑 月	腑 肉	*fǔ*	bowel /ˈbaʊəl/
35-n35	* 奇 大	奇 大	*qí*	extraordinary /ɪksˈtrɔːrdn̩ˌɛrɪ/
36-n36	恒 忄	恆 心	*héng*	*constant*
37-n37	* 肝 月	肝 肉	*gān*	liver /ˈlɪvɚ/
38-n38	* 心 心	心 心	*xīn*	heart /hɑrt/
39-n39	* 脾 月	脾 肉	*pí*	spleen /splin/
40-n40	* 肺 月	肺 肉	*fèi*	lung /lʌŋ/
41-n41	* 肾 月	腎 肉	*shèn*	kidney /ˈkɪdnɪ/
42-n42	包 勹	包 勹	*bāo*	*envelop, wrap*
43-n43	* 胆 月	膽 肉	*dǎn*	gallbladder /ˈgɔlblædɚ/
44-n44	* 小 小	小 小	*xiǎo*	small /smɔl/
45-n45	* 大 大	大 大	*dà*	large /lɑrdʒ/
46-n46	* 肠 月	腸 肉	*cháng*	intestine /ɪnˈtɛstin/
47-n47	* 胃 月	胃 肉	*wèi*	stomach /ˈstʌmək/
48-n48	* 脘 月	脘 肉	*wǎn*	stomach duct /dʌkt/

49-n49	*	膀 月	膀 肉	*páng*	bladder	/ˈblædəʳ/
50-n50	*	胱 月	胱 肉	*guāng*	bladder	/ˈblædəʳ/
51-n51	*	脬 月	脬 肉	*pāo*	bladder	/ˈblædəʳ/
52-n52	*	焦 隹	焦 火	*jiāo*	burner	/ˈbɝnəʳ/
53-n53	*	上 卜	上 一	*shàng*	upper	/ˈʌpəʳ/
54	*	中 中	中 丨	*zhōng*	center	/ˈsɛntəʳ/
					middle	/ˈmɪdl̩/
55-n54	*	下 卜	下 一	*xià*	lower	/loəʳ/
56-n55	*	脑 月	腦 肉	*nǎo*	brain	/bren/
57-n56	*	髓 骨	髓 骨	*suǐ*	marrow	/ˈmæro/
58-n57	*	骨 骨	骨 骨	*gǔ*	bone	/bon/
59-n58	*	脉 月	脈 肉	*mài*	vessel	/ˈvɛsl̩/
60-n59	*	胞 月	胞 肉	*bāo*	uterus	/ˈjutərəs/
61-n60	*	子 子	子 子	*zǐ*	child	/tʃaɪld/
62-n61	*	宫 宀	宮 宀	*gōng*	palace	/ˈpæləs/

注 Notes:

1. Chinese medicine, like modern Western medicine, conceives the body as comprising a number of organs and parts that each perform specific functions in the maintenance of health. Many of its theories concerning the functioning of organs—e.g., the lung's function of drawing in air, the stomach's function of preliminary processing of food, and the bladder's function of storing urine—are deduced from morphological characteristics of the organs themselves. Chinese medicine, however, differs from Western medicine in that it understands many other functions of the various components and the interrelationships between them through perceived yīn-yáng and five-phase correspondences. The attribution to the kidney of reproductive function as well as urinary function may partly be due to the fact that these functions have a partially shared morphological basis (Western medicine speaks of the 'genitourinary system'), and partly because of the macrocosmic associations of water (the phase associated with the kidney apparently on the basis of urinary function) with the notion of storage connoted by the corresponding season, winter.

The larger organs of the abdominothoracic cavity are central to the Chinese model. These are classed into two groups, the 五脏 *wǔ zàng* and 六腑 *liù fǔ*, here rendered as five viscera and six bowels. The five viscera—liver, heart, spleen, lung, and kidney—are said to produce and store essence (essence in a wider sense of qì, blood, essence, and spirit); the six bowels—gallbladder, small intestine, stomach, large intestine, bladder, and the triple burner—decompose food and convey waste. The viscera are considered yīn, while the bowels are considered yáng. In addition, there are the 奇恒之腑 *qí héng zhī fǔ*, the 'extraordinary organs', comprising the brain, marrow, bones, vessels, uterus, and gallbladder, so called because they are different from both the viscera and bowels. They are different from the bowels because they do not decompose food and convey waste, and from the viscera because they do not produce and store essence. The gallbladder is an exception, because it is classed both as a bowel and as an extraordinary organ (the extraordinary organs are so named because they fit into neither the category of the viscera nor into that of bowels).

Of all the organs, the five viscera are preeminent. Through the five phases, correspondences were established between each of the viscera and various aspect parts of the body (examples are shown in the table below). The viscera, as we shall see more clearly from various aspects of terminology, were considered to be power centers controlling these areas.

Five Phases in Man

Phase	Wood	Fire	Earth	Metal	Water
Viscus	Liver	Heart	Spleen	Lung	Kidney
Bowel	Gallbladder	Small intestine	Stomach	Large intestine	Bladder
Orifice	Eyes	Tongue	Mouth	Nose	Ears
Governing	Sinew	Vessels	Flesh	Skin & body hair	Bone
Mind	Anger	Joy	Thought	Sorrow	Fear
Humor	Tears	Sweat	Drool	Snivel	Spittle
Pulse	Stringlike	Surging	Moderate	Downy	Stone-like
Voice	Shouting	Laughing	Singing	Wailing	Moaning

2. The terms 脏 *zàng* (a simplified form of 臟), viscus (plural viscera), and 腑 *fǔ*, bowel, originally derived by metaphor from 藏 *zàng*, a storehouse, and 府 *fǔ*, a building in which official transactions take place. The use of these characters to denote places where grain was collected (府) and where it was stored (藏) apparently led to their application in the body to denote a group of organs that absorbed and processed food and another group that stored the nutrients extracted from food. These characters are used in certain early texts, but the addition of the flesh signific 月 has taken over completely. The compound term 脏腑 *zàng fǔ* is rendered in the present work as 'bowels and viscera' (rather than viscera and bowels), and sometimes as the 'organs' for brevity. In the term 奇恒之腑 *qí héng zhī fǔ*, the extraordinary organs, 奇恒 *qí héng* means 奇于恒 *qí yú héng*, different from the norm. The forms of the characters without flesh signific 月, which highlight the original metaphors, can be translated as as 'stores' and '(collection) houses'.

3. Most of the internal organs discussed in Chinese medicine are those that can be seen with the naked eye, and whose names are known to the lay (liver, kidney, heart, bladder etc.). Despite this some have argued that the regular English names should not be used on the grounds that the organs are

not understood to have the same functions in Chinese medicine as in Western medicine, and that Chinese medicine is concerned not with the physical organs, but only with functions. Guided by these thoughts, some have suggested that Pīnyīn names should be used instead, and Manfred Porkert has enshrined the functional view in a terminology in which liver appears as *orbs hepaticus*, heart as *orbs cardialis*, and spleen as *orbs lienalis*. The arguments in favor of such terms are faulted. Chinese medicine does indeed ascribe different functions to the organs than Western medicine, but the physical organs are the same. If the ancient Chinese had been concerned only with functions and not with physical identity, they would not have given them names of organs, and would not have deduced functions from organ morphology (e.g., the bladder storing urine). Furthermore, it would be wrong to assume that the English names of organs should be used only when the functions attributed to the organs in Chinese medicine are the same as those they are attributed in Western medicine. The English names for the organs concerned are very much older than the Western medical understanding, and survived the replacement of humoral pathology by modern medicine in the West precisely because both humoral pathology and modern medicine agreed on the physical referents of the terms.

4. The 三焦 *sān jiāo*, 'triple burner', is an entity whose identity has never been agreed on, some believing it to be an actual organ, and others assuming it to be a functional aspect of the five viscera and six bowels. The character 焦 literally means to burn or scorch. It has been suggested that it denotes an intangible counterpart of a physical organ called 膲 *jiāo* (the same character with the addition of the flesh signific 肉). It has also been suggested that it should be 樵, explained as meaning 槌 *chuí* in the sense of 'section', referring to the threefold division of this organ. P.U. Unschuld suggests that the name 焦 *jiāo* should be taken at face value and was chosen on the basis of an analogy to smelters and saltworks.[28]

5. In Chinese, names of organs are placed together in an additive sense, without any overt link, e.g., 肝脾 *gān pí*, the liver and spleen. When such combinations function as modifiers, they can be joined in English with a hyphen, e.g., 肝脾不和 *gān pí bù hé*, 'liver-spleen disharmony', meaning 'disharmony between the liver and spleen'.

6. The names of bowels and viscera can be combined with the names of the phases in order to indicate the organ as associated with the phase, e.g., 脾土 *pí tǔ*. In English, the compound is joined by a hyphen as 'spleen-earth'.

---

[28]*Medicine in China: A History of Ideas*, Unschuld, P.U., University of California Press, Berkeley, 1985, p. 81.

7. The character 胞 *bāo* is composed of 包, a bag or sack, combined with the flesh signific. It denotes various, more or less baglike structures including uterus, eyelid, bladder, or a mole discharged from the vagina. The meaning is clear from context: 眼胞 *yǎn bāo*, 'eyelid', 转胞 *zhuǎn bāo*, 'shifted bladder' (denoting frequent urination in pregnancy), 胞脉 *bāo mài*, 'uterine vessels', and 胞寒 *bāo hán*, 'uterine cold'. The uterus is more commonly referred to as 胞宫 *bāo gōng*, lit. 'uterine palace' or 子宫 *zǐ gōng*, lit. 'infant's palace'. The latter term is the most commonly used nowadays, and has been adopted by Western medicine. Note that 'uterus' has been chosen as the English equivalent in preference to 'womb' simply because it has a convenient adjectival form (uterine) that 'womb' does not have.

8. The compound 膀胱 *páng guáng*, which is never split, is the usual term for the bladder. The synonym 脬 *pāo* is comparatively rare.

9. The term 脘 *wǎn* (or *guǎn*), which is translated here as 'duct' or 'stomach duct', denotes the stomach cavity and adjoining parts of the gullet (esophagus) and small intestine. It is divided into three parts, the 上脘 *shàng wǎn*, 中脘 *zhōng wǎn*, and 下脘 *xià wǎn*, the upper, middle, and lower ducts. The term 'stomach duct' is also used to denote the area called the epigastrium in Western medicine, although in Chinese medicine distinction is sometimes made between the stomach duct and the small area just below the breast bone, which is referred to as 心下 *xīn xià*, '[region] below the heart'.

复合词 Compounds:

46. 五脏 *wǔ zàng*, five viscera
47. 六腑 *liù fǔ*, six bowels
48. 奇恒之腑 *qí héng zhī fǔ*, the extraordinary organs
49. 水脏 *shuǐ zàng*, water viscus (the kidney)
50. 心包 *xīn bāo*, pericardium
51. 五脏六腑 *wǔ zàng liù fǔ*, five viscera and six bowels
52. 脾肺 *pí fèi*, spleen and lung, spleen-lung
53. 肝肾 *gān shèn*, liver and kidney, liver-kidney
54. 肝阴 *gān yīn*, liver yīn
55. 胃肠 *wèi cháng*, stomach and intestines, gastrointestinal
56. 脾胃 *pí wèi*, spleen and stomach, spleen-stomach
57. 膀胱 *páng guāng*, bladder
58. 肝木 *gān mù*, liver-wood
59. 心火 *xīn huǒ*, heart-fire
60. 脾土 *pí tǔ*, spleen-earth
61. 肺金 *fèi jīn*, lung-metal

62. 肾水 *shèn shuǐ*, kidney-water
63. 三焦 *sān jiāo*, triple burner
64. 肝阳 *gān yáng*, liver yáng
65. 肝属木 *gān shǔ mù*, the liver belongs to earth
66. 上焦 *shàng jiāo*, upper burner
67. 脾在中焦 *pí zài zhōng jiāo*, the spleen is in the middle burner
68. 骨髓 *gǔ suǐ*, bone and marrow
69. 胞宫 *bāo gōng*, uterus
70. 子宫 *zǐ gōng*, uterus

习题 Exercise:

23. *liù fǔ* ....
24. heart yáng ....
25. 心阴 ....
26. *fèi jīn* ....
27. stomach and intestines, gastrointestinal ....
28. 心脾 ....
29. *xīn gān* ....
30. pericardium ....
31. 肺肾 ....
32. *xīn shèn* ....
33. liver and stomach, liver-stomach ....
34. 肝肾 ....
35. *gān pí* ....
36. liver yīn ....
37. 肾阴 ....
38. *shèn yáng* ....
39. the heart belongs to fire ....
40. 脾属土 ....
41. *fèi shǔ jīn* ....
42. the kidney belongs to water ....
43. 中焦 ....
44. *xià jiāo* ....
45. upper burner ....

46. 肺在上焦 ....

47. *wèi zài zhōng jiāo* ....

48. the kidney is in the lower burner ....

第一节　第六组   **SECTION 1: SET 6**

基本「元素」　　　　　　　　　Basic 'Elements'

63-n62	* 气 气	氣 气	*qì*	qì /tʃi/
64-n63	* 血 血	血 血	*xuè*	blood /blʌd/
65-n64	* 津 氵	津 水	*jīn*	liquid /ˈlɪkwɪd/
66-n65	* 液 氵	液 水	*yè*	humor /ˈhjumɚ/
67-n66	* 精 米	精 米	*jīng*	essence /ˈɛsəns/ *n.*
				essential /ɪˈsɛnʃəl/ *adj.*
68-n67	* 神 礻	神 示	*shén*	spirit /ˈspɪrɪt/

注 Notes:

1. The term 气 *qì* in its original form depicted rising vapors. The notion of vapor subsequently expanded to include air, breath, and invisible, or only vaguely visible forces. In most recent clinical literature, the term is rendered in its Pīnyīn translation. There is a lingering tendency to call it 'energy' or 'vital energy', although it is not clear whether their users are using 'energy' in a colloquial or strictly scientific sense (either of which bear little relation to the Chinese notion). Transliteration should be the translator's last resort because it obscures meaning from the foreign reader. Any English words matching the meaning of qì in any of its contexts cannot easily be used in other contexts, and so transliteration avoids the problem of too narrow an understanding, although P.U. Unschuld's '(finest matter) influences' is the closest approximation to the original sense yet found in the English language. However, the Chinese word was long ago adopted into the English language, and we have chosen to use the Pīnyīn transliteration 'qì' as a standard rendering. One major exception is the use of the word in the context of respiration (which will appear later in this text). The term 气短 *qì duǎn*, 'shortness of breath', uses qì to mean 'breath' in the verbal sense of breathing.

2. A distinction is made between 津 *jīn*, 'liquid', and 液 *yè*, 'humor', generally held to denote thin mobile and thick viscous fluids, respectively. The use of the terms in 黄帝内经 *Huáng Dì Nèi Jīng*, however, does not always reflect this distinction. For example, the term 五液 *wǔ yè*, 'five humors', includes thin mobile liquids.

3. The character 精 *jīng*, essence, means the nature of a thing or its most important constituent. In medicine, it denotes a substance responsible for growth, development, and reproduction, and determines the strength of the constitution, and is manifest physically in the male in the form of semen

(sometimes called 精气 *jīng qì*). It also denotes what is contained in food that is essential to human life (in this context often 精微 *jīng wēi*).

复合词 Compounds:

71. 气血 *qì xuè*, qì and blood, qì-blood
72. 津液 *jīn yè*, liquid and humor; fluids
73. 精神 *jīng shén*, essence-spirit
74. 气津 *qì jīn*, qì and liquid
75. 精血 *jīng xuè*, essence-blood
76. 精气 *jīng qì*, essential qì
77. 肝气 *gān qì*, liver qì
78. 心气 *xīn qì*, heart qì
79. 肺津 *fèi jīn*, lung liquid
80. 胃气 *wèi qì*, stomach qì

习题 Exercise:

49. 脾气　...
50. *fèi qì*　...
51. kidney qì　...
52. 肝血　...
53. *xīn xuè*　...

第一节　第七组 | **SECTION 1: SET 7**

五脏所主 | **The Governings of the Five Viscera**

69-n68	* 主王	主丶	*zhǔ*	govern	/ˈɡʌvɚn/
70-n69	所斤	所戶	*suǒ*	*what*	
71-n70	* 筋竹	筋竹	*jīn*	sinew	/ˈsɪnju/
72	* 脉月	脈肉	*mài*	vessel	/ˈvɛsl̩/
73-n71	* 肉冂	肉肉	*ròu*	flesh	/flɛʃ/
74-n72	* 肌月	肌肉	*jī*	flesh	/flɛʃ/
75-n73	* 皮皮	皮皮	*pí*	skin	/skɪn/
				cutaneous	/kjuˈteniəs/
76-n74	* 毛毛	毛毛	*máo*	[body] hair	/hɛr/
77	* 骨骨	骨骨	*gǔ*	bone	/bon/

注 **Notes:**

1. As has already been pointed out, the bowels and the viscera were originally considered to be storehouses or government offices. Another analogy portrays them as government officials said to 'govern' (主 *zhǔ*) various parts of the body and various activities: the spleen governs the flesh, the liver governs the sinews, the kidney governs the bone, etc.

2. The terms 肉 *ròu* and 肌 *jī* both mean flesh. If character composition faithfully reflects the original concepts represented by Chinese words, 肉 *ròu* originally meant meat, that is animal flesh intended for human consumption, since the original character is a pictograph of meat lumps of meat hanging, as in a butcher's shop. The character 肌 *jī* must have been devised later, since it includes 肉 as its signific. It denotes human flesh, flesh not intended for consumption. It is now used in Western medicine as the equivalent of muscle, but in Chinese medicine, it was synonymous with (though never actually completely displaced) 肉 as the word for flesh in general, including red flesh (muscle) and white flesh (fat).

3. The liver governs the 'sinews'. The term 筋 *jīn* is variously translated by different writers as 'tendon' or 'muscle and tendon', 'muscle', or 'sinew'. One of the earliest dictionaries of Chinese, the 说文解字 *Shuō Wén Jiě Zì*, defines 筋 *jīn* as 'the strength of the flesh', explains that the character is composed of the bamboo signific combined two other elements, one meaning flesh and the other meaning strength, and comments that bamboo is a thing that has a lot of *jīn*. The English words tendon and muscle denote narrowly defined anatomical entities. When the acupuncture point GB-31 (*fēng shì*, Wind Market) is described as being located between two *jīn*, we know that what is meant here in terms of Western anatomy is muscle not tendon. In other contexts, of course, tendon is meant. We have chosen 'sinew' to represent the concept in Chinese because in addition to denoting tendon, it has the connotations of strength that the Chinese term has. Since the English 'sinew' is virtually obsolete in Western medicine and is used in the everyday language to denote anything stringy and strong, it is easily endowed with the definition of *jīn*.

4. The term 五脏所主 *wǔ zàng suǒ zhǔ*, the governing of the five viscera, literally means 'what the five viscera govern', the specific parts of the body governed by the viscera. The heart governs the vessels; the lung governs the skin and [body] hair; the liver governs the sinew; the spleen governs the flesh; the kidney governs the bone.

复合词 **Compounds:**

81. 肝主筋 *gān zhǔ jīn*, the liver governs the sinews
82. 心主脉 *xīn zhǔ mài*, the heart governs the vessels

83. 脾主肉 *pí zhǔ ròu*, the spleen governs the flesh
84. 肺主皮毛 *fèi zhǔ pí máo*, the lung governs the skin and [body] hair
85. 肾主骨 *shèn zhǔ gǔ*, the kidney governs the bone
86. 皮毛 *pí máo*, skin and [body] hair
87. 筋骨 *jīn gǔ*, sinew and bone
88. 筋肉 *jīn ròu*, sinew and flesh
89. 骨髓 *gǔ suǐ*, bone and marrow; bone marrow

习题 Exercise:

54. skin and [body] hair ....

55. 筋骨 ....

56. *jīn ròu* ....

57. the liver belongs to earth and governs the sinews ....

58. 脾属土，主肌肉 ....

59. *fèi shǔ jīn, zhǔ pí máo* ....

60. the kidney belongs to water, and governs the bone ....

第一节　第八组				**SECTION 1: SET 8**

五官 　　　　　　　　　　　**The Five Offices**

78-n75	* 官 宀	官 宀	*guān*	official, office /ˈɔfɪs/
79-n76	* 目 目	目 目	*mù*	eye /aɪ/
80-n77	* 舌 舌	舌 舌	*shé*	tongue /tʌŋ/
81-n78	* 唇 辰	唇 口	*chún*	lip /lɪp/
82-n79	* 鼻 鼻	鼻 鼻	*bí*	nose /noz/
83-n80	* 耳 耳	耳 耳	*ěr*	ear /ɪr/
84-n81	之 丶	之 丿	*zhī*	*'s*
85-n82	者 耂	者 老	*zhě*	*a topic marker*
86-n83	也 ㇖	也 乙	*yě*	*statement-end marker*

注 Notes:

1. The Chinese 官 *guān* is an official or functionary, or the offices or functions that an official performs. The term 五官 *wǔ guān*, the five offices, denoting nose, eyes, lips, tongue, and ears, is one of the many bureaucratic metaphors in Chinese medicine. In the modern everyday language, 五官

wǔ guān is used loosely to refer to the features of the face, and in Western medicine 官 is used in several technical terms including 感官 *gǎn guān*, 'sense organ', and 器官 *qì guān*. Most speakers understand 'organ' to be a second meaning of 官, entirely separate from that of official. Few realize that parts of the body with specific physiological functions were originally so named because they were likened to officials performing important functions in the running of the state. In the early texts of Chinese medicine, the metaphor of 官—and that of many other Chinese medical terms—would have been very much alive. For this reason, we have translated the term 五官 *wǔ guān* literally 'five offices'.

2. The character 者 *zhě* in classical Chinese is sometimes placed after the subject of a statement to explicitly mark it as such. There is no equivalent marker in English, so it is not translated.

3. The character 之 *zhī* is a genitive particle in the classical language that corresponds to 的 *de* (in the neutral tone) in modern Mandarin. It is equivalent to *'s* or 'of' in English. Thus 心之官 *xīn zhī guān* is 'the heart's office' or 'the office of the heart'.

4. The character 也, most commonly used in the modern language in the sense of 'also', is here used in its classical sense of marking the end of a judgment or explanation. Like 者, it is an element of verbal punctuation characteristic of the classical language.

复合词 Compounds:

90. 目者，肝之官也 *mù zhě, gān zhī guān yě*, the eyes are the office of the liver

91. 舌者，心之官也 *shé zhě, xīn zhī guān yě*, the tongue is the office of the heart

92. 唇者，脾之官也 *chún zhě, pí zhī guān yě*, the lips are the office of the spleen

93. 鼻者，肺之官也 *bí zhě, fèi zhī guān yě*, the nose is the office of the lung

94. 耳者，肾之官也 *ěr zhě, shèn zhī guān yě*, the ears are the office of the kidney

---

第一节　第九组   **SECTION 1: SET 9**

五声   **Five Voices**

87-n84　＊声土　聲耳　　　*shēng*　voice /vɔɪs/

								sound /saʊnd/
88-n85	*	音	音	音	音	*yīn*	sound /saʊnd/
89-n86	*	呼	口	呼	口	*hū*	shouting /ˈʃaʊtɪŋ/
90-n87	*	笑	竹	笑	竹	*xiào*	laughing /ˈlæfɪŋ/
91-n88	*	歌	欠	歌	欠	*gē*	singing /ˈsɪŋɪŋ/
92-n89	*	哭	口	哭	口	*kū*	crying /ˈkraɪɪŋ/
93-n90	*	呻	口	呻	口	*shēn*	moaning /ˈmonɪŋ/

注 Note:

1. The Chinese 声 *shēng* means a human voice or any sound in general; 音 *yīn* means sound, note, or tone. The combination of the two characters 声音, like the single character 声, means either voice or sound in general.

复合词 Compounds:

95. 声音 *shēng yīn*, voice, sound

第一节　第十组	**SECTION 1: SET 10**

五色 — **Five Colors**

94-n91	*	色	刀	色	色	*sè*	color /ˈkʌlɚ/
95-n92	*	青	青	青	青	*qīng*	green-blue /ˈgrinˈblu/
96-n93	*	赤	赤	赤	赤	*chì*	red /rɛd/
97-n94	*	黄	壮	黄	黄	*huáng*	yellow /ˈjɛlo/
98-n95	*	白	白	白	白	*bái*	white /waɪt, hwaɪt/
99-n96	*	黑	黑	黑	黑	*hēi*	black /blæk/

注 Note:

The five colors 青、赤、黄、白、黑 *qīng, chì, huáng, bái, hēi* are considered to cover the full color spectrum, and at least two of them, 青 *qīng* and 黄 *huáng*, are wider in meaning than any corresponding English color word. Among the five colors, 青 *qīng* includes green and blue. It is classically described as 'the color of new shoots of grass', but in context of the complexion, for example, it is more often than not a color that would be more naturally described in English as blue, and hence is translated into English with the compound 'green-blue'. The 黄 *huáng* is here translated as yellow, but it must be borne in mind it actually includes light brown.

Under certain contexts, it might be possible to translate 青 *qīng* as green and 黄 *huáng* as brown. However, it is important to bear in mind that the five colors in Chinese medicine have five-phase correspondences (red belongs to fire, yellow to earth, white to metal, black to water, and green-blue to wood). Hence, the color words are technical terms with definite technical associations. They have to be consistently rendered with fixed terms. For this reason, we always render 青 *qīng* as green-blue, even if in the context it is clear whether it is green or blue.

第一节　第十一组					**SECTION 1: SET 11**

五臭					**Five Odors**
100-n97	* 臭 自	臭 自		*xiù*	smell /smɛl/
					odor /ˈodɚ/
101	* 臭 自	臭 自		*chòu*	malodor /ˈmælodɚ/
102-n98	* 臊 月	臊 肉		*sāo*	animal smell /ˈænɪml̩–smɛl/
103	* 焦 隹	焦 火		*jiāo*	burnt smell /ˈbɝnt–smɛl/
104-n99	* 香 香	香 香		*xiāng*	fragrant /ˈfregrənt/
105-n100	* 腥 月	腥 肉		*xīng*	fishy smell /ˈfɪʃɪ–smɛl/
106-n101	* 腐 广	腐 肉		*fŭ*	putrid smell /ˈpjutrɪd–smɛl/

注 Note:

1. The character 臭 is usually pronounced as *chòu* and means malodorous. Less commonly it is read as *xiù* in the meaning of a smell or odor. The character 臊 *sāo*, in denoting an odor, means the smell of urine. Outside the language of medicine, it is used in the latter sense and generally to denote unclean bodily smells. It also specifically denotes the smell of goats and goat meat, which strictly speaking is described as 羶、羴 *shān*.

2. The character 腥 *xīng* means uncooked meat, lard, foul smells in general, and the smell of fish in specific. Outside the technical language of medicine, it is used to describe the smells of uncooked fish or meat and of menstrual flow.

| 第一节　第十二组 | | | | **SECTION 1: SET 12** |

五味所入　　　　　　　　　　　**Five-Flavor Entries**

107-n102	* 入入	入入	*rù*	enter /ˈɛntɚ/ *vi.*
				entry /ˈɛntrɪ/ *n.*
108-n103	* 味口	味口	*wèi*	flavor /ˈflevɚ/
109-n104	* 酸酉	酸酉	*suān*	sour /saʊr/ *adj.*
				sourness /ˈsaʊrnɪss/ *n.*
110-n105	* 苦艹	苦艸	*kǔ*	bitter /ˈbɪtɚ/ *adj.*
				bitterness /ˈbɪtɚnɪs/ *n.*
111-n106	* 甘甘	甘甘	*gān*	sweet /swit/ *adj.*
				sweetness /ˈswitnɪs/ *n.*
112-n107	* 辛辛	辛辛	*xīn*	acrid /ˈækrɪd/ *adj.*
				acridity /æˈkrɪdɪtɪ/ *n.*
113-n108	* 咸戊	鹹鹵	*xián*	salty /ˈsɔltɪ/ *adj.*
				saltiness /ˈsɔltɪnɪs/ *n.*

注 Note:

Terms denoting flavors, like color terms, have five-phase correspondences, and hence are technical terms that should always be rendered with standard equivalents. In four cases, the translations are straightforward (sour, bitter, sweet, salty). 辛 *xīn* is here rendered as acrid; it is rendered by some writers as pungent.

复合词 Compounds:

96. 酸入肝 *suān rù gān*, sourness enters the liver
97. 苦入心 *kǔ rù xīn*, bitterness enters the heart
98. 甘入脾 *gān rù pí*, sweetness enters the spleen
99. 辛入肺 *xīn rù fèi*, acridity enters the lung
100. 咸入肾 *xián rù shèn*, saltiness enters the kidney

| 第一节　第十三组 | | | | **SECTION 1: SET 13** |

五液　　　　　　　　　　　　　**Five Humors**

114-n109	* 泪氵	淚水	*lèi*	tears /tɪrz/
115-n110	* 汗氵	汗水	*hàn*	sweat /swɛt/
116-n111	* 涎氵	涎水	*xián*	drool /drul/

117-n112	* 涕 氵	涕 水	*tì*	snivel /ˈsnɪvl̩/
118-n113	* 唾 口	唾 口	*tuò*	spittle /ˈspɪtl̩/

注 Note:

1. Saliva is traditionally considered to be two fluids, 涎 *xián*, drool, related to the spleen, and 唾 *tuò*, spittle, related to the kidney. Drool is thick and runs out of the mouth. It is said to collect in the spleen, and rise upward with qì; hence it called the humor of the spleen. Spittle is what is spat out of the mouth. It is sticky and foamy, and is said to be the humor of the kidney. Note that 涎 is composed of 延 *yán*, to stretch, with a water signific, reflecting the viscous quality especially associated with 涎 and drool in English. The latter character, 唾 *tuò*, is composed of 垂 *chuí*, hang down, with the mouth signific, which also suggests a viscous fluid.

第一节　第十四组　　　　　　　**SECTION 1: SET 14**

七情　　　　　　　**Seven Affects**

119-n114	* 情 忄	情 心	*qíng*	affect /ˈæfɛkt/
120-n115	* 志 士	志 心	*zhì*	mind /maɪnd/
121-n116	* 怒 心	怒 心	*nù*	anger /ˈæŋgɚ/
122-n117	* 喜 士	喜 口	*xǐ*	joy /dʒɔɪ/
123-n118	* 忧 忄	憂 心	*yōu*	anxiety /æŋˈzaɪətɪ/
124-n119	* 思 田	思 心	*sī*	thought /θɔt/
125-n120	* 悲 非	悲 心	*bēi*	sorrow /ˈsɑro/
126-n121	* 恐 恐	恐 心	*kǒng*	fear /fɪr/
127-n122	* 惊 忄	驚 馬	*jīng*	fright /fraɪt/

注 Note:

1. The 七情 *qī qíng*, seven affects, are anger, joy, anxiety, thought, sorrow, fear, and fright. Of these, anger, joy, anxiety, thought, and fear (associated with the liver, heart, lung, spleen, and kidney, respectively) are the 五志 *wǔ zhì*, 'five minds'. The term 情 *qíng*, rendered as 'affect', implies a state of mind. The term 志 *zhì*, implies will, determination, direction. The two are often combined as 情志 *qíng zhì*, 'affect-mind', to refer to emotional and mental states in general.

2. The terms denoting the seven affects have not been standardized. The word 'worry' has been variously used as the equivalent of both 思 *sī*, associated with the spleen, and 忧 *yōu*, associated with the lung.

复合词 Compounds:

101. 七情 *qī qíng*, the seven affects
102. 五志 *wǔ zhì*, the five 'minds'

第一节　第十五组　　　　　　SECTION 1: SET 15

比喻性字词　　　　　　　　Metaphorical Terms

128-n123	*	正 止	正 止	*zhèng*	right /raɪt/
129-n124	*	真 十	眞 目	*zhēn*	true /tru/
130-n125	*	元 二	元 儿	*yuán*	origin /ˈɔrɪdʒɪn/ *n.*
					original /əˈrɪdʒənl̩/ *adj.*
131-n126	*	原 厂	原 厂	*yuán*	source /sɔrs, sors/
132-n127	*	营 艹	營 火	*yíng*	construction /kənˈstrʌkʃən/
133-n128	*	卫 卩	衞 行	*wèi*	defense /dɪˈfɛns/
134-n129	*	源 氵	源 水	*yuán*	source /sɔrs, sors/
135-n130	*	天 天	天 大	*tiān*	heaven /ˈhɛvən/
136-n131	*	本 木	本 木	*běn*	root /rut/
137-n132	*	根 木	根 木	*gēn*	root /rut/
138-n133	*	帅 巾	帥 巾	*shuài*	commander /kəˈmændɚ/
139-n134	*	母 一	母 毋	*mǔ*	mother /ˈmʌðɚ/
140-n135	*	府 广	府 广	*fǔ*	house /haʊs/
141-n136	*	命 人	命 口	*mìng*	life /laɪf/
142-n137	*	门 门	門 門	*mén*	gate /get/
143-n138	*	海 氵	海 水	*hǎi*	sea /si/
144-n139	*	室 宀	室 宀	*shì*	chamber /ˈtʃembɚ/
145-n140	*	君 口	君 口	*jūn*	sovereign /ˈsɑvərɪn/
146	*	相 木	相 目	*xiàng*	minister /ˈmɪnɪstɚ/ *n.*
					ministerial /ˌmɪnɪˈstɪrɪəl/ *adj.*
147-n141	*	宗 宀	宗 宀	*zōng*	ancestor /ˈænsɛstɚ/ *n.*
					ancestral /ænˈsɛstrl̩/ *adj.*
148-n142	*	盖 羊	蓋 艸	*gài*	canopy /ˈkænəpɪ/
149-n143	*	华 十	華 艸	*huá*	bloom /blum/
					florid /ˈflɑrɪd/
150-n144	*	发 又	髮 髟	*fà*	hair [of the head] /hɛr/
151-n145	*	充 亠	充 儿	*chōng*	fullness /ˈfʊlnɪs/

152	* 子 子	子 子	*zǐ*	child /tʃaɪld/
153	* 宫 宀	宫 宀	*gōng*	palace /ˈpælɪs/
154	* 奇 大	奇 大	*qí*	extraordinary /ɪksˈtrɔrdnˌɛrɪ/
155-n146	先 儿	先 儿	*xiān*	*before, earlier*
156-n147	* 龙 龙	龍 龍	*lóng*	dragon /ˈdrægən/
157-n148	* 雷 雨	雷 雨	*léi*	thunder /ˈθʌndɚ/
158-n149	* 玉 玉	玉 玉	*yù*	jade /dʒed/
159-n150	* 宝 宀	寶 宀	*bǎo*	jewel /ˈjuəl/
160-n151	后 厂	後 彳	*hòu*	*after, later, post-*
161-n152	为 丶	爲 火	*wéi*	*to be; as; make as or into*

注 Notes:

1. Various kinds of metaphor have already been encountered in the five phases, and in the terms 脏腑 *zàng fǔ*, bowels and viscera, 五官 *wǔ guān*, the five offices, and 子宫 *zǐ gōng*, 'infant's palace' (the uterus). The terminology of Chinese medicine is rich in military, political, moral, natural, and religious metaphor, and a few notable examples are presented here. Militaristic terms include 'defense', 'construction', and 'commander'. Political terms include 'sovereign' and 'minister'. Natural images include 'root', 'bloom', 'mother', 'child', 'ancestor', 'thunder', 'jade', and 'sea'. Moral terms include 'right'. The term 门 *mén*, gate, and 室 *shì*, chamber, are two architectural metaphors that are used not only in Chinese medicine but also in the technical languages of many modern disciplines.

Metaphor reflecting the Chinese world view at the time of the 黄帝内经 *Huáng Dì Nèi Jīng* is seen in many aspects of Chinese medical terminology. Water and transportation metaphors are to be seen in the terminology of the channels. Military metaphors are also noted in terms in 'Repletion Terms' further ahead and in 'sovereign, minister, assistant, and courier' roles played by ingredients within a formula. Also, the names of acupuncture points are especially rich in metaphor (see Appendix 3).

2. The phrases 'the liver, its bloom is in the nails' and 'the heart, its bloom is in the face' are quotations from the 黄帝内经 *Huáng Dì Nèi Jīng*. The strangeness of the construction is due to missing text: 'the liver... its bloom is in the nails."

3. The character 宫 *gōng* denotes either the uterus or the heart.

复合词 Compounds:

103. 正气 *zhèng qì*, right qi
104. 真元 *zhēn yuán*, true origin

105. 原气 *yuán qì*, source qì
106. 元气 *yuán qì*, original qì
107. 宗气 *zōng qì*, ancestral qì
108. 君火 *jūn huǒ*, sovereign fire
109. 相火 *xiàng huǒ*, ministerial fire
110. 命门 *mìng mén*, life gate
111. 宗筋 *zōng jīn*, ancestral sinew
112. 肺为水之上源 *fèi wèi shuǐ zhī shàng yuán*, the lung is the upper source of water
113. 后天之本 *hòu tiān zhī běn*, the root of later heaven (acquired constitution)
114. 脾为后天之本 *pí wéi hòu tiān zhī běn*, the spleen is the root of later heaven (acquired constitution)
115. 肾为先天之本 *shèn wéi xiān tiān zhī běn*, the kidney is the root of earlier heaven (congenital constitution)
116. 肾为气之根 *shèn wéi qì zhī gēn*, the kidney is the root of qì
117. 气为血之帅 *qì wéi xuè zhī shuài*, qì is the commander of the blood
118. 血为气之母 *xuè wéi qì zhī mǔ*, blood is the mother of qì
119. 肝，其华在爪 *gān, qí huá zài zhǎo*, the liver, its bloom is in the nails
120. 心，其华在面 *xīn qí huá zài miàn*, the heart, its bloom is in the face
121. 脾，其华在唇 *pí qí huá zài chún*, the spleen, its bloom is in the lips
122. 肺，其华在毛 *fèi, qí huá zài máo*, the lung, its bloom is in the [body] hair
123. 肾，其华在发 *shèn, qí huá zài fà*, the kidney, its bloom is in the hair
124. 肝，其充在筋 *gān, qí chōng zài jīn*, the liver, its fullness is in the sinews
125. 心，其充在脉 *xīn, qí chōng zài mài*, the heart, its fullness is in the vessels
126. 脾，其充在肌 *pí, qí chōng zài jī*, the spleen, its fullness is in the flesh
127. 肺，其充在皮 *fèi, qí chōng zài pí*, the lung, its fullness is in the skin
128. 肾，其充在骨 *shèn, qí chōng zài gǔ*, the kidney, its fullness is in the bones
129. 肺为华盖 *fèi wéi huá gài*, the lung is the florid canopy
130. 肺为气之主 *fèi wèi qì zhī zhǔ*, the lung is the governor of qì
131. 肾为水脏 *shèn wéi shuǐ zàng*, the kidney is the water viscus
132. 血室 *xuè shì*, blood chamber
133. 髓海 *suǐ hǎi*, sea of marrow
134. 血海 *xuè hǎi*, sea of blood
135. 命门之火 *mìng mén zhī huǒ*, life gate fire

136. 龙雷之火 *lóng léi zhī huǒ*, dragon and thunder fire (i.e., the life gate fire)

137. 玉海 *yù hǎi*, sea of jade (i.e., the bladder)

习题 Exercise:

61. 正气 ....

62. *jūn huǒ* ....

63. ancestral qì ....

64. 宗筋 ....

65. *zhēn yuán* ....

66. source qì ....

67. 命门 ....

68. *fèi wèi shuǐ zhī shàng yuán* ....

69. the kidney is the root of earlier heaven (congenital constitution) ..

70. 气为血之帅 ....

71. *xuè wéi qì zhī mǔ* ....

72. 肾，其华在发 ....

第一节　第十六组				**SECTION 1: SET 16**

脏腑功能与相互关系用词				**Organ Functions & Interrelations**
162	* 主 王	主 丶	*zhǔ*	govern /ˈgʌvɚn/
163-n153	* 藏 艹	藏 艸	*cáng*	store /stɔr, stor/
164-n154	* 化 亻	化 匕	*huà*	transform /trænsˈfɔrm/
165-n155	* 运 辶	運 辵	*yùn*	move /muv/
166-n156	* 谷 谷	穀 禾	*gǔ*	grain /gren/
167-n157	* 统 纟	統 糸	*tǒng*	manage /ˈmænɪdʒ/ control /kənˈtrol/
168	* 上 卜	上 一	*shàng*	ascend /əˈsɛnd/
169	* 下 卜	下 一	*xià*	descend /dɪˈsɛnd/
170-n158	* 升 丿	升 十	*shēng*	upbear /ˈʌpbɛr/ bear upward /bɛr ˈʌpwɚd/
171-n159	* 降 阝	降 阜	*jiàng*	downbear /ˈdaʊnbɛr/ bear downward /bɛr ˈdaʊnwɚd/
172-n160	* 发 又	發 癶	*fā*	effuse /ɪˈfjuz/

173	相 木	相 目	*xiāng*	each other, mutual
174-n161	* 交 亠	交 亠	*jiāo*	inter(act) /ˈɪntɚ, ˌɪntəˈrækt/
175-n162	* 分 八	分 刀	*fēn*	separate /ˈsɛpəret/
176-n163	* 别 刂	别 刀	*bié*	separate /ˈsɛpəret/
177-n164	* 开 廾	開 門	*kāi*	open /ˈopən/
178-n165	* 窍 穴	竅 穴	*qiào*	orifice /ˈɔrəfɪs/
179-n166	* 肃	肅 聿	*sù*	depurate /ˈdɛpjuˌret/
180-n167	* 疏 マ	疏 疋	*shū*	course /kɔrs, kors/
181-n168	泄 氵	泄 水	*xiè*	flow, drain
182-n169	谋 讠	謀 言	*móu*	scheme
183-n170	虑 虍	慮 心	*lǜ*	worry
184-n171	* 余 人	餘 食	*yú*	surplus /ˈsɝpləs/
185-n172	* 受 爫	受 又	*shòu*	intake /ˈɪntek/
186-n173	* 纳 纟	納 糸	*nà*	intake /ˈɪntek/
187	* 腐 广	腐 肉	*fǔ*	rot /rɑt/
188-n174	* 熟 灬	熟 火	*shú*	ripen /ˈrɑɪ[ə]n/
189	* 精 米	精 米	*jīng*	essence /ˈɛsəns/ n.
190-n175	微 彳	微 彳	*wēi*	subtle
191-n176	糟 米	糟 米	*zāo*	distiller's grain
192-n177	粕 米	粕 米	*pò*	dregs, lee
193-n178	* 通 辶	通 辵	*tōng*	free /fri/
194-n179	* 调 讠	調 言	*tiáo*	regulate /ˈrɛgjəˌlet/ vt. regulation /ˌrɛgjəˈleʃən/ n.
195-n180	* 清 氵	清 水	*qīng*	clear /klɪr/
196-n181	* 浊 氵	濁 水	*zhuó*	turbid /ˈtɝbɪd/
197-n182	* 表 主	表 衣	*biǎo*	exterior /ɪksˈtɪrɪɚ/
198-n183	* 里 里	裡 衣	*lǐ*	interior /ɪnˈtɪrɪɚ/

注 Notes:

1. We have already noted that the bowels and viscera 'govern' various parts of the body. The notion of the function of an organ in Chinese medicine is traditionally expressed as the governing of activity. Thus, 胃主受纳 *wèi zhǔ shòu nà*, the stomach governs intake, means that the stomach has the function of taking in 'grain and water' (i.e., food and drink).

2. The term 糟粕 *zāo pò*, translated here as waste, is composed of two characters denoting solid matter drained off in the process of making liquor.

3. In expressions such as 肺开窍于鼻 *fèi kāi qiào yú bí*, literally 'the lung opens orifice at nose', the 窍 *qiào* is not rendered for reasons of English grammar.

4. The word 升 *shēng* means to 'rise', 'raise', and 'cause to rise'; 降 *jiàng* means to 'descend', 'lower', and 'cause to descend'. In Chinese medicine, both these words are used mainly in the first and last senses, i.e., in the intransitive and causative senses ('rise' and 'cause to rise', 'descend' and 'cause to descend'). English has no single verb that covers the two meanings, and usually expresses the causative notion by the addition of an verb (cause to rise). Simple though they are, these words actually cause problems that translators solve in different ways: some translators will go against English convention and use, for example, descend transitively ('descend the qì'); others rephrase the idea more naturally as 'direct the qì downwards'.

Since 升 *shēng* and 降 *jiàng* commonly appear in many compound Chinese medical terms, we have chosen to give them a fixed rendering, i.e., one that can be used consistently by the translator in all contexts. The English 'bear upward' and 'bear downward', which can be used in both the intransitive and causative senses, are adopted instead of the more obvious equivalents discussed above. For the sake of keeping the terminology neat and avoiding paraphrase, we use the terms as 'upbear' and 'downbear' in many contexts: 肺气降 *fèi qì jiàng*, 'lung qì bears downward', 降肺气 *jiàng fèi qì*, 'downbear lung qì'. This term choice enables us to translate the words 胜 *shēng* and 降 *jiàng* consistently in all contexts. Thus, 升阳益胃汤 *shēng yáng yì wèi tāng* can be rendered as Yáng-Upbearing Stomach-Boosting Decoction, whereas any rendering in which *shēng* is translated as 'direct the qì downward' would make the English name of this decoction periphrastic.

复合词 Compounds:

138. 心藏神 *xīn cáng shén*, the heart stores the spirit
139. 心主神 *xīn zhǔ shén*, the heart governs the spirit
140. 心主血脉 *xīn zhǔ xuè mài*, the heart governs the blood and vessels
141. 心开窍于舌 *xīn kāi qiào yú shé*, the heart opens into the tongue
142. 肺主气 *fèi zhǔ qì*, the lung governs qì
143. 肺开窍于鼻 *fèi kāi qiào yú bí*, the lung opens into the nose
144. 肺主肃降 *fèi zhǔ sù jiàng*, the lung governs depurative downbearing
145. 肺为气之主，肾为气之根 *fèi wéi qì zhī zhǔ, shèn wéi qì zhī gēn*, the lung is governor of qì; the kidney is the root of qì
146. 肺与大肠相为表里 *fèi yǔ dà cháng xiāng wéi biǎo lǐ*, the lung and large intestine stand in exterior-interior relationship to each other
147. 大肠主津 *dà cháng zhǔ jīn*, the large intestine governs liquid
148. 肺主气，心主血 *fèi zhǔ qì, xīn zhǔ xuè*, the lung governs qì, and the heart governs the blood
149. 肺主皮毛 *fèi zhǔ pí máo*, the lung governs the skin and [body] hair

150. 脾主运化水谷之精微 *pí zhǔ yùn huà shuǐ gǔ zhī jīng wēi*, spleen governs movement and transformation of the essence of grain and water

151. 水谷 *shuǐ gǔ*, grain and water (food and drink)

152. 精微 *jīng wēi*, essence

153. 脾统血 *pí tǒng xuè*, the spleen controls the blood

154. 脾藏营 *pí cáng yíng*, the spleen stores construction

155. 脾开窍于口 *pí kāi qiào yú kǒu*, the spleen opens into the mouth

156. 胃主受纳 *wèi zhǔ shòu nà*, the stomach governs intake

157. 胃主腐熟水谷 *wèi zhǔ fǔ shú shuǐ gǔ*, the stomach governs the rotting and ripening (or decomposition) of grain and water

158. 脾与胃相为表里 *pí yǔ wèi xiāng wéi biǎo lǐ*, the spleen and stomach stand in exterior-interior relationship to each other

159. 小肠主分别清浊 *xiǎo cháng zhǔ fēn bié qīng zhuó*, the small intestine governs the separation of the clear and turbid

160. 清阳 *qīng yáng*, clear yáng

161. 浊阴 *zhuó yīn*, turbid yīn

162. 清气 *qīng qì*, clear qì

163. 浊气 *zhuó qì*, turbid qì

164. 大肠主传化糟粕 *dà cháng zhǔ chuán huà zāo pò*, the large intestine governs the conveyance and transformation of waste

165. 肝主疏泄 *gān zhǔ shū xiè*, the liver governs free coursing

166. 肝藏血 *gān cáng xuè*, the liver stores the blood

167. 肝主筋 *gān zhǔ jīn*, the liver governs the sinews

168. 肝为刚脏 *gān wéi gāng zàng*, the liver is the unyielding viscus

169. 肝主谋虑 *gān zhǔ móu lǜ*, the liver governs the making of strategies

170. 肝藏魂 *gān cáng hún*, the liver stores the ethereal soul

171. 爪为筋之余 *zhuǎ (zhǎo) wéi jīn zhī yú*, the nails are the surplus of the sinews

172. 肝开窍于目 *gān kāi qiào yú mù*, the liver opens into the eyes

173. 胆主决断 *dǎn zhǔ jué duàn*, the gallbladder governs decision

174. 肾开窍于耳 *shèn kāi qiào yú ěr*, the kidney opens into the ears

175. 肾开窍于二阴 *shèn kāi qiào yú èr yīn*, the kidney opens into the two yīn

176. 肾藏精气 *shèn cáng jīng qì*, the kidney stores essential qì

177. 肾主骨生髓 *shèn zhǔ gǔ shēng suǐ*, the kidney governs the bone and engenders the marrow

178. 肾主开阖 *shèn zhǔ kāi hé*, kidney governs opening and closing

习题 Exercise:

73. *xīn cáng shén* ....
74. the heart governs the blood and vessels ....
75. 心开窍于舌 ....
76. *dà cháng zhǔ jīn* ....
77. the small intestine governs humor ....
78. 肾藏精 ....
79. *shèn zhǔ shuǐ* ....
80. the kidney opens into the ears ....
81. 肝开窍于目 ....
82. *wèi zhǔ shòu nà* ....
83. the kidney governs the bone and engenders the marrow ....
84. 脾主肉 ....

第一节　第十七组   **SECTION 1: SET 17**

人体部位   **Body Parts**

199-n184	* 人人	人人	*rén*	person /ˈpɜˈsən/ *n.*
				human /ˈhjumən/ *adj.*
200-n185	* 体亻	體骨	*tǐ*	body /ˈbɑdɪ/
201-n186	* 身身	身身	*shēn*	body /ˈbɑdɪ/
202-n187	* 形彡	形彡	*xíng*	body /ˈbɑdɪ/
203-n188	* 部阝	部邑	*bù*	part /pɑrt/
				region /ˈrɪdʒən/
204	* 位亻	位人	*wèi*	position /pəˈzɪʃən/
205	* 窍穴	竅穴	*qiào*	orifice /ˈɔrəfɪs/
206-n189	* 头大	頭頁	*tóu*	head /hɛd/
207-n190	* 颅页	顱頁	*lú*	skull /skʌl/
208-n191	* 面一	面面	*miàn*	face /fes/
209-n192	* 巅山	巔山	*diān*	vertex /ˈvɜˈtɛks/
210-n193	* 额页	額頁	*é*	forehead /ˈfɑrɪd, ˈfɔrhɛd/
211-n194	* 囟丿	囟口	*xìn*	fontanels /ˌfɑntəˈnɛlz/
212-n195	枕木	枕木	*zhěn*	*pillow*
213	* 目目	目目	*mù*	eye /aɪ/
214-n196	珠王	珠玉	*zhū*	*pearl, bead, ball*
215-n197	* 眼目	眼目	*yǎn*	eye /aɪ/

216-n198	*	睛 目	睛 目	*jīng*	eye /aɪ/
217-n199	*	瞳 目	瞳 目	*tóng*	pupil /ˈpjupl̩/
218-n200	*	睑 目	瞼 目	*jiǎn*	eyelid /ˈaɪlɪd/
219	*	胞 月	胞 肉	*bāo*	eyelid /ˈaɪlɪd/
220-n201		弦 弓	弦 弓	*xián*	*string of a bow or musical instrument*
221	*	舌 舌	舌 舌	*shé*	tongue /tʌŋ/
222-n202	*	口 口	口 口	*kǒu*	mouth /maʊθ/
223-n203	*	牙 牙	牙 牙	*yá*	tooth /tuθ/
224-n204	*	齿 齿	齒 齒	*chǐ*	tooth /tuθ/
225	*	鼻 鼻	鼻 鼻	*bí*	nose /noz/
226-n205		孔 子	孔 子	*kǒng*	*hole*
227	*	耳 耳	耳 耳	*ěr*	ear /ɪr/
228-n206		轮 车	輪 車	*lún*	*wheel*
229	*	唇 辰	唇 口	*chún*	lip /lɪp/
230-n207	*	角 角	角 角	*jiǎo*	corner /ˈkɔrnɚ/
231-n208	*	咽 口	咽 口	*yān*	pharynx /ˈfærɪŋks/ throat /θrot/
232-n209	*	喉 口	喉 口	*hóu*	larynx /ˈlærɪŋks/ throat /θrot/
233-n210	*	咙 口	嚨 口	*lóng*	throat /θrot/
234-n211	*	悬 心	懸 心	*xuán*	*hang, suspend*
235-n212	*	雍 一	雍 隹	*yōng*	*obstruct*
236-n213	*	颧 页	顴 頁	*quán*	cheek /tʃik/ (cheek bone region)
237-n214	*	颊 页	頰 頁	*jiá*	cheek /tʃik/
238-n215	*	腮 月	腮 肉	*sāi*	cheek /tʃik/
239-n216	*	颈 页	頸 頁	*jǐng*	neck /nɛk/
240-n217	*	项 页	項 頁	*xiàng*	nape /nep/
241-n218	*	肩 月	肩 肉	*jiān*	shoulder /ˈʃoldɚ/
242-n219	*	背 月	背 肉	*bèi*	back /bæk/ dorsum /ˈdɔrsəm/
243-n220	*	腰 月	腰 肉	*yāo*	lumbus /ˈlʌmbəs/
244-n221	*	胸 月	胸 肉	*xiōng*	chest /tʃɛst/
245-n222	*	膈 月	膈 肉	*gé*	diaphragm /ˈdaɪəˌfræm/
246-n223	*	乳 爫	乳 乙	*rǔ*	breast /brɛst/
247-n224	*	肋 月	肋 肉	*lè*	rib /rɪb/
248-n225	*	胁 月	脅 肉	*xié*	rib-side /ˈrɪbsaɪd/
249-n226	*	腹 月	腹 肉	*fù*	abdomen /ˈæbdəmən/
250	*	大 大	大 大	*dà*	greater /ˈgretɚ/
251	*	小 小	小 小	*xiǎo*	smaller /ˈsmɔlɚ/
252-n227	*	少 小	少 小	*shào*	lesser /ˈlɛsɚ/

253-n228	*	脐 月	臍 肉	*qí*	umbilicus /ʌmˈbɪlɪkəs, ˌʌmbɪˈlaɪkəs/ *n.*
					umbilical /ʌmˈbɪlɪkl̩/ *adj.*
254-n229		际 阝	際 阜	*jì*	*region, border, margin*
255-n230	*	茎 ⁺⁺	莖 艸	*jīng*	penis /ˈpinɪs/
256-n231	*	睾 丿	睪 目	*gāo*	testicle /ˈtɛstɪkl̩/
257-n232		丸 丸	丸 丶	*wán*	*ball, pill*
258-n233	*	囊 十	囊 口	*náng*	scrotum /ˈskrotəm/
259-n234	*	女 女	女 女	*nü*	woman /ˈwʊmən/ *n.*
					female /ˈfimel/ *adj.*
260	*	阴 阝	陰 阜	*yīn*	genital /ˈdʒɛnɪtl̩/ *adj.,*
					genitals *n. pl.*
					pudenda /pjuˈdɛndə/ *n.*
					pudendal /pjuˈdɛndl̩/ *adj.*
261-n235	*	产 立	產 生	*chǎn*	childbirth /ˈtʃaɪldbɝθ/
					birth /bɝθ/
262	*	门 门	門 門	*mén*	gate /get/
263-n236	*	户 戶	戶 戶	*hù*	door /dor, dɔr/
264-n237	*	肢 月	肢 肉	*zhī*	limb /lɪm/
265-n238	*	腋 月	腋 肉	*yè*	armpit /ˈarmpɪt/ *n.*
					axillary /æˈksɪlərɪ/ *adj.*
266-n239	*	手 手	手 手	*shǒu*	hand /hænd/
					arm /ɑrm/
					upper extremity /ˈʌpɚ ɪksˈtrɛmɪtɪ/
267-n240	*	臂 月	臂 肉	*bì, bèi*	arm (esp. upper arm) /arm/
268-n241	*	肘 月	肘 肉	*zhǒu*	elbow /ˈɛlbo/
269-n242	*	腕 月	腕 肉	*wàn*	wrist /rɪst/
270-n243	*	寸 寸	寸 寸	*cùn*	inch /ɪntʃ/
271-n244	*	关 丷	關 門	*guān*	bar /bar/
272-n245	*	尺 尺	尺 尸	*chǐ*	cubit /ˈkjubɪt/
273-n246	*	鱼 鱼	魚 魚	*yú*	fish /fɪʃ/
274-n247	*	指 足	指 手	*zhǐ*	finger /ˈfɪŋgɚ/
275-n248	*	足 足	足 足	*zú*	leg /lɛg/
					foot /fʊt/
					lower extremity /ˈloɚ ɪksˈtrɛmɪtɪ/
276-n249	*	脚 月	腳 肉	*jiǎo*	foot /fʊt/
277-n250	*	腿 月	腿 肉	*tuǐ*	leg /lɛg/
278-n251	*	股 月	股 肉	*gǔ*	thigh /θaɪ/
279-n252	*	膝 月	膝 肉	*xī*	knee /ni/
280-n253	*	膕 月	膕 肉	*guó*	back of the knee /bæk əv ðəni/
281-n254	*	胫 月	脛 肉	*jìng*	lower leg /ˈloɚ ˈlɛg/
282-n255	*	踝 足	踝 足	*huái*	ankle /ˈæŋkl̩/

283-n256	* 趾 足	趾 足	*zhǐ*	toe /to/
284-n257	* 胎 月	胎 肉	*tāi*	fetus /ˈfitəs/
285-n258	* 腠 月	腠 肉	*còu*	interstice /ˈɪntɚstɪs/
286-n259	理 王	理 玉	*lǐ*	veins (of stone), grain (of wood)
287-n260	* 鬼 鬼	鬼 鬼	*guǐ*	ghost /gost/
288	* 上 卜	上 一	*shàng*	upper body /ˈʌpɚˌbɑdɪ/
289	* 中 中	中 丨	*zhōng*	center /ˈsɛntɚ/
290	* 下 卜	下 一	*xià*	lower body /ˈloɚˌbɑdɪ/ *n.*
291-n261	* 内 冂	內 入	*nèi*	inner body /ˈɪnɚˌbɑdɪ/ *n.* internal /ɪnˈtɝnl̩/ *adj.*
292-n262	* 外 卜	外 夕	*wài*	outer body /ˈautɚˌbɑdɪ/ *n.* external /ɪksˈtɝnl̩/ *adj.*

注 Notes:

1. Body: The characters 身 *shēn*, 体 *tǐ*, and 形 *xíng* all mean body. The first, *shēn*, means person as well as body. The second, *tǐ*, means the body as an organic unity. The third, *xíng*, which has the general meaning of shape or form, means the body as a visible and tangible entity.

2. Eyes: Chinese has different characters for 'eye'. 目 *mù*, the classical expression, is usually used alone to mean eye, but also appears in compounds such as 目睛 *mù jīng*, 目珠 *mù zhū*, and 眼目 *yǎn mù*; 眼 and 睛 may be used individually, and the combination of the two, 眼睛, is the ordinary expression in modern spoken Mandarin. In Chinese medicine, the pupil is referred to as 瞳 *tóng*, a term which appears to have a similar origin to our own. The character contains the word 童, a child, alluding to the fact that one can see one's reflection in another's pupil but reduced to childlike proportions. In English, this part of the eye was named 'pupil' for the very same reason. In Chinese medical texts, the pupil is often referred to as 瞳神 *tóng shén*, "pupil spirit."

3. Teeth: Chinese has two characters for teeth, 牙 *yá* and 齿 *chǐ*. In their original forms, 牙 portrayed interlocking upper and lower teeth, while 齿 pictured (as the modern character still does) two rows of teeth. The character 牙 is used specifically in the sense of tusk, fang, and cutting teeth. Some traditional Chinese medical texts have said that 牙 means the upper teeth and 齿 the lower teeth, although this distinction seems to have gained little currency in medical literature. In modern spoken Mandarin, the two are combined as 牙齿; in the written language, the two characters can be combined either as 牙齿 or 齿牙, but are often used alone, e.g., 牙痛 *yá tòng* and 齿痛 *chǐ tòng*, both meaning 'toothache'. The character 牙 is often used to generally denote

the teeth and gums, and is sometimes translated as such, for example, 牙疔 *yá dīng*, a clove sore of the teeth and gum, is a sore that starts in the gum and then affects the teeth.

4. Cheek: Chinese has several expressions for cheek. 颊 *jiá* (most commonly in combination with 面 *miàn*, face, as 面颊 *miàn jiá*) is the general expression for the side of the face. 颧 *quán* is specifically the area of the cheek bone 颧骨 *quán gǔ*, but is often used as 颊. 腮 *sāi*, in the medical context, is seen in the compound 痄腮 *zhà sāi*, mumps, and also used in a colloquial expression for cheek, 腮帮子 *sāi bāng zǐ*.

5. Throat: Three characters denote the throat. In the technical context, 咽 *yān* is the upper part (pharynx), through which air and food pass, and 喉 *hóu* is the lower part (larynx), through which only air passes. The distinction, however, is often blurred. The colloquial term 喉咙 *hóu lóng* is only occasionally seen in medical literature.

The Chinese term 悬雍 *xuán yōng* is the uvula. The character 雍 means harmony, but with the addition of the earth signific 土, it becomes 壅, congest, accumulate, so that the name would reflect the uvula as a lump of flesh hanging in the back of the mouth. The English 'uvula' means little grape.

6. Chest and abdomen: 胸 *xiōng* is the chest, i.e., the part enclosed by the ribs; 胁 *xié*, the 'rib-side', is the side of the chest from the armpit to the bottom of the ribs. The abdomen is divided into the 大腹 *dà fù*, 'greater abdomen', the part above the umbilicus, and the 小腹 *xiǎo fù*, 'smaller abdomen', the part below the umbilicus. A small area just below the breastbone is called 心下 *xīn xià*, '[region] below the heart'; the part below this where the stomach can be felt is called 胃脘 *wèi wǎn*, the 'stomach duct' (a term that has already been introduced in another of its meanings, the physical stomach). The 小腹 *xiǎo fù*, smaller abdomen, is also called the 少腹 *shào fù*, the lesser abdomen, a term which is sometimes used specifically to mean the lateral regions of the smaller abdomen.

7. Extremities: Chinese has several expressions for the upper and lower extremities. Describing the upper extremities, 手 *shǒu* means specifically the hand or hand and arm; the upper arm is usually specifically referred to as 臂 *bì* (or *bèi*). Describing the lower extremities, 足 *zú* means leg or foot, and is used more commonly in the written language than in the spoken language; 脚 *jiǎo* is the foot, but is used in dialects also to mean leg; 腿 *tuǐ* means leg, and is divided into 大腿 *dà tuǐ*, the thigh, and 小腿 *xiǎo tuǐ*; the term 胫 *jìng* also denotes the lower leg. Since 手 *shǒu* and 足 *zú* mean both hand and arm, and foot and leg, respectively, they are often most accurately rendered as 'upper extremity' and 'lower extremity'. Note also that the characters denoting finger and toe, 指 and 趾, are both pronounced as *zhǐ*.

8. Lumbus: The Chinese 腰 *yāo* in this text is translated as 'lumbus'. Most speakers of modern English call this 'the lower back' (and pain in this area as 'low back pain'). In Chinese medicine, it is considered to be distinct from 背 *bèi*, 'back'. The lumbus is said to be the 'house of the kidney' and lumbar pain is usually considered to be a sign of kidney vacuity. The back, by contrast, is susceptible to external evils, and is more closely connected with lung. In former times, we might have translated 腰 *yāo* as 'loin', but this term is now ambiguous since it has also come to mean the genitals. Lumbus, the Latin word from which loin derives, retains the unequivocal meaning of the lower part of the back.

9. Interstices: The term 腠理 *còu lǐ*, interstices, refers to the 'grain' of the skin and flesh, that is, the linear spaces by which sweat leaves the body. Functionally, the 'interstices' would appear to correspond to sweat glands and ducts observed in Western anatomy, although Chinese medical theory states that they are found not only just below the skin, but through the flesh (muscle). The character 腠 *còu* with a water signific instead of a flesh signific (凑) means 'confluence', and it might be that the 腠理 *còu lǐ* are so named because they are streams that sweat flows into. The term 鬼门 *guǐ mén*, ghost gates, appears to refer to the sweat pores.

10. Umbilicus: 'Umbilicus' has been chosen as the English equivalent of 脐 *qí* in preference to 'navel'. The only reason for this is that 'umbilicus' has a convenient adjectival form (umbilical), whereas 'navel' does not.

11. Genitals: The character 茎 *jīng* is the stem of a plant. It is combined with 阴 as 阴茎 *yīn jīng* to mean penis, but is also used alone in this metaphorical meaning. 阴 *yīn* is also commonly used singly to denote the genitals.

复合词 Compounds:

179. 人体 *rén tǐ*, human body
180. 身体 *shén tǐ*, body
181. 形体 *xíng tǐ*, body
182. 部位 *bù wèi*, part, region
183. 九窍 *jiǔ qiào*, the nine orifices
184. 头面 *tóu miàn*, head and face
185. 囟门 *xìn mén*, fontanel
186. 枕骨 *zhěn gǔ*, pillow bone (the occipital bone)
187. 头身 *tóu shēn*, head and body
188. 面目 *miàn mù*, face and eyes
189. 眼睛 *yǎn jīng*, eye
190. 目睛 *mù jīng*, eye

191. 目珠 *mù zhū*, eyeball
192. 眼目 *yǎn mù*, eye
193. 二目 *èr mù*, both eyes
194. 胞睑 *bāo jiǎn*, eyelid
195. 眼弦 *yǎn xián*, eyelid rim
196. 耳目 *ěr mù*, ears and eyes
197. 耳轮 *ěr lún*, helix
198. 鼻子 *bí zǐ*, nose (the 子 is a colloquial addition to the character 鼻 that rarely appears in medical texts)
199. 鼻孔 *bí kǒng*, nostril
200. 人中 *rén zhōng*, human center; the philtrum
201. 牙齿 *yá chǐ*, teeth
202. 悬雍 *xuán yōng*, uvula
203. 颈项 *jǐng xiàng*, neck [and nape]
204. 心胸 *xīn xiōng*, heart [region] and chest
205. 心腹 *xīn fù*, heart [region] and abdomen
206. 胸腹 *xiōng fù*, chest and abdomen
207. 胁肋 *xié lè*, rib-side
208. 心下 *xīn xià*, [region] below the heart
209. 胃脘 *wèi wǎn*, stomach duct
210. 大腹 *dà fù*, greater abdomen
211. 少腹 *shào fù*, lesser abdomen
212. 小腹 *xiǎo fù*, smaller abdomen
213. 阴茎 *yīn jīng*, penis (lit. 'yīn stem')
214. 玉茎 *yù jīng*, jade stem (penis)
215. 睾丸 *gāo wán*, testicle
216. 毛际 *máo jì*, pubic hair region
217. 阴囊 *yīn náng*, scrotum; yīn sac
218. 阴头 *yīn tóu*, 'yīn head,' glans penis
219. 女阴 *nü yīn*, female pudenda
220. 产门 *chǎn mén*, birth gate (orificium vaginae)
221. 阴户 *yīn hù*, yīn door (orificium vaginae)
222. 玉门 *yù mén*, jade gate (orificium vaginae)
223. 腰膝 *yāo xī*, lumbus and knees
224. 腰背 *yāo bèi*, lumbus and back
225. 手足 *shǒu zú*, extremities
226. 手脚 *shǒu jiǎo*, extremities
227. 胸胁 *xiōng xié*, chest and rib-side
228. 肩背 *jiān bèi*, shoulder and back

229. 鱼际 *yú jì*, fish's margin (the thenar eminence)
230. 手指 *shǒu zhǐ*, finger
231. 表里 *biǎo lǐ*, exterior and interior
232. 口眼 *kǒu yǎn*, mouth and eyes
233. 口角 *kǒu jiǎo*, corner of the mouth
234. 股阴 *gǔ yīn*, yīn [aspect] of the thigh
235. 脚趾 *jiǎo zhǐ*, toe
236. 咽喉 *yān hóu*, throat
237. 喉咙 *hóu lóng*, throat
238. 四肢 *sì zhī*, [four] limbs
239. 肢体 *zhī tǐ*, limbs; limbs and body
240. 上肢 *shàng zhī*, upper limbs
241. 下肢 *xià zhī*, lower limbs
242. 足背 *zú bèi*, dorsum of the foot
243. 上焦 *shàng jiāo*, upper burner
244. 鬼门 *guǐ mén*, ghost gates
245. 腰者，肾之府 *yāo zhě, shèn zhī fǔ*, the lumbus is the house of the kidney
246. 膝者，筋之府 *xī zhě, jīn zhī fǔ*, the knee is the house of the sinews

习题 Exercise:

85. The character 胞 *bāo* appears in this section in the sense of eyelid. What other English equivalent has been previously encountered?

86. lesser abdomen　...

87. 小腹　...

88. *yān hóu*　...

89. exterior and interior　...

90. 牙齿　...

91. *chǐ yá*　...

92. lumbus and knees　...

93. 胸胁　...

94. *còu lǐ*　...

95. ghost gates　...

96. 腰者，肾之府　...

97. *yāo wéi shèn zhī fǔ*　...

98. the knee is the house of the sinews　...

第一节　第十八组　　　　　　　**SECTION 1: SET 18**

经络　　　　　　　　　　**Channels & Network Vessels**

293-n263	* 经 纟	經 糸	*jīng*	channel	/ˈtʃænl̩/
294-n264	* 络 纟	絡 糸	*luò*	net[work [vessel]]	/ˈnɛtwɝk–ˌvɛsl̩/
295-n265	* 太 大	太 大	*tài*	greater	/ˈgretɚ/
296	* 少 小	少 小	*shào*	lesser	/ˈlɛsɚ/
297-n266	* 明 日	明 日	*míng*	brightness	/ˈbraɪtnɪs/
298-n267	* 厥 厂	厥 厂	*jué*	reverting	/rɪˈvɝtɪŋ/
299-n268	* 督 目	督 目	*dū*	governing	/ˈgʌvənɪŋ/
300-n269	* 任 亻	任 人	*rèn*	controlling	/kənˈtrolɪŋ/
301-n270	* 冲 冫	衝 行	*chōng*	thoroughfare	/ˈθɝofɛr/
302-n271	* 带 巾	帶 巾	*dài*	girdling	/ˈgɝdlɪŋ/
303-n272	* 跷 足	蹺 足	*qiào*	springing	/ˈsprɪŋɪŋ/
304-n273	* 维 纟	維 糸	*wéi*	linking	/ˈlɪŋkɪŋ/
305	* 别 刂	別 刀	*bié*	divergence	/dəˈvɝdʒəns/
306-n274	* 孙 子	孫 子	*sūn*	grandchild	/ˈgrændtʃaɪld/
307-n275	* 浮 氵	浮 水	*fú*	superficial	/ˌsupɚˈfɪʃl̩/
308	* 开 廾	開 門	*kāi*	opening	/ˈopənɪŋ/
309-n276	* 枢 木	樞 木	*shū*	pivot	/ˈpɪvət/
310-n277	* 阖 门	闔 門	*hé*	closing	/ˈklozɪŋ/
311	* 皮 皮	皮 皮	*pí*	cutaneous	/kjuˈteniəs/
312	* 部 阝	部 邑	*bù*	region	/ˈpɑrt/
313-n278	* 多 夕	多 夕	*duō*	copious	/ˈkopɪəs/
314	* 少 小	少 小	*shǎo*	scant	/skænt/
315	* 属 尸	屬 尸	*shǔ*	home to	/hom tu/

注 Notes:

1. The term 经 *jīng* has been variously translated as 'meridian', 'channel', and 'conduit'. The Chinese originally meant a 'warp' of cloth, and came to be used as 'headrope' of a fishing net, 'a main line or axis', 'rule', 'line of longitude', and came to be used as an adjective, 'constant', and as a verb, 'to pass along', 'to endure', etc. Soulié de Morant says that the pathways of qi in the body are called 经 *jīng* because they were considered to be like the lines of north-south longitude used in astronomy. Translators who use the word 'channel' or 'conduit' favor the explanation that Chinese viewed the 经 *jīng* as being like waterways traversing the body. In *Medicine in China: A History of Ideas*, Paul U. Unschuld explains in great detail how the conceptions of those who charted the 经络 *jīng luò* must have been influenced by the notion

that the body must have a transportation system similar to the waterways upon which the life of the nascent Chinese empire depended. What we see here is not simply a metaphor for want of a name. The source of the metaphor (the rivers and canals used for transportation) may have prompted the notion of a channel system.

2. The 络脉 *luò mài*, network vessels, ramify through three levels. The first level is the 十五络 *shǐ wǔ luò*, the 'fifteen network vessels'; the second is the branches of these fifteen, which are referred to as 络 *luò*, 'network vessels'; and the third is the 孙络 *sūn luò*, 'grandchild network vessels', obviously named by geneological analogy.

3. The English names of the channels and vessels are systematically written followed parenthesized Pīnyīn of the yīn-yáng denomination, e.g., 'foot greater yáng (*tài yáng*) bladder channel', since some are more familiar with the Pīnyīn than with translated terms.

In the complex script, the character 衝 *chōng* means to hurtle or surge; in a now rare usage as a noun, it means thoroughfare. It partly overlaps in meaning with its homophone 沖 (with a water signific). In the simplified script, the 衝 has been replaced by 冲, a variant form of 沖. As a result, readers of the simplified script may be unaware of the original meaning of the term 冲脉 *chōng mài*, a vessel like a thoroughfare.

4. 属络 *shǔ luò*, homing and netting, are the relationships of the twelve channels to the bowels and viscera with which they are associated. For example, the foot greater yin (*tài yīn*) spleen channel homes to the spleen and nets the stomach.

复合词 Compounds:

247. 太阳 *tài yáng*, greater yáng (*tài yáng*)
248. 少阳 *shào yáng*, lesser yáng (*shào yáng*)
249. 阳明 *yáng míng*, yáng brightness (*yáng míng*)
250. 太阴 *tài yīn*, greater yīn (*tài yīn*)
251. 少阴 *shào yīn*, lesser yīn (*shào yīn*)
252. 厥阴 *jué yīn*, reverting yīn (*jué yīn*)
253. 太阳经 *tài yáng jīng*, greater yáng (*tài yáng*) channel
254. 少阳经 *shào yáng jīng*, lesser yáng (*shào yáng*) channel
255. 阳明经 *yáng míng jīng*, yáng brightness (*yáng míng*) channel
256. 太阴经 *tài yīn jīng*, greater yīn (*tài yīn*) channel
257. 少阴经 *shào yīn jīng*, lesser yīn (*shào yīn*) channel
258. 厥阴经 *jué yīn jīng*, reverting yīn (*jué yīn*) channel
259. 奇经八脉 *qí jīng bā mài*, eight extraordinary vessels

260. 督脉 *dū mài*, governing (*dū*) vessel
261. 任脉 *rèn mài*, controlling (*rèn*) vessel
262. 冲脉 *dū mài*, thoroughfare (*chōng*) vessel
263. 带脉 *dài mài*, girdling (*dài*) vessel
264. 阴蹻脉 *yīn qiāo mài*, yīn springing (*yīn qiāo*) vessel
265. 阳蹻脉 *yáng qiāo mài*, yáng springing (*yáng qiāo*) vessel
266. 阴维脉 *yīn wéi mài*, yīn linking (*yīn wéi*) vessel
267. 阳维脉 *yáng wéi mài*, yáng linking (*yáng wéi*) vessel
268. 孙络 *sūn luò*, grandchild network vessels
269. 浮络 *fú luò*, superficial network vessels
270. 手太阳经 *shǒu tài yáng jīng*, hand greater yáng (*tài yáng*) channel
271. 太阳为开 *tài yáng wéi kāi*, greater yáng (*tài yáng*) is the opening
272. 少阳为枢 *shào yáng wéi shū*, lesser yáng (*shào yáng*) is the pivot
273. 阳明为阖 *yáng míng wéi hé*, yáng brightness (*yáng míng*) is the closing
274. 太阴为开 *tài yīn wéi kāi*, greater yīn (*tài yīn*) is the opening
275. 少阴为枢 *shào yīn wéi shū*, lesser yīn (*shào yīn*) is the pivot
276. 厥阴为阖 *jué yīn wéi hé*, reverting yīn (*jué yīn*) is the closing
277. 属络 *shǔ luò*, homing and netting
278. 十二经筋 *shí èr jīng jīn*, the twelve channel sinews
279. 十二皮部 *shí èr pí bù*, the twelve cutaneous regions
280. 阳脉 *yáng mài*, yáng vessel
281. 八脉 *bā mài*, the eight vessels
282. 经络之气 *jīng luò zhī qì*, qì of the channels and network vessels
283. 经气 *jīng qì*, channel qì
284. 少阳多气少血 *shào yáng duō qì shǎo xuè*, the lesser yáng (*shào yáng*) has copious qì and scant blood
285. 太阳多血少气 *tài yáng duō xuè shǎo qì*, the greater yáng (*tài yáng*) has copious blood and scant qì
286. 阳明多气多血 *yáng míng duō qì duō xuè*, the yáng brightness (*yáng míng*) has copious blood and copious qì

习题 Exercise:

99. hand lesser yáng (*shào yáng*) channel ....
100. 手阳明经 ....
101. *shǒu tài yīn jīng* ....
102. hand lesser yīn (*shào yīn*) channel ....
103. 手厥阴经 ....
104. *zú tài yáng jīng* ....

105. foot lesser yáng (*shào yáng*) channel ....

106. 足阳明经 ....

107. *zú tài yīn jīng* ....

108. foot lesser yīn (*shào yīn*) channel ....

109. 足厥阴经 ....

110. *gān jīng* ....

111. heart channel ....

112. 脾经 ....

113. *fèi jīng* ....

114. kidney channel ....

115. stomach channel ....

116. 少阴多气少血 ....

117. *jué yīn duō xuè shǎo qì* ....

118. the greater yīn (*tài yīn*) has copious qì and copious blood ....

| 第一节　第十九组 | | SECTION 1: SET 19 |

穴位   Points

316-n279	* 穴 穴	穴 穴	*xué*	hole /hol/	
				point /pɔɪnt/	
317	位 亻	位 人	*wèi*	*position*	
318-n280	道 辶	道 辵	*dào*	*way, dao*	
319-n281	* 俞 人	俞 入	*shū*	point /pɔɪnt/	
				hole /hol/	
				transport (point)	
				/ˈtrænspɔrt, -pɔrt/	
320-n282	* 腧 月	腧 肉	*shū*	point /pɔɪnt/	
				hole /hol/	
321-n283	* 输 车	輸 車	*shū*	point /pɔɪnt/	
				hole /hol/	
				transport (point)	
				/ˈtrænspɔrt, -pɔrt/	
322-n284	* 井 二	井 二	*jǐng*	well /wɛl/	
323-n285	* 荥 艹	滎 水	*yíng*	brook /bruk/	
324	* 经 纟	經 糸	*jīng*	river /rɪvɚ/	
				channel /ˈtʃænl̩/	

325-n286	* 合 人	合 口	*hé*	uniting /juˈnaɪtɪŋ/
326-n287	* 募 ⺾	募 艸	*mù*	alarm /əˈlɑrm/
327-n288	* 会 人	會 曰	*huì*	meeting /ˈmitɪŋ/
328	* 交 ⼇	交 ⼇	*jiāo*	intersection /ˌɪntɚˈsɛkʃən/
329-n289	* 总 纟	總 糸	*zǒng*	command /kəˈmænd/
330	* 原 厂	原 厂	*yuán*	source /sɔrs, sors/
331	* 络 纟	絡 糸	*luò*	network /ˈnɛtwɝˈk/
332-n290	* 郄 阝	郄 邑	*xī*	cleft /klɛft/

注 Notes:

1. The Chinese 穴 *xué*, (acupuncture) point, has the literal meaning of cave or hole. It therefore reflects the concept of palpable gaps in body tissues. The term 'point' that is now almost universally used among English speakers does not reflect such a conception. In writing, the term 穴 *xué* is used either alone or in the combination 穴位 *xué wèi*. The combination 穴道 *xué dào* is considered to be colloquial.

2. The characters 俞, 腧, and 输 are all read as *shū* and all have the general meaning of acupuncture point. The last of them has the cart signific 车 *chē* and in its normal usage outside acupuncture means 'transport'. These three characters are seen most commonly in the names of point groups. The term 五输穴 *wǔ shū xué*, the five transporting points, is always written with 输, transport. Amongst these five points is one called the 俞, the stream point, which by convention is not usually written in either of the other two forms, and which is traditionally explained as meaning 注 *zhù*, to pour, flow, or stream. A term denoting another group of points, the 背输穴 *bèi shū xué*, is now usually written with 输, transport, but in the *Nèi Jīng*, which first introduced these points, it was written as 俞. The *Nàn Jīng* followed the *Nèi Jīng* in writing this character as 俞, but notes 扁鹊 Biǎn Què (in writings now lost) had written it as 输, making explicit the notion of transportation associated with the function of these points.

3. The terminology of the 五输穴 *wǔ shū xué*, the five transporting points (e.g., 'well points' and 'brook points'), reflects the conception of the channels as a system of waterways and a transportation system. 经穴 *jīng xué* is often referred to in English as the 'river point', but outside the context of the five transport points, the same term means 'channel point'. 合穴 *hé xué* is rendered in this text literally as 'uniting point'; it is often referred to as the 'sea point'.

4. The term 募穴 *mù xué*, denoting points located on the chest, are rendered in this text as 'alarm points'. The character 募 actually means to muster.

复合词 Compounds:

287. 穴位 *xué wèi*, point, hole
288. 穴道 *xué dào*, point, hole
289. 五输穴 *wǔ shū xué*, five transport points
290. 井穴 *jǐng xué*, well point
291. 荥穴 *yíng xué*, brook point
292. 俞穴 *shū xué*, stream point
293. 经穴 *jīng xué*, river point
294. 合穴 *hé xué*, uniting point
295. 下合穴 *xià hé xué*, lower uniting point
296. 背输穴 *bèi shū xué*, back transport points
297. 募穴 *mù xué*, alarm point
298. 原穴 *yuán xué*, source point
299. 郄穴 *xī xué*, cleft point
300. 络穴 *luò xué*, network point
301. 交会穴 *jiāo huì xué*, intersection point
302. 会穴 *huì xué*, meeting point
303. 气会 *qì huì*, meeting point of the qì
304. 血会 *xuè huì*, meeting point of the blood
305. 脏会 *zàng huì*, meeting point of the viscera
306. 腑会 *fǔ huì*, meeting point of the bowels
307. 筋会 *jīn huì*, meeting point of the sinew
308. 骨会 *gǔ huì*, meeting point of the bone
309. 髓会 *suǐ huì*, meeting point of the marrow
310. 八会穴 *bā huì xué*, eight meeting points
311. 四总穴 *sì zǒng xué*, four command points

习题 Exercise:

119. 八会穴 ....
120. *jiāo huì xué* ....
121. lower uniting point ....
122. 背输穴 ....
123. *mù xuè* ....
124. meeting point ....
125. 五输穴 ....
126. *yíng xué* ....
127. meeting point of the qì ....

第一节　第二十组	**SECTION 1: SET 20**

病因   **Causes of Disease**

333-n291	* 病疒	病疒	*bìng*	disease /dɪˈziz/
334-n292	* 因囗	因囗	*yīn*	cause /kɔz/
335	* 内冂	內入	*nèi*	internal /ɪnˈtɜ˞nl̩/
336	* 外夕	外卜	*wài*	external /ɪksˈtɜ˞nl̩/
337-n293	* 邪阝	邪邑	*xié*	evil /ˈivl̩/
338-n294	* 淫氵	淫水	*yín*	excess /ɪkˈsɛs/
339-n295	* 风风	風風	*fēng*	wind /wɪnd/
340-n296	* 寒宀	寒宀	*hán*	cold /kold/
341-n297	* 暑日	暑日	*shǔ*	summerheat /ˈsʌmə˞ˌhit/
342-n298	* 湿氵	濕水	*shī*	dampness /ˈdæmpnɪs/
343-n299	* 燥火	燥火	*zào*	dryness /ˈdraɪnɪs/
344	* 火火	火火	*huǒ*	fire /faɪr/
345-n300	* 热灬	熱火	*rè*	heat /hit/
346-n301	* 温氵	溫水	*wēn*	warmth /wɔrmθ/ *n.*
				warm /wɔrm/ *adj.*
347-n302	* 凉氵	涼水	*liáng*	cool /kul/ *adj.*
348-n303	* 冷冫	冷冫	*lěng*	cold /kold/
349-n304	* 疠疒	癘疒	*lì*	pestilence /ˈpɛstɪləns/
350-n305	* 山山	山山	*shān*	mountain /ˈmaʊntɪn/
351-n306	岚山	嵐山	*lán*	*mist, vapor*
352-n307	* 瘴疒	瘴疒	*zhàng*	miasma /maɪˈæzmə/ *n.*,
				miasmic /maɪˈæzmɪk/ *adj.*
353-n308	* 痰疒	痰疒	*tán*	phlegm /flɛm/
354-n309	* 饮饣	飲食	*yǐn*	rheum /rum/
355-n310	* 虫虫	蟲虫	*chóng*	worm /wɜ˞m/
				insect /ˈɪnsɛkt/
356-n311	* 毒丰	毒毋	*dú*	toxin /ˈtɑksɪn/
357-n312	* 瘀疒	瘀疒	*yū*	static blood /ˌstætɪk blʌd/
				stasis /ˈstesɪs/
358-n313	* 伤亻	傷人	*shāng*	damage /ˈdæmɪdʒ/
				injury /ˈɪndʒəri/

359	饮 亻	飲 食	*yǐn*	drink
360-n314	食 食	食 食	*shí*	eat
361-n315	* 过 辶	過 辵	*guò*	excessive /ɪkˈsɛsɪv/
362-n316	贪 貝	貪 貝	*tān*	*rapacious, greed*
363-n317	* 洁 氵	潔 水	*jié*	clean /klin/
364-n318	* 酒 氵	酒 水	*jiǔ*	liquor /ˈlɪkɚ/
365-n319	* 暴 日	暴 日	*bào*	voracious /vəˈreʃəs/
366	* 生 丿	生 生	*shēng*	raw /rɔ/
367-n320	* 肥 月	肥 肉	*féi*	fat /fæt/ *n.*
				fatty /ˈfætɪ/ *adj.*
368-n321	* 辣 辛	辣 辛	*là*	spicy-hot /ˈspɑɪsɪ–hɑt/ *adj.*
369-n322	失 丿	失 大	*shī*	lose
370	* 调 讠	調 言	*tiáo*	regulate /ˈrɛɡjəˌlet/ *vt.*
				regulation /rɛɡjəˈleʃən/ *n.*
371-n323	* 劳 卝	勞 力	*láo*	taxation /tæksˈeʃən/
372-n324	房 戶	房 戶	*fáng*	*room, bedroom, sexual activity*
373	室 宀	室 宀	*shì*	*room, bedroom*
374-n325	* 节 竹	節 竹	*jié*	temper(ance) /ˈtɛmpər(əns)/
375-n326	* 慎 忄	愼 心	*shèn*	careful /ˈkɛrful/
376-n327	* 蛇 虫	蛇 虫	*shé*	snake /snek/
377-n328	* 咬 口	咬 口	*yǎo*	bite /baɪt/

注 Notes:

1. The causes of disease 因 *yīn* or 病因 *bìng yīn*, were first classified as external, internal, and neutral by the Sòng dynasty physician Chén Wú-Zé (陈无择) in his *Sān Yīn Jí Yī Bìng Zhèng Fāng Lùn* (三因极一病症方论 "A Unified Treatise on Diseases, Patterns, and Remedies According to the Three Causes"), which was published in A.D. 1174. External causes are the six excesses. Internal causes are the seven affects. Neutral causes (literally "non-external-internal") include eating too much or too little, taxation fatigue, knocks and falls, crushing, drowning, and animal, insect, and reptile injuries. The classification may seem somewhat unusual until it is realized that external, internal, and neutral correspond to heaven, man, and earth, respectively.

2. In Chinese medical texts, 六淫 *liù yín*, the six excesses, are among the causes of disease most commonly mentioned. Most of these have obvious equivalents in English (cold, wind, fire, dryness). 暑 *shǔ*, the torrid heat of summer, has no single-word equivalent in English; we have coined 'summer-heat' to meet the need. 湿 *shī* in its general usage corresponds to 'wetness', 'moisture', 'dampness', and 'humidity'. 'Wetness', and to a certain degree

'moisture' also imply water in its liquid form. 'Humidity', other than in the meteorological sense of 'degree of dampness', generally has connotations of heat ('hot and humid'). 'Dampness' is a general term, but in practice tends to have connotations of cold ('cold and damp'). In the medical context, 'humidity' and 'dampness' would appear to have the most appropriate connotations, and since 湿 is said to be a yīn evil, we choose 'dampness'. Note that 'dampness' means either the quality of dampness or the degree of dampness. In everyday English, all-pervasive health-threatening moisture is usually referred to as 'damp' rather than 'dampness' (and it is 'damp', not 'dampness', of course, that rots our floor boards). However, in the Chinese medical context 'damp-drying medicinal', especially if the hyphen were omitted, would not be as clear as 'dampness-drying medicinal'. 'Damp-heat' is a quite firmly established compound. No-one seems to write 'dampness-heat."

3. The characters 寒 *hán* and 冷 *lěng* are both rendered as cold. In modern Mandarin, the latter is the most commonly used word for cold. In Chinese medical usage, 寒 denotes the disease evil cold and the cold nature of drugs and certain diseases. The character 冷, most commonly used as an adjective, tends to denote cold immediately felt by the thermal sense (cold hands, cold drinks).

4. Attention should be paid to the technical distinctions between 'fire', 'summerheat', and 'heat'. Of these, only 'fire' and 'summerheat' appear among the six excesses. Here, 'fire' usually denotes any unseasonal form of heat outside the summer months. However, 'fire' also denotes a certain form of heat arising internally in the body, and manifesting in upper-body (head) signs, such as dizziness, sore throat, or mouth sores. 'Heat' is a generic term for summerheat and either form of fire, as used in pattern identification. Translators should be careful not to substitute one of these terms for another in translation.

5. The term 痰 *tán*, 'phlegm', denotes a thick viscous fluid, which is understood to arise either when the spleen fails to transform the fluids or when heat condenses the fluids of the body. Phlegm collects in the lung (the 'lung is the collecting place of phlegm'). However, it is also held to be capable of affecting other parts of the body, causing a variety of different diseases. The English term phlegm (from the Greek *phlegein*, to burn) and the Chinese 痰 (which contains 炎, flaming), possibly both reflect an original conception of a humor resulting from heat. Phlegm is thick and sticky, and stands in opposition to 饮 *yǐn*, which literally means 'drink', but which in the medical context means a pathological accumulation of thin fluid in the body. Both phlegm and rheum are both products of disease and causes of disease.

6. The Chinese 瘴 *zhàng*, miasma, is a vapor to which some forms of malaria are attributed. It often appears in the combination 瘴气 *zhàng qì*, 'miasmic qì', and most commonly in the four-character compound 山岚瘴气 *shān lán zhàng qì*, literally 'mountain-mist miasmic qì', hinting that in China miasma is observed in forest mountain areas.

7. The Chinese 虫 *chóng* includes insects, spiders, worms, and reptiles.

8. The Chinese 伤 *shāng* is rendered as 'injury' in 外伤 *wài shāng*, external injury. In other contexts, when the offending agent is a disease evil, it is rendered as 'damage', e.g., 伤寒 *shāng hán*, cold damage.

9. The Chinese 劳 *láo* in the Chinese medical context denotes various strains on the body. It does not necessarily imply active 'over-exertion', a term often used in English.

10. In this book, combinations of disease evils are written with a hyphen, e.g., 'damp-heat', meaning dampness in combination with heat. Where the name of one evil qualifies that of another, the names are written without a hyphen, e.g., 'heat phlegm', meaning phlegm having the qualities of heat.

复合词 Compounds:

312. 病因 *bìng yīn*, cause of disease
313. 内因 *nèi yīn*, internal cause
314. 外因 *wài yīn*, external cause
315. 不内外因 *bù nèi wài yīn*, neutral cause
316. 六淫 *liù yín*, six excesses
317. 病邪 *bìng xié*, disease evil
318. 风寒 *fēng hán*, wind-cold
319. 暑湿 *shǔ shī*, summerheat-damp
320. 暑热 *shǔ rè*, summerheat-heat
321. 温燥 *wēn zào*, warm dryness
322. 凉燥 *liáng zào*, cool dryness
323. 痰饮 *tán yǐn*, phlegm-rheum
324. 痰热 *tán rè*, phlegm-heat
325. 痰火 *tán huǒ*, phlegm-fire
326. 风痰 *fēng tán*, wind phlegm
327. 寒痰 *hán tán*, cold phlegm
328. 热痰 *rè tán*, heat phlegm
329. 燥痰 *zào tán*, dryness phlegm
330. 湿痰 *shī tán*, damp phlegm
331. 痰湿 *tán shī*, phlegm-damp
332. 血瘀 *xuè yū*, blood stasis

333. 瘀血 *yū xuè*, static blood
334. 风水 *fēng shuǐ*, wind water
335. 热毒 *rè dú*, heat toxin
336. 邪气 *xié qì*, evil qi
337. 火气 *huǒ qì*, fire qi
338. 湿气 *shī qì*, damp qì
339. 湿毒 *shī dú*, damp toxin
340. 温热 *wēn rè*, warm heat
341. 湿热 *shī rè*, damp-heat
342. 血燥 *xuè zào*, blood dryness
343. 伤寒 *shāng hán*, cold damage
344. 伤暑 *shāng shǔ*, summerheat damage
345. 温邪 *wēn xié*, warm evil
346. 疠气 *lì qì*, pestilential qì
347. 山岚瘴气 *shān lán zhàng qì*, miasma, miasmic qì
348. 外伤 *wài shāng*, external injury
349. 饮食 *yǐn shí*, food and drink; diet
350. 饮食失调 *yǐn shí shī tiáo*, dietary irregularity
351. 内伤七情 *nèi shāng qī qíng*, internal damage by the seven affects, affect damage
352. 暴饮暴食 *bào yǐn bào shí*, voracious eating and drinking
353. 贪凉饮冷 *tān liáng yǐn lěng*, overconsumption of cold foods and drinks
354. 劳倦 *láo juàn*, taxation fatigue
355. 五劳 *wǔ láo*, five taxations
356. 过食肥甘 *guò shí féi gān*, excessive consumption of sweet and fatty foods
357. 过食生冷 *guò shí shēng lěng*, excessive consumption of raw and cold foods
358. 过食辛辣 *guò shí xīn là*, excessive consumption of hot-spicy foods
359. 伤酒 *shāng jiǔ*, liquor damage
360. 房室过多 *fáng shì guò duō*, excessive sexual activity
361. 房室不节 *fáng shì bù jié*, sexual intemperance
362. 房劳 *fáng láo*, sexual taxation
363. 起居不慎 *qǐ jū bú shèn*, careless living
364. 蛇咬 *shé yǎo*, snake bite
365. 虫咬 *chóng yǎo*, insect bite

习题 Exercise:

131. What are the two meanings of 饮 *yǐn*? ....

132. *wài yīn* ....
133. wind-heat ....
134. 肝火 ....
135. *shāng yīn* ....
136. food damage ....
137. 伤酒 ....
138. *shāng fēng* ....
139. excessive drinking (of liquor) ....
140. 蛇咬 ....
141. *chóng yǎo* ....
142. cause of disease ....
143. 山岚瘴气 ....
144. *tán huǒ* ....
145. phlegm-rheum ....
146. 暴饮暴食 ....
147. *guò shí féi gān* ....

第二节：四诊
Section 2: The Four Examinations

This section introduces diagnostic terminology. The material is presented in the traditional categories of the four examinations: inspection, listening and smelling (together considered as one), inquiry, and palpation. This is perhaps not ideal, since many phenomena are the subject of more than one of the four. Stool, for example, is dealt with in inspection and listening and smelling, and much of the information that either of these two examinations would render is often replaced by data gathered through inquiry.

第二节　第一组				**SECTION 2: SET 1**

四诊				**Four Examinations**
378-n329	* 诊 讠	診 言	*zhěn*	examine /ɪgzˈæmɪn/ *vt.*
				examination /ɪgzæməˈneʃən/ *n.*
379-n330	* 望 王	望 月	*wàng*	inspect /ɪnˈspɛkt/ *vt.*
				inspection /ɪnˈspɛkʃən/ *n.*
380-n331	* 闻 门	聞 耳	*wén*	listen /ˈlɪsən/ *vi.*
				listening /ˈlɪsn̩ɪŋ/ *n.*
				smell /smɛl/ *vi.*
				smelling /ˈsmɛlɪŋ/ *n.*
381-n332	* 问 门	問 口	*wèn*	inquire /ɪnˈkwaɪr/ *vi.*
				inquiry /ɪnˈkwaɪrɪ/ *n.*
382-n333	* 切 刀	切 刀	*qiè*	palpate /pælˈpet/ *vt.*
				palpation /pælpˈeʃən/ *n.*

注 Notes:

1. The character 闻 *wén* means both to listen (hear) and to smell. Its signific\nific is the 耳 *ěr*, which suggests that to hear was the original meaning. In the 黄帝内经 *Huáng Dì Nèi Jīng*, the term referred to listening, not smelling. It was only later that identification of smells was developed.

2. Palpation, 切诊 *qiē zhěn*, includes 脉诊 *mài zhěn*, pulse-taking, and 按诊 *àn zhěn*, body palpation.

复合词 Compounds:

366. 望诊 *wàng zhěn*, inspection

367. 闻诊 *wén zhěn*, listening and smelling
368. 问诊 *wèn zhěn*, inquiry
369. 切诊 *qì zhěn*, palpation

望诊
Inspection

第二节 第二组				**SECTION 2: SET 2**

望神				**Inspection of the Spirit**
383	* 神 礻	神 示	*shén*	spirit /ˈspɪrɪt/
384-n334	得 彳	得 彳	*dé*	*get, obtain*
385	失 丿	失 大	*shī*	*lose*
386-n335	无 尢	無 火	*wú*	*have not; there is not, there are not*
387-n336	* 假 亻	假 人	*jiǎ*	false /fɔls/
388-n337	* 乱 舌	亂 乙	*luàn*	deranged /dɪˈrendʒd/
389	* 少 小	少 小	*shǎo*	little /ˈlɪtl/
390-n338	* 昏 氏	昏 日	*hūn*	cloud /ˈklaʊd/

注 Notes:

1. 望神 *wàng shén*, 'inspection of the spirit', means looking at the patient to find general signs of vitality. Here, 'spirit' is wider in meaning than the spirit stored by the heart, the principle of consciousness. It means not only the heart spirit as manifest in mental vigor, but also general physical vitality.

2. The term 望神 *wàng shén* is a verb + object construction, 'look at spirit', used as a noun construction, 'looking at the spirit' or 'inspection of the spirit'.

复合词 Compounds:

370. 得神 *dé shén*, spiritedness
371. 失神 *shī shén*, spiritlessness
372. 无神 *wú shén*, spiritlessness
373. 假神 *jiǎ shén*, false spiritedness
374. 少神 *shǎo shén*, little spirit
375. 神乱 *shén luàn*, deranged spirit
376. 神昏 *shén hūn*, clouded spirit

第二节　第三组	**SECTION 2: SET 3**

望形体 — Inspection of the Physical Body

391	* 肥 月	肥 肉	*féi*	fat /fæt/ *adj.*
				fatness /ˈfætnɪs/ *n.*
				obese /oˈbis/ *adj.*
				obesity /əˈbizɪtɪ/ *n.*
392-n339	* 胖 月	胖 肉	*pàng*	fat /fæt/ *adj.*
				fatness /ˈfætnɪs/ *n.*
				obese /oˈbis/ *adj.*
				obesity /əˈbizɪtɪ/ *n.*
393-n340	消 氵	消 水	*xiāo*	*wasted*
394-n341	* 瘦 疒	瘦 疒	*shòu*	thin /θɪn/
				emaciated /ɪˈmeʃɪˌetɪd/
395	* 浮 氵	浮 水	*fú*	puffy /ˈpʌfɪ/
396-n342	* 肿 月	腫 肉	*zhǒng*	swelling /ˈswɛlɪŋ/

复合词 Compounds:

377. 肥胖 *féi pàng*, fatness; obesity
378. 消瘦 *xiāo shòu*, emaciation
379. 浮肿 *fú zhǒng*, puffy swelling

第二节　第四组	**SECTION 2: SET 4**

望姿态、动态 — Inspection of the Posture & Bearing

397-n343	* 姿 女	姿 女	*zī*	posture /ˈpɑstʃɚ/
398-n344	动 力	動 力	*dòng*	*move, stir*
399-n345	态 心	態 心	*tài*	*state*
400-n346	向 丿	向 口	*xiàng*	*toward*
401	里 里	裡 衣	*lǐ*	*inside*
402-n347	* 蜷 足	踡 足	*quán*	curled /kɝld/
403-n348	* 卧 臣	臥 臣	*wò*	lie /laɪ/
404-n349	* 坐 土	坐 土	*zuò*	sit /sɪt/
405	得 彳	得 彳	*dé*	*can, able*
406-n350	* 半 丨	半 十	*bàn*	half /hæf/
				hemi- /ˈhɛmɪ/

407-n351	遂 辶	遂 辵	*suì*	follow, obey
408-n352 *	撒 扌	撒 手	*sā*	limp /lɪmp/
409	角 角	角 角	*jiǎo*	horn
410-n353	弓 弓	弓 弓	*gōng*	bow
411	反 厂	反 又	*fǎn*	backward, reversed, counter
412-n354	张 弓	張 弓	*zhāng*	stretch
413-n355 *	拘 扌	拘 手	*jū*	hypertonicity /ˌhaɪpɚtəˈnɪsɪtɪ/
414-n356 *	急 心	急 心	*jí*	tension /ˈtɛnʃən/
				hypertonicity /ˌhaɪpɚtəˈnɪsɪtɪ/
415-n357 *	挛 心	攣 心	*luán*	hypertonicity /ˌhaɪpɚtəˈnɪsɪtɪ/
416-n358 *	强 弓	強 弓	*jiàng*	rigidity /rɪˈdʒɪdətɪ/
417-n359 *	瘈 疒	瘈 疒	*jì*	tugging /ˈtʌgɪŋ/
418-n360 *	瘲 疒	瘲 疒	*zòng*	slackening /ˈslækənɪŋ/
419-n361	直 十	直 目	*zhí*	straight
420-n362	舞 ㇒	舞 舛	*wǔ*	dance
421-n363	蹈 足	蹈 足	*dào*	dance
422-n364	扬 扌	揚 手	*yáng*	lift
423-n365	踯 足	躑 足	*zhí*	move to and fro
424-n366 *	颤 页	顫 頁	*chàn, zhàn*	shaking /ˈʃəkɪŋ/
425-n367 *	抽 扌	抽 手	*chōu*	tug /tʌg/
426-n368 *	搐 扌	搐 手	*chù*	convulsion /kənˈvʌlʃən/
427-n369 *	用 用	用 用	*yòng*	use /jus/ *n.*
428-n370 *	撮 扌	撮 手	*cuō*	grope /grop/
429-n371	空 穴	空 穴	*kōng*	empty space, air
430	理 王	理 玉	*lǐ*	order
431-n372 *	线 纟	線 糸	*xiàn*	thread /θrɛd/
432-n373	循 彳	循 彳	*xún*	feel along, follow with the hands
433-n374	衣 衣	衣 衣	*yī*	clothes, clothing
434-n375	摸 扌	摸 手	*mō*	rub, caress
435-n376 *	床 广	床 广	*chuáng*	bed /bɛd/
436-n377 *	痿 疒	痿 疒	*wěi*	wilt /wɪlt/
437-n378 *	废 广	廢 广	*fèi*	disabled /dɪˈsɛbl̩d/
438-n379	惕 忄	惕 心	*tì*	cautious; 'jumpy'
439-n380 *	腘 月	腘 肉	*rùn*	twitch /twɪtʃ/
440-n381 *	蠕 虫	蠕 虫	*rú*	wriggle /ˈrɪgl̩/
441-n382 *	举 丶	舉 臼	*jǔ*	raise /rez/

1. The term 角弓反张 *jiǎo gōng fǎn zhāng* literally means 'horn bow backward stretch', and refers to spasm of the muscles causing the head, neck,

and spine to arch backwards. In Western medicine, it is formally known by the awe-inspiring term 'opisthotonos' (from the Greek *opisthen*, behind, and *tonos*, stretch). It occurs in lockjaw and fright wind.

2. The terms 拘急 *jū jí* and 拘挛 *jū luán*, 'hypertonicity', and 筋急 *jīn jí* and 筋挛 *jīn luán*, 'hypertonicity of the sinews', refer to stiffness and tension in the limbs inhibiting normal bending and stretching, usually attributable to wind, and occurring, for example, in impediment *bì* patterns and in wind stroke. 瘛瘲 *jì zòng* is alternating tensing and relaxation of the sinews (clonic spasm), often observed in externally contracted febrile (heat) disease, epilepsy, and lockjaw. 瘛 *jì*, tugging, means a tensing and contraction, whereas 瘲 *zòng*, slackening, is a relaxation and stretching. The terms 抽风 *chōu fēng*, tugging wind, and 四肢抽搐 *sì zhī chōu chù*, convulsion of the limbs, are synonyms of tugging and slackening.

3. 撮空理线 *cuō kōng lǐ xiàn* groping in the air and pulling at [invisible] threads, and 循衣摸床 *xún yī mō chuáng*, picking at bedclothes, both refer to the unconscious groping of critically ill patients. In Western medicine, this is called carphology (from the Greek *karphos*, straw + *legein*, collect).

复合词 Compounds:

380. 姿态 *zī tài*, posture
381. 动态 *dòng tài*, bearing
382. 向里蜷卧 *xiàng lǐ quán wò*, lying in curled-up posture (lit. 'lying curled toward the inside')
383. 坐而不得卧 *zuò ér bù dé wò*, ability to sit but not to lie down
384. 半身不遂 *bàn shēn bú suì*, hemiplegia
385. 手撒口开 *shǒu sā kǒu kāi*, limp hands and open mouth
386. 角弓反张 *jiǎo gōng fǎn zhāng*, arched-back rigidity
387. 四肢 *sì zhī*, four limbs, limbs
388. 拘急 *jū jí*, hypertonicity
389. 拘挛 *jū luán*, hypertonicity
390. 挛急 *luán jí*, hypertonicity
391. 强直 *jiàng zhí*, rigidity
392. 抽风 *chōu fēng*, tugging wind
393. 脚挛急 *jiǎo luán jí*, hypertonicity of the foot
394. 筋急 *jīn jí*, sinew hypertonicity
395. 筋挛 *jīn luán*, hypertonicity of the sinews
396. 手指挛急 *shǒu zhǐ luán jí*, hypertonicity of the fingers
397. 四肢拘急 *sì zhī jū jí*, hypertonicity of the limbs
398. 四肢强直 *sì zhī jiàng zhí*, rigidity of the limbs

399. 四肢抽搐 *sì zhī chōu chù*, convulsion of the limbs
400. 手舞足蹈 *shǒu wǔ zú dào*, flailing of the limbs
401. 扬手踯足 *yáng shǒu zhí zú*, flailing of the limbs
402. 足颤 *zú zhàn*, shaking feet
403. 手颤 *shǒu chàn*, tremor of the hand
404. 手指挛急 *shǒu zhǐ luán jí*, hypertonicity of the fingers
405. 筋惕肉瞤 *jīn tì ròu rùn*, jerking sinews and twitching flesh
406. 手足蠕动 *shǒu zú rú dòng*, wriggling of the extremities
407. 四肢不用 *sì zhī bù yòng*, loss of use of the limbs
408. 四肢不举 *sì zhī bù jǔ*, inability to lift the limbs
409. 四肢不收 *sì zhī bù shōu*, loss of use of the limbs
410. 肢体痿癖 *zhī tǐ wěi fèi*, disabled wilted limbs
411. 肩不举 *jiān bù jǔ*, inability to raise the shoulder
412. 手足不遂 *shǒu zú bù suì*, paralysis of the limbs
413. 撮空理线 *cuō kōng lǐ xiàn*, groping in the air and pulling at [invisible] threads (lit. 'groping [in] empty [space and] ordering threads')
414. 循衣摸床 *xún yī mō chuáng*, picking at bedclothes; carphology (lit. fumbling with clothes and stroking the bed)

第二节　第五组				**SECTION 2: SET 5**

望面色				**Inspection of the Facial Complexion**
442	* 面一	面 面	*miàn*	face /fes/
443	* 色刀	色 色	*sè*	color /ˈkʌlɚ/
				complexion /kəmˈplɛkʃən/
444	* 无 尢	無 火	*wú*	-less /lɪs/
445-n383	* 泽 氵	澤 水	*zé*	sheen /ʃin/
446	* 青 青	青 青	*qīng*	green-blue /grin blu/
447	* 赤 赤	赤 赤	*chì*	red /rɛd/
448-n384	* 红 纟	紅 糸	*hóng*	red /rɛd/
449	* 黄 土	黃 黃	*huáng*	yellow /ˈjɛlo/
450	* 白 白	白 白	*bái*	white /waɪt, hwaɪt/
451	* 黑 黑	黑 黑	*hēi*	black /blæk/
452-n385	* 紫 纟	紫 糸	*zǐ*	purple /ˈpɝpl̩/
453-n386	* 涂 氵	途 土	*tú*	smear /smir/
454-n387	妆 丬	粧 米	*zhuāng*	makeup
455-n388	* 油 氵	油 水	*yóu*	oil /ɔɪl/

456-n389	彩 彡	彩 彡	*cǎi*	*color*
457-n390	* 泛 氵	泛 水	*fàn*	floating /ˈfloʊtɪŋ/
458-n391	* 潮 氵	潮 水	*cháo*	tidal /ˈtaɪdl̩/
459-n392	黧 黑	黧 黑	*lí*	*very dark*
460-n393	* 晦 日	晦 日	*huì*	dark /dɑrk/
				somber /ˈsɑmbɚ/
461-n394	* 暗 日	暗 日	*àn*	dark /dɑrk/
462-n395	* 苍 艹	蒼 艸	*cāng*	somber /ˈsɑmbɚ/
463-n396	* 淡 氵	淡 水	*dàn*	pale /pel/
464-n397	* 㿠 白	㿠 白	*huǎng*	bright /braɪt/
465-n398	* 萎 艹	萎 艸	*wěi*	withered /ˈwɪðɚd/
466-n399	* 华 艹	華 艸	*huá*	luster /ˈlʌstɚ/

注 Notes:

1. A distinction is made between three types of 'white' complexion: 苍白 *cāng bái*, 'somber white', is associated with fulminant desertion of yáng qì or contraction of exterior wind-cold; 淡白 *dàn bái*, 'pale white', is associated with blood vacuity; and 㿠白 *huǎng bái*, 'bright white', is associated with yáng qì vacuity.

2. 两颧泛红如妆 *liǎng quán fàn hóng rú zhuāng*, cheeks a floating red color as if dabbed with rouge, is a complexion seen in severe illness and is a sign of vacuous yáng floating upward.

复合词 Compounds:

415. 色泽 *sè zé*, complexion
416. 面青 *miàn qīng*, green-blue face
417. 面赤 *miàn chì*, red face
418. 面黄 *miàn huáng*, yellow face
419. 面白 *miàn bái*, white face
420. 面黑 *miàn hēi*, black face
421. 面色白 *miàn sè bái*, white facial complexion
422. 面色苍白 *miàn sè cāng bái*, somber white facial complexion
423. 面色淡白 *miàn sè dàn bái*, pale white facial complexion
424. 面色㿠白 *miàn sè huǎng bái*, bright white facial complexion
425. 面色红 *miàn sè hóng*, red facial complexion
426. 面色红赤 *miàn sè hóng chì*, red facial complexion
427. 两颧红色如涂油彩 *liǎng quán hóng sè rú tú yóu cǎi*, cheeks red as if smeared with oil paint

428. 两颧泛红如妆 *liǎng quán fàn hóng rú zhuāng*, cheeks a floating red color as if dabbed with rouge

429. 面色潮红 *miàn sè cháo hóng*, tidal reddening of the face

430. 面色萎黄 *miàn sè wěi huáng*, withered-yellow complexion

431. 面色青 *miàn sè qīng*, green-blue facial complexion

432. 面色青紫 *miàn sè qīng zǐ*, green-blue or purple facial complexion; purplish green-blue facial complexion

433. 面色青紫晦暗 *miàn sè qīng zǐ huì àn*, dark purplish green-blue facial complexion

434. 面色黧黑 *miàn sè lí hēi*, soot-black facial complexion

435. 面色无华 *miàn sè wú huá*, lusterless complexion

第二节　第六组	**SECTION 2: SET 6**

望头面				**Inspection of the Head & Face**
467-n400	* 陷 阝	陷 阜	*xiàn*	sunken /ˈsʌŋkən/
468	* 高 高	高 高	*gāo*	high
469-n401	* 凸 凵	凸 凵	*tú*	bulging /ˈbʌldʒɪŋ/
470-n402	能 厶	能 肉	*néng*	*can, able*
471-n403	* 摇 扌	搖 手	*yáo*	shake /ʃek/
472-n404	缝 纟	縫 糸	*fèng*	*seam*
473-n405	* 焮 火	焮 火	*xìn*	scorch /skɔrtʃ/
474	* 浮 氵	浮 水	*fú*	puffy /ˈpʌfɪ/
475-n406	甲 田	甲 田	*jiǎ*	*scale*
476-n407	错 钅	錯 金	*cuò*	*wrong, deranged*
477-n408	* 枯 木	枯 木	*kū*	dry /draɪ/
				withered /ˈwɪðəd/
478-n409	* 胀 月	脹 肉	*zhàng*	distention /dɪsˈtɛnʃən/
479-n410	须 彡	鬚 髟	*xū*	*whiskers*
480-n411	* 早 日	早 日	*zǎo*	premature /ˈprɛmətʃɚ/
481-n412	脱 月	脫 肉	*tuō*	*shed, lose*
482-n413	* 稀 禾	稀 禾	*xī*	thin /θɪn/
483	疏 マ	疏 疋	*shū*	*far apart, thinly spread*
484-n414	润 氵	潤 水	*rùn*	*moist, glossy, lustrous*
485	* 泽 氵	澤 水	*zé*	sheen /ʃin/
486-n415	穗 禾	穗 禾	*suì*	*awn*
487	* 干 干	乾 乙	*gān*	dry /draɪ/
488-n416	光 光	光 儿	*guāng*	*light*
489	彩 彡	彩 彡	*cǎi*	*bright, splendid*

490-n417	* 视 ネ	視 示	*shì*	look /lʊk/
491	* 上 卜	上 一	*shàng*	upward /ˈʌpwəˈd/
492	直 十	直 目	*zhí*	*straight*
493-n418	* 眵 目	眵 目	*chī*	eye discharge /aɪ ˈdɪstʃɑrdʒ/
494-n419	窠 宀	窠 宀	*kē*	*nest*
495	* 卧 臣	臥 臣	*wò*	lie /laɪ/
496-n420	* 蚕 天	蠶 虫	*cán*	silk moth /ˈsɪlkmɑθ/
497-n421	* 突 宀	突 宀	*tú*	protrude /proˈtrud/ *vi.*
				protruding /proˈtrudɪŋ/ *adj.*
498-n422	* 槁 木	槁 木	*gǎo*	desiccated /ˈdɛsɪˌketɪd/
499-n423	煽 火	煽 火	*shàn*	*fan*
500-n424	作 亻	作 人	*zuò*	*do, make; act; produce (an effect); occur*
501-n425	* 裂 衣	裂 衣	*liè*	cracked /krækt/
502-n426	* 深 氵	深 水	*shēn*	deep /dip/
503-n427	闭 门	閉 門	*bì*	*close*
504-n428	* 喎 口	喎 口	*wāi*	deviated /ˈdivɪˌetɪd/
505-n429	* 斜 斗	斜 斗	*xié*	deviated /ˈdivɪˌetɪd/
506-n430	* 僻 亻	僻 人	*pì*	deviated /ˈdivɪˌetɪd/
507-n431	* 噤 口	噤 口	*jìn*	clenched (of the jaw) /klɛntʃt/
508-n432	* 振 扌	振 手	*zhèn*	tremble /ˈtrɛmbl̩/
509-n433	短 矢	短 矢	*duǎn*	*short*
510-n434	* 缩 纟	縮 糸	*suō*	shrunken /ˈʃrʌŋkən/
511-n435	结 纟	結 糸	*jié*	*form into*
512-n436	* 瓣 辛	瓣 瓜	*bàn*	petal /ˈpɛtl̩/
				gaping /ˈgepɪŋ/
513-n437	* 啮 口	嚙 口	*niè*	bite /baɪt/
514-n438	烂 火	爛 火	*làn*	*rotten, disintegrated, ulcerated*

注 Notes:

1. The character 胀 *zhàng*, distention, sometimes denotes a subjective sensation and sometimes a visible or tangible expansion. In the example of 面部 焮红肿胀 *miàn bù xìn hóng zhǒng zhàng*, 'scorching red distended swollen face', it denotes a sensation. In the context of the abdomen, it is often (but not necessarily) used to mean a visible enlargement in contrast to the subjective sensation 满 *mǎn*, fullness.

2. The characters 凸 and 突 are both read as *tú*, and both mean to protrude or stick out. 突 *tú* also means sudden.

3. The character 振 *zhèn* is here used in the sense of trembling. Further ahead, it is used in the sense of 'vitalize' (often in the negative as 不振 *bú*

zhèn, 'devitalized'). In the sense of trembling, it is the same as 颤 *chàn* (or *zhàn*).

复合词 Compounds:

436. 囟门下陷 *xìn mén xià xiàn*, depressed fontanels
437. 囟门高凸 *xìn mén gāo tú*, bulging fontanels
438. 摇头不能自主 *yáo tóu bù néng zì zhǔ*, uncontrollable shaking of the head
439. 头摇 *tóu yáo*, shaking of the head
440. 头缝不合 *tóu fèng bù hé*, non-closure of the fontanels
441. 头大面肿 *tóu dà miàn zhǒng*, massive head and swollen face
442. 面部焮红肿胀 *miàn bù xìn hóng zhǒng zhàng*, scorching red distended swollen face
443. 头面红肿 *tóu miàn hóng zhǒng*, red swollen head and face
444. 面浮 *miàn fú*, puffy face
445. 腮肿 *sāi zhǒng*, swollen cheeks
446. 头发润泽 *tóu fà rùn zé*, glossy hair
447. 须发早白 *xū fà zǎo bái*, premature graying
448. 头发稀疏 *tóu fà xī shū*, thin hair
449. 头发干枯 *tóu fà gān kū*, dry hair
450. 发结如穗 *fà jié rú suì*, hair knotted in awns
451. 脱发 *tuō fà*, hair loss
452. 眼无光彩 *yǎn wú guāng cǎi*, dull eyes
453. 两目上视 *liǎng mù shàng shì*, both eyes looking upward
454. 斜视 *xié shì*, squint
455. 直视 *zhí shì*, forward-staring eyes
456. 眼睛发红多眵 *yǎn jīng fā hóng duō chī*, reddening of the eyes with copious discharge
457. 眼睛红肿痛 *yǎn jīng hóng zhǒng tòng*, red sore swollen eyes
458. 目赤 *mù chì*, red eyes
459. 目黄 *mù huáng*, yellowing of the eyes
460. 目窠内陷 *mù kē nèi xiàn*, sunken eyes
461. 眼球外突 *yǎn qiú wài tú*, protruding eyes; bulging eyes
462. 目下有卧蚕 *mù xià yǒu wò cán*, sleeping silkworms beneath the eyes
463. 耳轮肿胀 *ěr lún zhǒng zhàng*, distended swollen helices
464. 耳轮甲错 *ěr lún jiǎ cuò*, encrusted helices
465. 耳轮枯焦 *ěr lún kū jiāo*, withered helices
466. 鼻色赤 *bí sè chì*, red nose
467. 鼻色青 *bí sè qīng*, green-blue nose

468. 鼻色枯槁 *bí sè kū gǎo*, desiccated nose
469. 鼻孔作煽 *bí kǒng zuò shàn*, flaring of the nostrils
470. 鼻煽 *bí shàn*, flaring of the nostrils
471. 鼻孔干燥 *bí kǒng gān zào*, dry nostrils
472. 鼻衄 *bí nü*, nosebleed
473. 人中短缩 *rén zhōng duǎn suō*, shrunken philtrum
474. 唇色淡红 *chún sè dàn hóng*, pale red lips
475. 唇色深红 *chún sè shēn hóng*, deep red lips
476. 口唇青紫 *kǒu chún qīng zǐ*, purplish green-blue lips
477. 唇肿 *chún zhǒng*, swollen lips
478. 口唇干燥 *kǒu chún gān zào*, dry lips
479. 唇燥裂 *chún zào liè*, dry cracked lips
480. 唇裂 *chún liè*, cracked lips
481. 口角不闭 *kǒu jiǎo bú bì*, gaping corners of the mouth
482. 口角流涎 *kǒu jiǎo liú xián*, drooling from the corners of the mouth
483. 口眼喎斜 *kǒu yǎn wāi xié*, deviated eyes and mouth
484. 口张不闭 *kōu zhāng bú bì*, gaping mouth
485. 口噤 *kǒu jìn*, clenched jaw
486. 撮口 *cuō kǒu*, pursed mouth
487. 口僻 *kǒu pì*, deviated mouth
488. 口振 *kǒu zhèn*, trembling mouth
489. 齿黄 *chǐ huáng*, yellow teeth
490. 齿黑 *chǐ hēi*, black teeth
491. 齿燥如枯骨 *chǐ zào rú kū gǔ*, teeth dry as desiccated bone
492. 牙齿干燥如枯骨 *yá chǐ gān zào rú kū gǔ*, teeth dry as desiccated bone
493. 齿疏 *chī shū*, sparse teeth
494. 齿龈红肿 *chǐ yín hóng*, red swollen gums
495. 齿龈溃烂 *chǐ yín kuì làn*, ulcerated gums
496. 齿龈结瓣 *chǐ yín jié bàn*, petaled gums
497. 牙宣 *yá xuān*, gaping gums
498. 咽肿 *yān zhǒng*, swollen throat; swollen pharynx
499. 咽喉红肿痛 *yān hóu hóng zhǒng tòng*, red sore swollen throat
500. 咽喉腐烂 *yān hóu fǔ làn*, putrefying throat
501. 咽喉白腐 *yān hóu bái fǔ*, white putrid throat

第二节　第七组　　　　　　　　**SECTION 2: SET 7**

望胸腹　　　　　　　　　　Inspection of the Chest &
　　　　　　　　　　　　　　　　Abdomen

515	* 胸 月	胸 肉	*xiōng*	chest /tʃɛst/
516	* 腹 月	腹 肉	*fù*	abdomen /ˈæbdəmən/
517-n439	* 扁 户	扁 户	*biǎn*	flat /flæt/ (low and broad)
518-n440	平 一	平 干	*píng*	*flat, even, smooth*
519	* 大 大	大 大	*dà*	large /lɑrdʒ/
520-n441	* 鼓 鼓	鼓 鼓	*gǔ*	drum /drʌm/
521-n442	* 单 丷	單 口	*dān*	simple /ˈsɪmpl̩/
522	暴 日	暴 日	*pù*	*expose*
523-n443	凹 丨	凹 凵	*āo*	*indented, concave*
524-n444	* 舟 舟	舟 舟	*zhōu*	boat /bot/
525	* 突 宀	突 宀	*tú*	protrude /proˈtrud/ *vi.*
				protruding /proˈtrudɪŋ/ *adj.*
				protrusion /proˈtruʒən/ *adj.*
526	* 筋 竹	筋 竹	*jīn*	vein /ven/

注 Notes:

1. The term 筋 *jīn*, previously introduced as 'sinews', is used in the phrase 腹露青筋 *fù lù qīng jīn* 'prominent [green-blue] abdominal veins' to mean the visible markings under the skin, i.e., veins.

2. The character 凹 *āo*, to 'cave in', is the opposite of 凸 *tú*, to 'stick out', previously introduced.

复合词 Compounds:

502. 胸部扁平 *xiōng bù biǎn píng*, flat chest
503. 腹皮拘急 *fù pí jū jí*, tense abdominal skin
504. 腹大如鼓 *fù dà rú gǔ*, abdomen large as a drum
505. 单腹胀大 *dān fù zhàng dà*, simple abdominal distention (without swelling of the limbs)
506. 腹露青筋 *fù lù qīng jīn*, prominent [green-blue] abdominal veins
507. 腹皮青筋暴露 *fù pí qīng jīn pù lù*, prominent green-blue veins on the abdominal skin
508. 腹部凹陷如舟 *fù bù āo xiàn rú zhōu*, abdomen hollow like a boat
509. 脐突 *qí tú*, protrusion of the umbilicus

第二节　第八组	SECTION 2: SET 8

望斑疹

Inspection of the Macules & Papules

527-n445	* 斑 王	斑 文	*bān*	macules /ˈmækjulz/
528-n446	* 疹 疒	疹 疒	*zhěn*	papules /ˈpæpjulz/
529	发 又	發 癶	*fā*	*develop; put forth; effuse*
530	* 枯 木	枯 木	*kū*	dry /draɪ/
531-n447	* 痦 疒	痦 疒	*péi*	miliaria /ˌmɪlɪˈɛrɪə/

复合词 Compounds:

510. 红疹 *hóng zhěn*, red papules
511. 发斑 *fā bān*, macular eruption
512. 白痦 *bái péi*, miliaria alba
513. 枯痦 *kū péi*, dry miliaria

第二节　第九组	SECTION 2: SET 9

望舌质

Inspection of the Tongue Body

532	* 舌 舌	舌 舌	*shé*	tongue /tʌŋ/
533-n448	质 厂	質 貝	*zhì*	*substance*
534-n449	* 胖 月	胖 肉	*pàng*	enlarged /ɪnˈlardʒd/
535	* 大 大	大 大	*dà*	enlarged /ɪnˈlardʒd/
536	* 瘦 疒	瘦 疒	*shòu*	thin /θɪn/
537-n450	* 瘪 疒	瘪 疒	*biě*	thin /θɪn/
538-n451	* 边 辶	邊 辶	*biān*	margin /ˈmardʒɪn/
539-n452	* 痕 疒	痕 疒	*hén*	impression /ɪmˈprɛʃən/
540-n453	* 嫩 女	嫩 女	*nèn*	tender-soft /ˈtɛndɚ-sɔft/
541-n454	* 老 耂	老 老	*lǎo*	tough /tʌf/
542	* 裂 衣	裂 衣	*liè*	fissured /ˈfɪʃɚd/
543-n455	* 纵 纟	縱 糸	*zòng*	protracted /proˈtræktɪd/
544-n456	* 滑 氵	滑 水	*huá*	smooth /smuð/
545-n457	* 卷	卷 卩	*juǎn*	curled /kɝld/
546	* 强 弓	強 弓	*jiàng*	stiff /stɪf/
547-n458	* 歪 不	歪 止	*wāi*	deviated /ˈdivɪˌetɪd/
548-n459	* 弄 王	弄 廾	*nòng*	worrying /ˈwɝɪŋ/

549	* 颤页	顫頁	*chàn, zhàn*	trembling /ˈtrɛmblɪŋ/
550	* 萎艹	萎艸	*wěi*	limp /lɪmp/
551	* 淡氵	淡水	*dàn*	pale /pel/
552	* 红纟	紅糸	*hóng*	red /rɛd/
553-n460	* 绛纟	絳糸	*jiàng*	crimson /ˈkrɪmzn̩/
554-n461	* 点灬	點黑	*diǎn*	speckles /ˈspɛkl̩z/ *n.* speckled /ˈspɛkl̩d/ *adj.*
555-n462	* 刺刂	刺刀	*cì*	prickles /ˈprɪkl̩z/ *n.* prickly /ˈprɪklɪ/ *adj.*
556-n463	芒艹	芒艸	*máng*	*awn, spike*
557-n464	* 荣芾	榮火	*róng*	luxuriant /lʌgˈʒʊriənt/ luxuriance /lʌgˈʒʊriəns/
558	* 枯木	枯木	*kū*	withered /ˈwɪðəd/ witheredness /ˈwɪðədnɪs/

复合词 Compounds:

514. 舌裂 *shé liè*, fissured tongue
515. 舌萎 *shé wěi*, limp tongue
516. 舌肿 *shé zhǒng*, swollen tongue
517. 舌胖 *shé pàng*, enlarged tongue
518. 舌纵 *shé zòng*, protracted tongue
519. 舌卷 *shé juǎn*, curled tongue
520. 舌强 *shé jiàng*, stiff tongue
521. 舌歪 *shé wāi*, deviated tongue
522. 舌颤 *shé chàn*, trembling tongue
523. 弄舌 *nòng shé*, worrying tongue
524. 啮舌 *niè shé*, tongue biting
525. 舌疮 *shé chuāng*, tongue sore
526. 舌上出血 *shé shàng chū xuè*, bleeding from the upper surface of the tongue
527. 舌生芒刺 *shé shēng máng cì*, prickly tongue
528. 舌生瘀斑 *shé shēng yū bān*, stasis macules on the tongue
529. 舌边齿痕 *shé biān chǐ hén*, tooth marks on the margins of the tongue
530. 舌红绛 *shé hóng jiàng*, red or crimson tongue
531. 舌干 *shé gān*, dry tongue
532. 舌淡白 *shé dàn bái*, pale tongue
533. 舌红 *shé hóng*, red tongue

534. 舌绛 *shé jiàng*, crimson tongue

535. 舌质红绛 *shé zhí hóng jiàng*, red or crimson tongue

536. 舌紫 *shé zǐ*, purple tongue

537. 舌青 *shé qīng*, green-blue tongue

538. 舌质荣枯 *shé zhí róng kū*, luxuriance and witheredness of the tongue (two general states of the tongue)

第二节　第十组				**SECTION 2: SET 10**

望舌苔				**Inspection of the Tongue Fur**
559-n465	* 苔 ⁺⁺	苔 艸	*tāi*	fur /fɝ/
560	* 润 氵	潤 水	*rùn*	moist /mɔɪst/
561	* 滑 氵	滑 水	*huá*	glossy /ˈɡlɔsɪ/
562	* 燥 火	燥 火	*zào*	dry /draɪ/
563-n466	* 糙 米	糙 米	*cāo*	rough /rʌf/
564-n467	* 厚 厂	厚 厂	*hòu*	thick /θɪk/
565-n468	* 薄 竹	薄 竹	*bó*	thin /θɪn/
566-n469	* 净 氵	淨 水	*jìng*	clean /klin/
567-n470	* 腻 月	膩 肉	*nì*	slimy /ˈslaɪmɪ/
568-n471	* 垢 土	垢 土	*gòu*	grimy /ˈɡraɪmɪ/
569-n472	* 剥 刂	剝 刀	*bō*	peeling /ˈpilɪŋ/
570	* 光 光	光 儿	*guāng*	bare /bɛr/
571-n473	* 镜 钅	鏡 金	*jìng*	mirror /ˈmɪrɚ/
572	* 老 耂	老 老	*lǎo*	old /old/
573	* 焦 隹	焦 火	*jiāo*	burnt /bɝnt/
574-n474	* 灰 火	灰 火	*huī*	gray /gre/

注 Notes:

1. The character 苔 has the grass signific ⁺⁺. In its original meaning of moss, it is read as *tái* in the second tone; in its meaning of tongue fur or tongue coating, it is read as *tāi* in the first tone. While Chinese uses a metaphor from the plant world, English uses one from the animal world (fur).

2. The Chinese 腻 *nì* is rendered in this terminology as 'slimy'. Inelegant though this word may be, it corresponds closely to the Chinese. Many people refer to this condition of the tongue fur as 'greasy', although greasy misleadingly suggests the presence of oil.

3. In the compounds that follow, we see both verb + noun and noun + verb phrases, e.g., 白苔 *bái tāi* and 苔白 *bāi tāi*. The difference between the two is that the verb + noun compounds are all noun phrases composed of qualifier and head, while the noun + verb phrases are subject subject + predicate phrases that may also serve as noun phrases. The verb + noun phrases are usually the name of a condition while noun + verb phrases may serve as the name of a condition (e.g., 腹痛), or may be descriptive 舌苔黄腻 *shé tāi huáng nì*, literally, 'tongue fur [is] yellow and slimy'. In verb + noun phrases, there is usually only one verb, while noun + verb phrases serving a descriptive purpose may include multiple verbs. Since English allows a head noun to be qualified by multiple adjectives, and conventionally uses this kind of construction in describing patients' symptoms, we have followed this format in the translation of descriptive phrases (e.g., 'slimy yellow tongue fur'). 'Also, we have adopted the slightly unorthodox practice of not separating the English qualifiers by commas. In multiple diagnostic enumerations such as 'thick sticky yellow phlegm, a slimy yellow tongue fur, and a slippery rapid pulse," this practice makes for clearer presentation of the information.

复合词 Compounds:

539. 剥苔 *bō tāi*, peeled fur
540. 舌光 *shé guāng*, smooth bare tongue
541. 镜面舌 *jìng miàn shé*, mirror tongue
542. 糙苔 *cāo tāi*, rough tongue fur
543. 垢腻苔 *gòu nì tāi*, grimy slimy tongue fur
544. 浊腻苔 *zhuó nì tāi*, turbid slimy tongue fur
545. 舌净 *shé jìng*, clean tongue
546. 苔化 *tāi huà*, transforming tongue fur
547. 滑苔 *huá tāi*, glossy tongue fur
548. 舌苔白 *shé tāi bái*, white tongue fur
549. 白苔 *bái tāi*, white fur
550. 黄苔 *huáng tāi*, yellow fur
551. 舌苔黄 *shé tāi huáng*, yellow tongue fur
552. 舌苔灰黑 *shé tāi huī hēi*, gray-black tongue fur
553. 舌苔腐垢 *shé tāi fǔ gòu*, putrid grimy tongue fur
554. 舌苔黄腻 *shé tāi huáng nì*, slimy yellow tongue fur
555. 舌苔白腻 *shé tāi bái nì*, slimy white tongue fur
556. 舌苔白如积粉 *shé tāi bái rú jī fěn*, mealy white tongue fur
557. 舌苔干燥 *shé tāi gān zào*, dry tongue fur
558. 舌苔焦黄 *shé tāi jiāo huáng*, burnt-yellow tongue fur
559. 舌苔焦黑 *shé tāi jiāo hēi*, burnt-black tongue fur

560. 舌苔白厚 *shé tāi bái hòu*, thick white tongue fur
561. 舌苔薄白 *shé tāi bó bái*, thin white tongue fur
562. 舌苔黄糙 *shé tāi huáng cāo*, rough yellow tongue fur
563. 舌苔焦黄 *shé tāi jiāo huáng*, burnt-yellow tongue fur
564. 舌苔老黄 *shé tāi lǎo huáng*, old-yellow tongue fur
565. 舌苔燥如沙 *shé tāi zào rú shā*, tongue fur dry as sand

第二节　第十一组	**SECTION 2: SET 11**

望痰、涎、涕、唾	**Inspection of Phlegm, Drool, Tears & Spittle**

575	* 痰 疒	痰 疒	*tán*	phlegm /flɛm/
576	* 涎 氵	涎 水	*xián*	drool /drul/
577	* 涕 氵	涕 水	*tì*	snivel /ˈsnɪvl̩/
578	* 唾 口	唾 口	*tuò*	spittle /ˈspɪtl̩/
579	* 多 夕	多 夕	*duō*	copious /ˈkopɪəs/
580	* 少 小	少 小	*shǎo*	scant /skænt/
581	* 清 氵	清 水	*qīng*	clear /klɪr/
582	* 浊 氵	濁 水	*zhuó*	turbid /ˈtɝbɪd/
583	* 稀 禾	稀 禾	*xī*	thin /θɪn/
584	* 薄 艹	薄 艸	*bó*	thin /θɪn/
585-n475	* 黏 禾	黏 黍	*nián*	sticky /ˈstɪkɪ/
586-n476	* 稠 禾	稠 禾	*chóu*	thick /θɪk/
587-n477	* 胶 月	膠 肉	*jiāo*	glue /glu/
588-n478	* 块 土	塊 土	*kuài*	lump /lʌmp/
589-n479	泡 氵	泡 水	*pào*	*bubble, soak*
590-n480	* 沫 氵	沫 水	*mò*	foam /fom/ *n.* foamy /ˈfomɪ/ *adj.*
591-n481	* 败 贝	敗 攴	*bài*	rotten /ˈrɑtn̩/
592-n482	* 絮 糸	絮 糸	*xù*	wadding /ˈwɑdɪŋ/
593-n483	* 咳 口	咳 口	*ké*	cough /kɔf/
594-n484	* 吐 口	吐 口	*tǔ*	spit /spɪt/
595-n485	* 咯 口	咯 口	*kǎ*	expectorate /ɪksˈpɛktəˌret/
596-n486	* 流 氵	流 水	*liú*	run /rʌn/
597-n487	* 难 又	難 隹	*nán*	difficult /ˈdɪfɪkʌlt/
598-n488	* 脓 月	膿 肉	*nóng*	pus /pʌs/

复合词 Compounds:

566. 痰多 *tán duō*, copious phlegm
567. 痰少 *tán shǎo*, scant phlegm
568. 无痰 *wú tán*, no phlegm; absence of phlegm
569. 痰白清稀 *tán bái qīng xī*, clear thin white phlegm
570. 痰清白稀薄 *tán qīng bái xī bó*, clear thin white phlegm
571. 痰黄黏稠 *tán huáng nián chóu*, thick sticky yellow phlegm
572. 痰黏稠如胶 *tán nián chóu rú jiāo*, gluey thick sticky phlegm
573. 痰少而黏 *tán shǎo ér nián*, scant sticky phlegm
574. 痰黄浊黏稠 *tán huáng zhuó nián chóu*, thick sticky turbid yellow phlegm
575. 痰色青，清稀而多泡沫 *tán sè qīng, qīng xī ér duō pào mò*, foamy thin clear green-blue phlegm
576. 泡沫 *pào mò*, foam
577. 痰如败絮 *tán rú bài xù*, phlegm like rotten wadding
578. 吐痰清稀白 *tú tán qīng xī bái*, spitting of clear thin white phlegm
579. 咳痰 *ké tán*, coughing of phlegm
580. 咳痰清稀 *ké tán qīng xī*, coughing of thin clear phlegm
581. 咳痰黄稠 *ké tán huáng chóu*, coughing of thick yellow phlegm
582. 咳痰黏稠 *ké tán nián chóu*, coughing of thick sticky phlegm
583. 咳血 *ké xuè*, coughing of blood
584. 咳吐脓血 *ké tǔ nóng xuè*, coughing of pus and blood
585. 痰中带血丝 *tán zhōng dài xuè sī*, phlegm streaked with blood
586. 清涕 *qīng tì*, clear snivel
587. 口角流涎 *kǒu jiǎo liú xián*, drooling from the corner of the mouth
588. 多唾 *duō tuò*, copious spittle
589. 浊涕 *zhuó tì*, turbid snivel
590. 鼻流浊涕 *bí liú zhuó tì*, runny nose with turbid snivel
591. 流涎清稀 *liú xián qīng xī*, thin clear drool
592. 口出黏涎 *kǒu chū nián xián*, thick drool running from the mouth

第二节　第十二组				**SECTION 2: SET 12**

望呕吐物   **Inspection of Vomitus**

599-n489	* 呕 口 嘔 口		*ǒu*	retching /ˈrɛtʃɪŋ/
600	* 吐 口 吐 口		*tù*	vomiting /ˈvɑmɪtɪŋ/
601-n490	物 牛 物 牛		*wù*	*matter*

602-n491	* 秽 禾	穢 禾	*huì*	foul /faʊl/
603-n492	* 绿 纟	綠 糸	*lü*	green /grin/
604-n493	鲜 鱼	鮮 魚	*xiān*	*fresh; bright (of colors)*

注 Note:

The Chinese 呕吐 *ǒu tù* means vomiting; 呕 *ǒu* is explained as 'producing sound without matter' (dry retching) while 吐 *tù* is explained as 'producing matter without sound' (actual vomiting). In practice, both characters are used individually in their specific senses and in the broad sense of the compound. The character 吐 *tù* is used in a wider sense of ejecting matter through the mouth, and is not necessarily limited to matter brought up from the stomach. Read as *tǔ* (in the third tone), it means to spit. In Chinese medicine, 吐血 *tù xuè* means vomiting or spitting of blood, and 吐法 *tù fǎ* is a method of treatment that involves bringing food up from the stomach or expelling phlegm from the throat. In this broader meaning, *tù* is translated in this text as ejection.

复合词 Compounds:

593. 呕吐清水 *ǒu tù qīng shuǐ*, vomiting of clear water
594. 呕吐物清稀 *ǒu tù wù qīng xī*, clear thin vomitus
595. 呕吐物秽浊 *ǒu tù wù huì zhuó*, foul turbid vomitus
596. 呕吐痰涎 *ǒu tù tán xián*, vomiting of phlegm-drool
597. 呕吐黄绿苦水 *ǒu tù huáng lü kǔ shuǐ*, vomiting of yellow-green bitter water
598. 吐血鲜红 *ǒu xuè xiān hóng*, vomiting of bright red blood
599. 吐血紫暗 *ǒu xuè zǐ àn*, vomiting of dark purple blood

| 第二节　第十三组 | **SECTION 2: SET 13** |

望大便 | **Inspection of the Stool**

605		大 大	大 大	*dà*	*greater*
606-n494	*	便 亻	便 人	*biàn*	stool /stul/
607-n495	*	粪 米	糞 米	*fèn*	stool /stul/
608-n496	*	溏 氵	溏 水	*táng*	sloppy /ˈslɑpɪ/
609	*	薄 艹	薄 艸	*bó*	thin /θɪn/
610-n497	*	鸭 鸟	鴨 鳥	*yā*	duck /ˈdʌk/
611-n498	*	羊 羊	羊 羊	*yáng*	sheep /ʃip/
612-n499		状 丬	狀 犬	*zhuàng*	*appearance*

613	* 脓 月	膿 肉	*nóng*	pus /pʌs/
614-n500	完 宀	完 宀	*wán*	finish; completely
615	* 干 干	乾 乙	*gān*	dry /draɪ/
616	* 结 纟	結 糸	*jié*	bound /baʊnd/

注 Note:

1. The compound 大便 *dà biàn*, stool or feces, actually means 'greater convenience', and stands in contrast to 小便 *xiǎo biàn*, which literally means 'lesser convenience'. These metaphors are virtually dead, much as the English 'stool' (which originally referred to the toilet as a thing on which one sits), and in the spoken language both terms are also understood as verb + object constructions, producing sentences such as 小便小不出来 *xiǎo biàn xiǎo bù chū lái*, cannot urinate. The character 便 *biàn* is often used alone specifically to refer to stool in particular.

2. 便溏 *biàn táng*, sloppy stool, denotes semiliquid excrement, which is often likened to duck's droppings.

复合词 Compounds:

600. 大便色黄 *dà biàn sè huáng*, yellow stool
601. 大便色黑 *dà biàn sè hēi*, black stool
602. 大便色绿 *dà biàn sè lü*, green stool
603. 大便色赤 *dà biàn sè chì*, red stool
604. 大便干结 *dà biàn gān jié*, dry bound stool
605. 粪便干燥 *fèn biàn gān zào*, dry stool
606. 大便如羊屎状 *dà biàn rú yáng shǐ zhuàng*, stool like sheep's droppings
607. 大便软 *dà biàn ruǎn*, soft stool
608. 大便黏稠 *dà biàn nián chóu*, thick sticky stool
609. 大便溏薄 *dà biàn táng bó*, thin sloppy stool
610. 大便稀溏 *dà biàn xī táng*, thin sloppy stool
611. 大便清稀 *dà biàn qīng xī*, clear thin stool
612. 鸭溏 *yā táng*, duck's slop
613. 完谷不化 *wán gǔ bú huà*, untransformed food (stool containing undigested food)
614. 便脓血 *biàn nóng xuè*, pus and blood in the stool
615. 大便带血 *dà biàn dài xuè*, stool containing blood
616. 便血鲜红 *biàn xuè xiān hóng*, bright red blood in the stool
617. 便血黑 *biàn xuè hēi*, black blood in the stool

第二节　第十四组   **SECTION 2: SET 14**

望小便   **Inspection of the Urine**

617		小 小	小 小	*xiǎo*	*lesser*
618-n501	*	尿 尸	尿 尸	*niào*	urine /ˈjurɪn/
619-n502		浑 氵	渾 水	*hún*	*murky, turbid*
620	*	浊 氵	濁 水	*zhuó*	turbid /ˈtɜ·bɪd/
621-n503		澄 氵	澄 水	*chéng*	*clear, transparent*
622-n504		澈 氵	澈 水	*chè*	*clear, diaphanous*
623-n505	*	泔 氵	泔 水	*gān*	rice water /ˈraɪs–wɔtɚ/

注 Notes:

1. The term 小便 *xiǎo biàn*, lit. 'lesser convenience', is the same in meaning as the non-metaphorical expression 尿 *niào*. The choice between the two expressions often depends on where the accompanying description is one character or two, as is seen in the list of terms below.

2. Urine described as 赤 *chì*, lit. 'red', is a deep color rather like that of tea, and is usually a sign of heat. In English, it is rendered as 'reddish', since 'red urine' might suggest a bright redness that is observed in bloody urine.

复合词 Compounds:

618. 小便 *xiǎo biàn*, urine
619. 小便黄赤 *xiǎo biàn huáng chì*, yellow or reddish urine; reddish yellow urine
620. 小便色赤 *xiǎo biàn sè chì*, reddish urine
621. 小便色如浓茶 *xiǎo biàn sè rú nóng chá*, urine the color of strong tea
622. 小便色黑 *xiǎo biàn sè hēi*, black urine
623. 小便清澈 *xiǎo biàn qīng chè*, clear urine
624. 小便澄澈 *xiǎo biàn chéng chè*, clear urine
625. 小便浑浊 *xiǎo biàn hún zhuó*, turbid urine
626. 尿浊 *niào zhuó*, urinary turbidity
627. 小便如米泔状 *xiǎo biàn rú mǐ gān zhuàng*, urine like rice water
628. 小便多泡沫 *xiǎo biàn duō pào mò*, foamy urine
629. 尿血 *niào xuè*, bloody urine
630. 尿精 *niào jīng*, semen in the urine

习题 Exercise:

148. spiritedness   ....

149. 无神 ....
150. *jiǎ shén* ....
151. fatness; obesity ....
152. 口眼喎斜 ....
153. *kǒu jìn* ....
154. hemiplegia ....
155. 角弓反张 ....
156. *jū jí* ....
157. hypertonicity ....
158. 筋急 ....
159. *sì zhī jū jí* ....
160. flailing of the limbs ....
161. 四肢抽搐 ....
162. *shǒu zú rú dòng* ....
163. inability to raise the shoulder ....
164. 撮空理线 ....
165. *xún yī mō chuáng* ....
166. red swollen head and face ....
167. 面浮 ....
168. *kǒu jìn* ....
169. red face ....
170. 面黄 ....
171. *miàn sè huǎng bái* ....
172. pale white facial complexion ....
173. 面色苍白 ....
174. *miàn sè wěi huáng* ....
175. lusterless complexion ....
176. 斑疹 ....
177. *bái péi* ....
178. fissured tongue ....
179. 舌胖 ....
180. *shé wāi* ....
181. tongue sore ....

182. 芒刺 ....

183. *shé shēng máng cì* ....

184. tooth marks on the margins of the tongue ....

185. 舌光 ....

186. *shé gān* ....

187. pale tongue ....

188. 舌淡白 ....

189. *shé hóng* ....

190. crimson tongue ....

191. 舌紫 ....

192. *bái tāi* ....

193. yellow fur ....

194. 舌苔黄腻 ....

195. *shé tāi jiāo huáng* ....

196. old-yellow tongue fur ....

197. 舌苔白如积粉 ....

198. *shé tāi jiāo hēi* ....

199. thin white tongue fur ....

200. 无痰 ....

201. *tán qīng bái xī bó* ....

202. thick sticky yellow phlegm ....

203. 痰黄浊黏稠 ....

204. *tán rú bài xù* ....

205. coughing of thin clear phlegm ....

206. 咳痰黏稠 ....

207. *tán zhōng dài xuè sī* ....

208. thin clear drool ....

209. 鼻流浊涕 ....

210. *ǒu tù tán xián* ....

211. vomiting of yellow-green bitter water ....

212. 吐血紫暗 ....

213. *dà biàn sè hēi* ....

214. dry stool ....

215. 大便黏稠　．．．

216. *dà biàn xī táng*　．．．．．．．．．．．．．．．．．．．．．．．．．．．．．．．．．．．．．．．

217. untransformed food　．．．．．．．．．．．．．．．．．．．．．．．．．．．．．．．．

218. 大便带血　．．．

219. *biàn xuè hēi*　．．．

220. urine　．．

221. 小便色赤　．．．

222. *xiǎo biàn hún zhuó*　．．．．．．．．．．．．．．．．．．．．．．．．．．．．．．．

223. urine like rice water　．．．．．．．．．．．．．．．．．．．．．．．．．．．．．．

224. 尿精　．．．

闻诊
Listening and Smelling

听声音　Listening to Sounds

第二节　第十五组　　　　　　SECTION 2: SET 15

闻发声异常　　　　　　　　　　Abnormalities of Voice

624	* 声 土	聲 耳	*shēng*	voice /vɔɪs/ sound /saʊnd/
625	* 音 音	音 音	*yīn*	sound /saʊnd/
626-n506	* 轻 车	輕 車	*qīng*	light /laɪt/
627	* 微 彳	微 彳	*wēi*	faint /fent/
628-n507	* 细 纟	細 糸	*xì*	fine /faɪn/
629-n508	* 怯 忄	怯 心	*qiè*	timid /ˈtɪmɪd/
630-n509	* 弱 弓	弱 弓	*ruò*	weak /wik/
631-n510	* 低 亻	低 人	*dī*	low /lo/
632-n511	* 重 丿	重 里	*zhòng*	heavy /ˈhɛvɪ/
633	* 浊 氵	濁 水	*zhuó*	turbid /ˈtɜˑbɪd/
634-n512	* 嘶 口	嘶 口	*sī*	hoarse /hɔrs, hors/
635-n513	* 嗄 口	嗄 口	*shà*	hoarse /hɔrs, hors/
636-n514	哑 口	啞 口	*yǎ*	*mute, voiceless*
637-n515	* 喑 口	喑 口	*yīn*	loss of voice /lɔs əv vɔɪs/
638-n516	沙 氵	沙 水	*shā*	*gritty*
639	* 呻 口	呻 口	*shēn*	moan /mon/
640-n517	吟 口	吟 口	*yín*	*wail*

注 **Note:**

The Chinese 怯, timid, implies lack of vigor as well as fearfulness.

复合词 Compounds:

631. 声音嘶哑 *shēng yīn sī yǎ*, hoarse voice
632. 声音轻微细弱 *shēng yīn qīng wēi xì ruò*, faint light fine voice
633. 声音沙哑 *shēng yīn shā yǎ*, gritty voice
634. 声音粗哑 *shēng yīn cū yǎ*, hoarse voice (lit. rough and mute voice — the roughness being created by interruptions in the sound of the voice)
635. 声音低微 *shēng yīn dī wēi*, low faint voice
636. 声音低怯 *shēng yīn dī qiè*, low timid voice
637. 声音重浊 *shēng yīn zhòng zhuó*, heavy turbid voice
638. 声重 *shēng zhòng*, heavy voice
639. 呻吟 *shēn yín*, moaning
640. 失音 *shī yīn*, loss of voice
641. 喑哑 *yīn yǎ*, loss of voice

第二节　第十六组　　　　　　　　　**SECTION 2: SET 16**

闻语言异常　　　　　　　　　　**Abnormalities of Speech**

641-n518	* 语 讠	語 言	*yǔ*	speech /spitʃ/
642-n519	* 言 讠	言 言	*yán*	speech /spitʃ/
643-n520	* 谵 讠	譫 言	*zhān*	delirium /dəˈlɪrɪəm/ *n.*
				delirious /dəˈlɪrɪəs/ *adj.*
644-n521	郑 阝	鄭 邑	*zhèng*	*repetitive*
645-n522	独 犭	獨 犬	*dú*	*alone, solitary*
646	错 钅	錯 金	*cuò*	*wrong, deranged*
647-n523	伦 亻	倫 人	*lùn*	*order*
648-n524	次 冫	次 欠	*cì*	*order*
649	* 乱 舌	亂 乙	*luàn*	deranged /dɪˈrendʒd/
650-n525	妄 亡	妄 女	*wàng*	*wild, deranged*
651-n526	* 癫 疒	癲 疒	*diān*	withdrawal /wɪðˈdrɔəl/
652-n527	* 狂 犭	狂 犬	*kuáng*	mania /ˈmenɪə/ *n.*
				manic /ˈmænɪk/ *adj.*
653-n528	* 謇 讠	謇 言	*jiǎn*	sluggish /ˈslʌgɪʃ/
654-n529	* 蹇 足	蹇 足	*jiǎn*	sluggish /ˈslʌgɪʃ/
655-n530	涩 氵	澀 水	*sè*	*rough*

复合词 Compounds:

642. 谵语 *zhān yǔ*, delirious speech
643. 郑声 *zhèng shēng*, muttering
644. 错语 *cuò yǔ*, confused speech
645. 语无伦次 *yǔ wú lún cì*, incoherent speech (lit. speech without order)
646. 言语错乱 *yán yǔ cuò luàn*, deranged speech
647. 错言妄语 *cuò yán wàng yǔ*, deranged speech
648. 狂言 *kuáng yán*, manic speech
649. 癫语 *diān yǔ*, withdrawal speech (i.e., speech associated with patients suffering from withdrawal disease. See the Diseases section ahead.)
650. 语言謇 (蹇) 涩 *yǔ yán jiǎn sè*, difficult sluggish speech

第二节　第十七组	**SECTION 2: SET 17**

闻呼吸异常与咳嗽	**Breathing Abnormalities & Cough**

656	*	呼 口	呼 口	*hū*	exhale /ɛksˈhel/
657-n531	*	吸 口	吸 口	*xī*	inhale /ɪnˈhel/
658	*	气 气	氣 气	*qì*	breathing /ˈbriðɪŋ/
659-n532	*	息 自	息 心	*xī*	breathing /ˈbriðɪŋ/
660	*	微 彳	微 彳	*wēi*	faint /fent/
661	*	急 心	急 心	*jí*	rapid /ˈræpɪd/
662-n533	*	促 亻	促 人	*cù*	hasty /ˈhestɪ/
663-n534	*	逆 辶	逆 辵	*nì*	counterflow /ˈkaʊntɚˌflo/
664-n535	*	粗 米	粗 米	*cū*	rough /rʌf/
665	*	短 矢	短 矢	*duǎn*	shortness /ˈʃɔrtnɪs/
666-n536	*	喘 口	喘 口	*chuǎn*	panting /ˈpæntɪŋ/
667-n537	*	哮 口	哮 口	*xiāo*	wheezing /ˈwizɪŋ, ˈhwizɪŋ/
668	*	咳 口	咳 口	*ké*	cough /kɔf/ (sonorous)
669-n538	*	嗽 口	嗽 口	*sòu*	cough /kɔf/ (productive)
670-n539	*	鸣 口	鳴 口	*míng*	rale /rɑl/
671-n540	*	呵 口	呵 口	*hē*	yawn /jɔn/
672-n541	*	欠 欠	欠 欠	*qiàn*	yawn /jɔn/
673-n542	*	鼾 鼻	鼾 鼻	*hān*	snoring /ˈsnorɪŋ/
674-n543	*	叹 口	嘆 口	*tàn*	sigh /saɪ/
675		太 大	太 大	*tài*	*great*
676-n544		喷 口	噴 口	*pēn*	*spray*
677-n545	*	嚏 口	嚏 口	*tì*	sneeze /sniz/

678-n546　*　衄血　衄血　　*nü*　　spontaneous external bleeding
　　　　　　　　　　　　　　　　　/spɑnˈtenɪəs ɪksˈtɜ˞nļ ˈblidɪŋ/
　　　　　　　　　　　　　　　　　bleed /blid/

注 Notes:

1. The Chinese 喘 *chuǎn* literally means 'panting' and generally denotes breathing difficulties. Although it is often translated as 'asthma' (which in Greek also means 'panting'), it is not as specific. What is known as 'asthma' in Western medicine is traditionally called 哮喘 *xiāo chuǎn*, 'wheezing and panting'.

2. The Chinese language has two words for cough, 咳 *ké* and 嗽 *sòu*. According to the 黄帝内经 *Huáng Dì Nèi Jīng*, these two characters are the same in meaning, and this usage prevailed until the Sòng Dynasty (A.D. 960-1279), when 刘完素 Liú Wán-Sù (c. A.D. 1120-1200) introduced a distinction: "咳 *ké* means a cough that produces sound but no matter, and arises when lung qì is damaged and loses its clarity; 嗽 *sòu* is a cough that produces matter without sound, and is attributed to spleen dampness stirring to form phlegm; 咳嗽 *ké sòu* is a cough with phlegm and sound, and arises when damage to lung qì stirs dampness in the spleen, so that the *ké* becomes *sòu*." From that time on, some followed the 黄帝内经 *Huáng Dì Nèi Jīng* in treating the characters as synonymous, whereas others adopted the distinction made by Liú Wán-Sù. In modern literature, the distinct forms are often referred to as 干咳 *gān ké*, dry cough, and 痰咳 *tán ké,* phlegm cough, and both together are referred to together by the combined form 咳嗽 *ké sòu*.

3. 衄 *nü* or 衄血 *nü xuè*, spontaneous external bleeding, refers to bleeding of any kind not attributable to external injury. It tends to refer to nosebleed, which is the most common form, but there is also spontaneous bleeding of the breast, ear, flesh, gum, and tongue. The term 吐衄 *tǔ nü* is a contracted combination 吐血 *tù xuè* and 衄血 *nü xuè* meaning blood ejection and spontaneous external bleeding.

复合词 Compounds:

651. 呼吸 *hū xī*, breathing
652. 气微 *qì wēi*, faint breathing
653. 气粗 *qì cū*, rough breathing
654. 气短 *qì duǎn*, shortness of breath
655. 短气 *duǎn qì*, shortness of breath
656. 气急 *qì jí*, rapid breathing
657. 气喘 *qì chuǎn*, panting

658. 喘息 *chuǎn xí*, panting
659. 喘不得卧 *chuǎn bù dé wò*, panting with inability to lie down
660. 哮 *xiāo*, wheezing
661. 哮喘 *xiāo chuǎn*, wheezing and panting
662. 咳喘 *ké chuǎn*, cough and panting
663. 咳逆上气 *ké nì shàng qì*, cough and counterflow qì ascent
664. 咳嗽 *ké sòu*, cough
665. 咳嗽无力 *ké sòu wú lì*, forceless cough
666. 咳声重浊 *ké shēng zhòng zhuó*, heavy turbid cough
667. 喉中痰鸣 *hóu zhōng tán míng*, phlegm rale in the throat
668. 鼻鼾 *bí hān*, snoring
669. 呵欠 *hē qiàn*, yawning
670. 叹息 *tàn xī*, sighing
671. 善太息 *shàn tài xī*, frequent sighing (lit. tendency to great breathing)
672. 喷嚏 *pēn tì*, sneezing

嗅气味   Smelling Odors

第二节　第十八组　　　　　　　　SECTION 2: SET 18

嗅气味 | Odors

679-n547	* 嗅口	嗅口	*xiù*	smell	/smɛl/
680	* 臭自	臭自	*chòu*	malodorous	/mæˈlodərəs/
681	* 酸酉	酸酉	*suān*	sour	/saur/
682	* 腐广	腐肉	*fǔ*	putrid	/ˈpjutrɪd/
683	* 秽禾	穢禾	*huì*	foul	/faul/
684	* 腥月	腥肉	*xīng*	fishy	/fɪʃɪ/
685	* 败贝	败攴	*bài*	rotten	/rɑtn̩/
686-n548	* 嗳口	嗳口	*ài*	belching	/ˈbɛltʃɪŋ/
687-n549	矢矢	矢矢	*shǐ*	*stool*	

注 Notes:

1. The term 臭 *chòu*, malodorous, is a general word describing bad smells. The term 腐 *fǔ*, putrid, commonly describes the breath, often in combination with 酸 *suān*, sour. The term 秽 *huì*, foul, describes highly unpleasant smells such as are sometimes associated with the stool. As previously mentioned, the

term 腥 *xīng*, fishy, describes the smell like fish or blood associated especially with phlegm or menstrual flow.

2. The Chinese 矢 *shǐ* means arrow, but in Chinese medicine it is often used euphemistically in place of its vulgar-sounding homophone 屎 *shǐ*, shit, feces, especially in the term 矢气 *shǐ qì*, 'fecal qi', i.e., flatus expelled from the anus.

复合词 Compounds:

673. 气味腥臭 *qì wèi xīng chòu*, fishy smell
674. 气味酸臭 *qì wèi suān chòu*, sour smell
675. 气味秽臭 *qì wèi huì chòu*, foul smell
676. 气味腐臭 *qì wèi fǔ chòu*, putrid smell
677. 汗气 *hàn qì*, smell of sweat
678. 嗳气酸腐 *ài qì suān fǔ*, belching of sour putrid qì
679. 嗳腐 *ài fǔ*, putrid belching
680. 大便奇臭如败卵 *dà biàn qí chòu rú bài luǎn*, stool smelling extraordinarily of rotten eggs
681. 矢气秽臭 *shǐ qì huì chòu*, foul-smelling flatus
682. 小便味腥 *xiǎo biàn wèi xīng*, fishy-smelling urine
683. 口臭 *kǒu chòu*, bad breath
684. 口腥 *kǒu xìng*, fishy-smelling breath
685. 鼻臭 *bí chòu*, malodorous nasal breath
686. 呕吐腥臭 *ǒu tù xīng chòu*, fishy-smelling vomitus
687. 呕吐酸臭 *ǒu tù suān chòu*, sour-smelling vomitus

习题 Exercise:

225. *shēng yīn sī yǎ* ....
226. faint light fine voice ....
227. 声音粗哑 ....
228. *shēng yīn dī qiè* ....
229. moaning ....
230. 失音 ....
231. *zhān yǔ* ....
232. muttering ....
233. 错语 ....
234. *yǔ wú lún cì* ....
235. deranged speech ....

问诊
Inquiry

第二节　第十九组　　　　　　　**SECTION 2: SET 19**

问寒热　　　　　　　　　　　**Inquiry About Heat & Cold**

688	* 寒 宀	寒 宀	*hán*	cold /kold/
689	* 热 灬	熱 火	*rè*	heat /hit/
				heat [effusion] /ˈhit ɪˌfjuʒən/
690-n550	烧 火	燒 火	*shāo*	burn; hot
691-n551	但 亻	但 人	*dàn*	only
692	* 风 风	風 風	*fēng*	wind /wɪnd/
693-n552	* 恶 亚	惡 心	*wù*	aversion to /əˈvɚʒn̩ tu/
694-n553	* 怕 忄	怕 心	*pà*	fear /fɪr/
695-n554	* 畏 田	畏 田	*wèi*	fear /fɪr/
696-n555	* 憎 忄	憎 心	*zēng*	abhor /əbˈhɔr/ vi.
				abhorrence /əbˈhɔrəns/ n.
697-n556	* 战 戈	戰 戈	*zhàn*	shiver /ˈʃɪvɚ/
698	* 冷 冫	冷 冫	*lěng*	cold /kold/
699	* 形 彡	形 彡	*xíng*	physical /ˈfɪzɪkl̩/
700-n557	* 壮 丬	壯 爿	*zhuàng*	vigorous /ˈvɪgərəs/
701-n558	* 烘 火	烘 火	*hōng*	baking /ˈbekɪŋ/
702	* 暴 日	暴 日	*bào*	fulminant /ˈfʌlmɪnənt/

703-n559	往 彳	往 彳	*wǎng*	go; in the direction of
704-n560	* 烦 火	煩 火	*fán*	vexation /vɛksˈeʃən/
705	* 潮 氵	潮 水	*cháo*	tidal /ˈtaɪdl̩/
706	* 骨 骨	骨 骨	*gǔ*	bone /bon/
707-n561	* 蒸 艹	蒸 艸	*zhēng*	steam /stim/
708	* 劳 艹	勞 力	*láo*	taxation /tæksˈeʃən/
709-n562	日 日	日 日	*rì*	sun, day
710-n563	* 晡 日	晡 日	*bū*	late afternoon /let ˌæftɚˈnun/

注 Notes:

1. Heat [effusion] (fever): The Chinese 热 *rè* means 'heat' as a cause of disease. It also means palpable bodily heat that we normally refer to as 'fever', and which modern medicine measures objectively within the body by means of a thermometer. Chinese medicine traditionally had no objective way of measuring temperature, and used the word 'heat' to describe hot states whether palpable or subjective. 'Heat' in this sense, as distinct from a cause of illness, is often distinguished by the compound 发热 *fā rè*, putting out or 'effusing' heat. It would be difficult to argue that 'fever' is categorically a mistranslation of 发热 *fā rè* (or simply 热 *rè*), but it is clear that, whether it is used in the colloquial sense or the stricter modern medical sense, it is not as broad in meaning as the Chinese terms. For this reason, we have chosen 'heat effusion', writing this often as 'heat [effusion]', when the Chinese use simply the word 热 *rè* in this sense.

Traditionally, heat [effusion] is described in purely qualitative terms ('vigorous', 'baking', 'tidal'), although 高热 *gāo rè*, 'high heat [effusion]', which is commonly seen in modern Chinese medical texts, reflects the Western medical tendency to quantify.

但热不寒 *dàn rè bù hán* 'heat (only) without cold', means heat effusion only, without aversion to cold.

2. Cold: A subjective feeling of cold is called 恶寒 *wù hán*, 'aversion to cold'. The term 恶寒 *wù hán* appears often to be translated as 'chills', but in actual fact, the Chinese term is wider in meaning. It means an acute sensation of cold experienced in external contractions, and a less acute condition experienced in yáng vacuity. Only the former can be represented by the English word chills. For this reason, we speak of 'aversion to cold', rather than 'chills'. In some cases, the Chinese 寒 *hán*, 'cold', stands for this as distinct from cold as a cause of illness. In such cases, we write '[aversion to] cold'. The Chinese 恶风 *wù fēng*, aversion to wind, is a feeling of cold experienced by exposure to wind or drafts. The term 憎寒 *zēng hán*, abhorrence of cold, denotes exter-

nal shivering with internal heat vexation arising when a deep-lying internal heat evil blocks yáng qì and prevents it from reaching the exterior.

In the Chinese term 形寒肢冷 *xíng hán zhī lěng*, physical cold and cold limbs, 形 means body in the visible or tangible sense; hence 形寒 is a coldness of the body that can be felt with the hand and seen in the posture assumed by the patient. Chinese medicine holds that 'when yáng is vacuous, there is external cold' (阳虚则外寒 *yáng xū zé wài hán*), i.e., visible and tangible externalized manifestations of cold.

复合词 Compounds:

688. 恶风 *wù fēng*, aversion to wind
689. 怕冷 *pà lěng*, fear of cold
690. 畏冷 *wèi lěng*, fear of cold
691. 憎寒 *zēng hán*, abhorrence of cold
692. 发热 *fā rè*, heat [effusion]
693. 壮热 *zhuàng rè*, vigorous heat [effusion]
694. 憎寒壮热 *zēng hán zhuàng rè*, abhorrence of cold and vigorous heat [effusion]
695. 烘热 *hōng rè*, baking heat [effusion]
696. 暴热 *bào rè*, fulminant heat [effusion]
697. 畏恶风寒 *wèi wù fēng hán*, aversion to wind and cold
698. 寒战 *hán zhàn*, shivering
699. 身热肢寒 *shēn rè zhī hán*, hot body and cold limbs
700. 形寒肢冷 *xíng hán zhī lěng*, physical cold and cold limbs
701. 恶寒发热 *wù hán fā rè*, aversion to cold with heat [effusion]
702. 寒热往来 *hán rè wǎng lái*, alternating heat [effusion] and [aversion to] cold
703. 但热不寒 *dàn rè bù hán*, heat without cold
704. 五心烦热 *wǔ xīn fán rè*, vexing heat in the five hearts
705. 潮热 *cháo rè*, tidal heat [effusion]
706. 骨蒸劳热 *gǔ zhēng láo rè*, steaming bone taxation heat [effusion]
707. 日晡潮热 *rì bū cháo rè*, late afternoon tidal heat [effusion]

第二节　第二十组	**SECTION 2: SET 20**

问汗   **Inquiry About Sweating**

711	* 汗 氵 汗 水	*hàn*	sweat /swɛt/
			sweating /ˈswɛtɪŋ/

712-n564	盗 皿	盗 皿		*dào*	*thief, robber*
713-n565	* 自 自	自 自		*zì*	*spontaneous* /spɑnˈtenɪəs/
714-n566	偏 亻	偏 人		*piān*	*tend, biased*
715-n567	* 溅 氵	溅 水		*jí*	*drizzle* /ˈdrɪzl̩/
716-n568	* 绝 纟	絕 糸		*jué*	*expiration* /ˌɛkspəˈreʃən/

注 Notes:

1. The term 盗汗 *dào hàn*, translated as 'night sweating', literally means a 'thief sweat' reflecting the fact that it 'steals' its appearance unbeknown to the patient as he sleeps. The term 'night sweating' is not ideal, because it suggests sweating at night only, whereas 盗汗 *dào hàn* means sweating during sleep.

2. The term 汗多 *hàn duō*, 'copious sweat', means a large amount of sweat; 多汗 *duō hàn*, 'profuse sweating', implies that the patient sweats regularly in large amounts.

3. 战汗 *zhàn hàn*, shiver sweating, is sweating accompanied by pronounced shivering and is a sign of the struggle between evil and right in externally contracted febrile (heat) diseases.

复合词 Compounds:

708. 无汗 *wú hàn*, absence of sweating

709. 汗出 *hàn chū*, sweating

710. 汗多 *hàn duō*, copious sweat

711. 多汗 *duō hàn*, profuse sweating

712. 大汗 *dà hàn*, great sweating

713. 战汗 *zhàn hàn*, shiver sweating

714. 自汗 *zì hàn*, spontaneous sweating

715. 盗汗 *dào hàn*, night sweating

716. 绝汗 *jué hàn*, expiration sweating

717. 黄汗 *huáng hàn*, yellow sweat

718. 头汗 *tóu hàn*, sweating head

719. 心胸汗出 *xīn xiōng hàn chū*, sweating from the chest and heart [region]

720. 腋汗 *yè hàn*, sweating armpits

721. 手足汗出 *shǒu zú hàn chū*, sweating hands and feet

722. 手足溅溅汗出 *shǒu zú jí jí hàn chū*, streaming sweating of the hands and feet

第二节　第二十一组　　　　　SECTION 2: SET 21

问头项　　　　　　　　　　　Inquiry About Head & Neck

717	* 头 大	頭 頁	*tóu*	head /hɛd/
718	* 面 一	面 面	*miàn*	face /fes/
719	* 胀 月	脹 肉	*zhàng*	distention /dɪsˈtɛnʃən/
720	* 重 丿	重 里	*zhòng*	heavy /ˈhɛvɪ/
721-n569	* 晕 日	暈 日	*yūn*	dizzy /ˈdɪzɪ/ *adj.*
				dizziness /ˈdɪzɪnɪs/ *n.*
722-n570	* 眩 目	眩 目	*xuàn*	dizzy /ˈdɪzɪ/ *adj.*
				dizziness /ˈdɪzɪnɪs/ *n.*
723-n571	* 裹 一	裹 衣	*guǒ*	swathe /sweð/
724-n572	* 掣 手	掣 手	*chè*	pulling /ˈpʊlɪŋ/
725-n573	* 倾 亻	傾 人	*qīng*	bowed /baʊd/
726	* 鸣 口	鳴 口	*míng*	ringing /ˈrɪŋɪŋ/
727-n574	* 啮 口	嚙 口	*niè*	grind /graɪnd/ (the teeth)
728-n575	* 齘 齿	齘 齒	*xiè*	grind /graɪnd/ (the teeth)
729	粗 米	粗 米	*cū*	*fat, thick*
730-n576	* 久 丿	久 丿	*jiǔ*	enduring /ɪnˈdjurɪŋ/

注 Notes:

1. 眩晕 *xuàn yūn*, dizziness, is visual distortion with a whirling sensation in the head that in severe cases can upset the sense of balance. In some literature, flowery vision (blurred vision) giving rise to dizziness is known as 'dizzy vision', whereas dizziness giving rise to flowery vision is called 'dizzy head'. In practice, this distinction is not observed much.

2. 昏厥 *hūn jué*, clouding reversal, is sudden loss of consciousness and collapse, sometimes accompanied by reversal cold of the limbs. Clouding reversal is usually of short duration as in various reversal patterns; the patient returns to consciousness without hemiplegia or deviation of the eyes and mouth as occurs in wind stroke. In rare cases, it continues, as in deathlike reversal. Clouding reversal of short duration corresponds to syncope in Western medical terminology. However, a literal translation of the term has been chosen in view of the importance of the term 厥 *jué* in Chinese etiological descriptions, since loss of consciousness is understood as a reversal or disruption in the movement of qì.

复合词 Compounds:

723. 头晕 *tóu yūn*, dizzy head

724. 目眩 *mù xuàn*, dizzy vision

725. 头晕目眩 *tóu yūn mù xuàn*, dizzy head and vision

726. 眩晕 *xuàn yūn*, dizziness

727. 头昏 *tóu hūn*, clouded head

728. 昏厥 *hūn jué*, clouding reversal

729. 头重 *tóu zhòng*, heavy-headedness

730. 头重如裹 *tóu zhòng rú guǒ*, head heavy as if swathed

731. 头痛 *tóu tòng*, headache

732. 久头痛 *jiǔ tóu tòng*, enduring headache

733. 头痛如掣 *tóu tòng rú chè*, headache with pulling sensation, iron-band headache

734. 偏头痛 *piān tóu tòng*, hemilateral headache

735. 头胀 *tóu zhàng*, distention in the head

736. 面部疼痛 *miàn bù téng tòng*, facial pain

737. 头冷 *tóu lěng*, cold head

738. 头热 *tóu rè*, hot head

739. 头皮麻木 *tóu pí má mù*, numbness of the scalp

740. 头倾 *tóu qīng*, bowed head

741. 头摇 *tóu yáo*, shaking of the head

742. 脑鸣 *nǎo míng*, ringing in the brain

743. 啮齿 *niè chǐ*, grinding of the teeth

744. 齘齿 *xiè chǐ*, grinding of the teeth

745. 项强 *xiàng jiàng*, rigidity of the neck

746. 颈粗 *jǐng cū*, fat neck

747. 颈项痛 *jǐng xiàng tòng*, neck pain

第二节　第二十二组				**SECTION 2: SET 22**

问五官				**Inquiry About the Five Offices**
731	* 官 宀	官 宀	*guān*	office /ˈɔfɪs/
732-n577	* 塞 宀	塞 土	*sāi*	congest /kənˈdʒɛst/ *vt.*
				congestion /kənˈdʒɛstʃən/ *n.*
733	* 酸 酉	酸 酉	*suān*	sour-sore /ˈsaʊr ˈsɔr, -sor/
734-n578	* 花 艹	花 艸	*huā*	flowery /ˈflaʊrɪ, ˈflaʊərɪ/
735	* 痒 疒	癢 疒	*yǎng*	itch /ɪtʃ/
736-n579	羞 羊	羞 羊	*xiū*	*shy*
737	* 怕 忄	怕 心	*pà*	fear /fɪr/
738-n580	* 近 辶	近 辵	*jìn*	close /klos/ *adj.*

739-n581	*	远辶	遠辵	*yuǎn*	distant /ˈdɪstənt/
740-n582	*	聋龙	聾耳	*lóng*	deafness /ˈdɛfnɪs/
741	*	鸣口	鳴口	*míng*	tinnitus /tɪˈnaɪtəs, ˈtɪnɪtəs/
742		流氵	流水	*liú*	*flow, run*
743	*	泪氵	淚水	*lèi*	tears /tɪrz/
744-n583	*	眵目	眵目	*chī*	eye discharge /ˈaɪ–ˌdɪstʃɑrdʒ/

注 Note:

Most of the terms in this section are self-explanatory. 眼花 *yǎn huā* and 目花 *mù huā*, here translated literally as 'flowery vision', means any kind of blurring of vision or floaters.

复合词 Compounds:

748. 目痛 *mù tòng*, eye pain
749. 眼花 *yǎn huā*, flowery vision
750. 目花 *mù huā*, flowery vision
751. 目珠夜痛 *mù zhū yè tòng*, night-time eyeball pain
752. 头目胀痛 *tóu mù zhàng tòng*, distention and pain of the head and eyes
753. 目眩 *mù xuàn*, dizzy vision
754. 目痒 *mù yǎng*, itchy eyes
755. 目涩 *mù sè*, dry eyes
756. 目干涩 *mù gān sè*, dry eyes
757. 羞明怕热 *xiū míng pà rè*, aversion to light and fear of heat
758. 视物如蒙 *shì wù rú méng*, seeing things as clouded
759. 视物如双 *shì wù rú shuāng*, double vision
760. 视一为二 *shì yī wéi èr*, seeing one as two
761. 视物变形 *shì wù biàn xíng*, visual distortion of objects
762. 不能远视 *bù néng yuǎn shì*, inability to see distant objects
763. 不能近视 *bù néng jìn shì*, inability to see close objects
764. 流泪 *liú lèi*, tearing
765. 迎风流泪 *yíng fēng liú lèi*, tearing on exposure to wind
766. 重听 *zhòng tīng*, hearing impairment (lit. 'heavy hearing', inability to hear sounds clearly)
767. 耳聋 *ěr lóng*, deafness
768. 耳鸣 *ěr míng*, tinnitus
769. 耳鸣如蝉声 *ěr míng rú chán shēng*, tinnitus like the sound of cicadas
770. 耳痛 *ěr tòng*, ear pain
771. 耳痒 *ěr yǎng*, itchy ears

772. 鼻干 *bí gān*, dry nose
773. 鼻痛 *bí tòng*, pain in the nose
774. 鼻痒 *bí yǎng*, itchy nose
775. 鼻塞 *bí sāi*, nasal congestion
776. 鼻流涕 *bí liú tì*, running nose
777. 鼻酸 *bí suān*, sour-sore nose
778. 唇痒 *chún yǎng*, itchy lips
779. 唇干 *chún gān*, dry lips
780. 唇麻 *chún má*, numb lips
781. 舌痛 *shé tòng*, painful tongue
782. 舌麻 *shé má*, numb tongue
783. 舌痒 *shé yǎng*, itchy tongue
784. 喉痒 *hóu yǎng*, itchy throat
785. 咽干 *yān gān*, dry throat; dry pharynx
786. 喉咙肿痛 *hóu lóng zhǒng tòng*, sore swollen throat
787. 喉咙痛 *hóu lóng tòng*, sore throat
788. 咽喉痛 *yān hóu tòng*, sore throat
789. 喉中梗阻 *hóu zhōng gěng zǔ*, blockage of the throat
790. 目多眵 *mù duō chī*, copious eye discharge

第二节　第二十三组	**SECTION 2: SET 23**

问周身　　　　　　　　　　**Inquiry About the Body**

745-n584	* 周 冂	周 口	*zhōu*	whole /hol/
746-n585	* 倦 亻	倦 人	*juàn*	fatigue /fə'tig/
747-n586	* 疲 疒	疲 疒	*pí*	fatigue /fə'tig/
748-n587	* 怠 心	怠 心	*dài*	fatigue /fə'tig/
749-n588	* 乏 丿	乏 丿	*fá*	lack /læk/
750-n589	* 力 力	力 力	*lì*	strength /strɛŋθ/
751-n590	顿 页	頓 頁	*dùn*	*fatigue*
752	* 重 丿	重 里	*zhòng*	heaviness /'hɛvɪnɪs/
753-n591	* 困 口	困 口	*kùn*	cumbersome /'kʌmbɚsəm/
754-n592	* 痛 疒	痛 疒	*tòng*	pain /pen/
755-n593	* 疼 疒	疼 疒	*téng*	pain /pen/
756-n594	* 楚 木	楚 木	*chǔ*	pain /pen/
757-n595	* 酸 疒	痠 疒	*suān*	aching /'ekɪŋ/
758-n596	* 游 氵	遊 辵	*yóu*	wandering /'wɑndərɪŋ/
759-n597	走 走	走 走	*zǒu*	*go, run*

760-n598	* 麻 麻　麻 麻	*má*	numbness /ˈnʌmnɪs/	
			tingling /ˈtɪŋglɪŋ/	
761	* 木 木　木 木	*mù*	numbness /ˈnʌmnɪs/	
762-n599	* 躁 足　躁 足	*zào*	agitation /ˌædʒɪˈteʃən/	

注 Notes:

1. Of the two words for pain, 痛 *tòng* is much more commonly seen than 疼 *téng*. The latter is most commonly used together with the former, as in 全身疼痛 *quán shēn téng tòng*.

2. The Chinese 麻 *má* means 'hemp', 'linen', or 'sackcloth'. Its use in the meaning of 'tingling' or 'numbness' is probably derived from an analogy to the effect of sackcloth or linen on the skin.

3. Note the large variety of terms meaning 'fatigue'.

4. 身重 *shēn zhòng*, 'generalized heaviness', is a subjective feeling of heaviness.

复合词 Compounds:

791. 倦怠 *juàn dài*, fatigue
792. 疲倦 *pí juàn*, fatigue
793. 疲劳 *pí láo*, fatigue
794. 疲乏 *pí fá*, fatigue, fatigue and lack of strength
795. 倦怠乏力 *juàn dài fá lì*, fatigue and lack of strength
796. 疲乏无力 *pí fá wú lì*, fatigue and lack of strength
797. 疲倦乏力 *pí juàn fá lì*, fatigue and lack of strength
798. 无力倦怠 *wú lì juàn dài*, fatigue and lack of strength
799. 身疲 *shēn pí*, fatigued body
800. 身倦乏力 *shēn juàn fá lì*, fatigued body and lack of strength
801. 体倦乏力 *tǐ juàn fá lì*, fatigued body and lack of strength
802. 体倦无力 *tǐ juàn wú lì*, fatigued body and lack of strength
803. 形倦神怠 *xíng juàn shén dài*, physical fatigue and lassitude of spirit
804. 神疲 *shén pí*, fatigued spirit
805. 神疲乏力 *shén pí fá lì*, fatigued spirit and lack of strength
806. 形倦神疲 *xíng juàn shén pí*, physical fatigue and lassitude of spirit
807. 食后困顿 *shí hòu kùn dùn*, drowsiness after eating
808. 身重 *shēn zhòng*, generalized heaviness
809. 身痛 *shēn tòng*, generalized pain
810. 周身酸楚 *zhōu shēn suān chǔ*, generalized pain

811. 游走疼痛 *yóu zǒu téng tòng*, wandering pain
812. 全身疼痛 *quán shēn téng tòng*, generalized pain
813. 身振摇 *shēn zhèn yáo*, generalized shaking
814. 半身麻木 *bàn shēn má mù*, hemilateral numbness
815. 四肢倦怠 *sì zhī juàn dài*, fatigued limbs
816. 四肢困倦 *sì zhī kùn juàn*, fatigued cumbersome limbs
817. 肢倦乏力 *zhī juàn fá lì*, fatigued limbs and lack of strength
818. 肢倦 *zhī juàn*, fatigued limbs

第二节　第二十四组				**SECTION 2: SET 24**

问背腰				**Inquiry About the Back & Lumbus**
763	* 背 月	背 肉	*bèi*	back /bæk/
764	* 腰 月	腰 肉	*yāo*	lumbus /ˈlʌmbəs/
765	* 力 力	力 力	*lì*	strength /strɛŋθ/
766-n600	* 软 车	軟 車	*ruǎn*	limp /lɪmp/
767-n601	* 脊 肉	脊 肉	*jí*	spine /spaɪn/
768-n602	* 绳 纟	繩 糸	*shéng*	rope /rop/
769-n603	* 束 束	束 木	*shù*	girthed /gɜˑθt/

注 Note:

Lumbar pain is sometimes associated with limpness of the knees; both signs are associated with kidney vacuity.

复合词 Compounds:

819. 肩背拘急 *jiān bèi jù jí*, hypertonicity of the shoulder and back
820. 背痛 *bèi tòng*, back pain
821. 背冷 *bèi lěng*, cold in the back
822. 背热 *bèi rè*, hot back
823. 腰脊痛 *yāo jǐ tòng*, pain in the lumbar spine
824. 腰酸 *yāo suān*, aching lumbus
825. 腰冷重 *yāo lěng zhòng*, coldness and heaviness in the lumbar region
826. 腰膝无力 *yāo xī wú lì*, lack of strength in the lumbus and knees
827. 腰如绳束 *yāo rú shéng shù*, waist as if girthed with a rope
828. 腰膝酸软 *yāo xī suān ruǎn*, limp aching lumbus and knees

第二节　第二十五组   SECTION 2: SET 25

问胸胁   Inquiry About Chest & Rib-Side

770	* 胸 月	胸 肉	*xiōng*	chest /tʃɛst/
771	* 胁 肉	脅 肉	*xié*	rib-side /ˈrɪbsaɪd/
772-n604	* 闷 门	悶 心	*mèn*	oppression /əˈprɛʃən/
773-n605	* 满 氵	滿 水	*mǎn*	fullness /ˈfʊlnɪs/
774-n606	* 痞 疒	痞 疒	*pǐ*	glomus /ˈgloməs/
775	* 苦 艹	苦 艸	*kǔ*	suffer /ˈsʌfəˈ/
776	* 烦 火	煩 火	*fán*	vexation /vɛksˈeʃən/
777-n607	* 懊 忄	懊 心	*ào*	anguish /ˈæŋgwɪʃ/
778-n608	* 恼 忄	惱 心	*nóng*	anguish /ˈæŋgwɪʃ/
779-n609	* 悸 忄	悸 心	*jì*	palpitation /ˌpælpəˈteʃən/
780-n610	* 隐 阝	隱 邑	*yǐn*	dull /dʌl/
781-n611	* 灼 火	灼 火	*zhuó*	scorching /ˈskɔrtʃɪŋ/
782-n612	* 支 十	支 支	*zhī*	propping /ˈprɑpɪŋ/

注 **Notes:**

1. The term 痞 *pǐ*, 'glomus', is composed of the illness signific 疒 with 否 meaning negation. It is used in the sense of a local sensation of fullness and blockage and, especially in the combination 痞块 *pǐ kuài*, in the sense of a palpable lump. The translation glomus was coined by us from the Latin glomus, a ball or lump, which has also given rise to the English word conglomeration.

2. The term 烦 *fán* means a subjective feeling of restlessness in the heart and chest; 躁 *zào* means physical agitation.

3. The term 心中懊恼 *xīn zhōng ào nóng*, anguish in the heart, a symptom first described in the *Shāng Hán Lùn*, is a feeling of heat and clamoring stomach (which is explained in the next set). It arises when, after exterior patterns have been treated inappropriately by sweating or draining precipitation, the external evil enters the interior and lodges in the chest and diaphragm, thus harassing the stomach.

4. In the term 胸胁苦满 *xiōng xié kǔ mǎn*, 苦 is interpreted to mean to suffer ('suffering from fullness in the chest and rib-side') rather than bitterness.

5. 胸胁支满 *xiōng xié zhī mǎn*, 'propping fullness in the chest and rib-side', is a feeling of fullness that gives the patient the sensation of being propped up.

复合词 Compounds:

829. 胸痛 *xiōng tòng*, chest pain

830. 胸闷 *xiōng mèn*, oppression in the chest

831. 胸满胁痛 *xiōng mǎn xié tòng*, fullness in the chest and pain in the rib-side, thoracic fullness and rib-side pain

832. 胸胁苦满 *xiōng xié kǔ mǎn*, fullness in the chest and rib-side

833. 胸胁满 *xiōng xié mǎn*, chest and rib-side fullness

834. 胸胁逆满 *xiōng xié nì mǎn*, counterflow fullness in the chest and rib-side

835. 胸胁痛 *xiōng xié tòng*, chest and rib-side pain

836. 胸胁胀满 *xiōng xié zhàng mǎn*, painful distention in the chest and rib-side

837. 胸胁支满 *xiōng xié zhī mǎn*, propping fullness in the chest and rib-side

838. 胁痛 *xié tòng*, rib-side pain

839. 腋胁痛 *yè xié tòng*, axillary and rib-side pain

840. 胁肋疼痛 *xié lè téng tòng*, rib-side pain

841. 胁肋隐痛 *xié lè yǐn tòng*, dull rib-side pain

842. 胁肋胀痛 *xié lè zhàng tòng*, rib-side distention and pain, rib-side distending pain

843. 胁胀 *xié zhàng*, rib-side distention

844. 两胁拘急 *liǎng xié jū jí*, hypertonicity of both rib-sides; tension in both rib-sides

845. 两胁灼痛 *liǎng xié zhuó tòng*, scorching pain in both rib-sides

846. 心烦 *xīn fán*, vexation

847. 心中懊恼 *xīn zhōng ào nóng*, anguish in the heart

848. 心悸 *xīn jì*, palpitation

849. 烦躁 *fán zào*, vexation and agitation

第二节　第二十六组				**SECTION 2: SET 26**

问腹部   **Inquiry About the Abdomen**

783	* 嗳 口	嗳 口	*ài*	belching /ˈbɛltʃɪŋ/
784-n613	* 呃 口	呃 口	*è*	hiccup /ˈhɪkʌp/
785-n614	* 嘈 口	嘈 口	*cáo*	clamor /ˈklæmɚ/
786-n615	杂 木	雜 隹	*zá*	*sundry; confused*
787-n616	* 吞 天	吞 口	*tūn*	swallow /ˈswɑlo/
788-n617	* 泛 氵	泛 水	*fàn*	upflow /ˈʌpflo/
789	* 酸 酉	酸 酉	*suān*	sour /saʊr/ *adj.*

					acid /ˈæsɪd/ *adj., n.*
790	* 恶 亚	惡 心	*ě*		nausea /ˈnɔʃ(ɪ)ə, ˈnɔʒ(ɪ)ə/ *n.*
					nauseous /ˈnɔʃ(ɪ)ə/ *adj.*
791	* 呕 口	嘔 口	*ǒu*		retching /ˈrɛtʃɪŋ/
792	* 吐 口	吐 口	*tù*		vomiting /ˈvɑmɪtɪŋ/
					ejection /ɪˈdʒɛkʃən/
793-n618	即 艮	即 卩	*jí*		*then, immediately*
794-n619	* 蛕 虫	蛕 虫	*huí*		roundworm /ˈraʊndwɝm/
795-n620	* 蛔 虫	蛔 虫	*huí*		roundworm /ˈraʊndwɝm/
796-n621	* 刀 刀	刀 刀	*dāo*		knife /naɪf/
797-n622	* 针 钅	針 金	*zhēn*		needle /ˈnidl̩/
798-n623	* 锥 钅	錐 金	*zhuī*		awl /ɔl/
799-n624	* 割 刂	割 刀	*gē*		cut /kʌt/
800	* 刺 刂	刺 刀	*cì*		stab /stæb/
801-n625	* 窜 穴	竄 穴	*cuàn*		scurry /ˈskɝɪ/
802-n626	* 定 宀	定 宀	*dìng*		fixed /fɪkst/
803-n627	* 处 夂	處 虍	*chù*		location /ləˈkeʃən, loˈkeʃən/
804-n628	露 雨	露 雨	*lù*		*expose*
805	* 单 丷	單 口	*dān*		simple /ˈsɪmpl̩/
806	* 鸣 口	鳴 口	*míng*		rumbling /ˈrʌmblɪŋ/

注 Notes:

1. The Chinese 嘈杂 *cáo záo* literally means 'noise confusion'. The term is defined as a sensation in the stomach described as being pain but unlike pain, and like hunger but unlike hunger; hence 'noise' is used in a figurative sense. The term is rendered in English as 'clamoring stomach'.

2. In the term 恶心 *ě xīn*, nausea, 恶 is read as *ě* in the third tone. Western medicine uses the same term, but writes 噁 with the mouth signific. The character 恶 is pronounced as *wù* when it means fear or aversion to, and as *è* when it means malign.

3. The term 吐酸 *tù suān*, 'acid vomiting', means the expulsion of sour fluid or matter from the stomach through the mouth; 吞酸 *tūn suān*, 'acid swallowing' or 'acid regurgitation', means bringing up acid fluid from the stomach and swallowing it before one can spit it out; 泛酸 *fàn suān*, 'acid upflow', is a broader term denoting either of the former.

4. The character 蛕 *huí* is synonymous and homophonic with 蛔. The latter is now more common, and has been adopted by Western medicine as the equivalent of ascaris.

5. The origin of blood expelled from the mouth was not always clearly understood by Chinese doctors. The term 吐血 *tù xuè*, for example, could mean the expulsion of blood from either the stomach or the lung. For this reason, we have chosen the more generic rendering of 'blood ejection'. Most translators probably take 吐 *tù* at face value and render the term as 'vomiting of blood'. That, however, is not the meaning in all texts.

6. We have already encountered the terms 小腹 *xiǎo fù*, the smaller abdomen, and 少腹 *shào fù*, the lesser abdomen. In the terms 小腹痛 *xiǎo fù tòng*, smaller-abdominal pain, and 少腹痛 *shào fù tòng*, lesser-abdominal pain, we encounter their adjectival forms, which in English we have hyphenated for clarity.

复合词 Compounds:

850. 心下悸 *xīn xià jì*, palpitation below the heart
851. 心下痞 *xīn xià pǐ*, glomus below the heart
852. 嗳气 *ài qì*, belching
853. 吐酸 *tù suān*, acid vomiting
854. 吞酸 *tūn suān*, acid swallowing, acid regurgitation
855. 泛酸 *fàn suān*, acid upflow
856. 食入即吐 *shí rù jí tù*, immediate vomiting of ingested food
857. 呃逆 *è nì*, hiccup
858. 嘈杂 *cáo zá*, clamoring stomach
859. 恶心 *ě xīn*, nausea
860. 干呕 *gān ǒu*, dry retching
861. 呕吐 *ǒu tù*, vomiting
862. 吐血 *tù xuè*, blood ejection
863. 吐衄 *tǔ nü*, blood ejection and spontaneous external bleeding
864. 吐蚘 *tù huí*, vomiting of roundworm
865. 胃脘痛 *wèi wǎn tòng*, stomach duct pain
866. 腹痛 *fù tòng*, abdominal pain
867. 痛有定处 *tòng yǒu dìng chù*, pain of fixed location
868. 痛如刀刺 *tòng rú dāo cì*, pain like the stabbing of a knife
869. 痛如刀割 *tòng rú dāo gē*, pain like the cutting of a knife
870. 痛如针刺 *tòng rú zhēn cì*, pain like the stabbing of a needle
871. 痛如锥刺 *tòng rú zhuī cì*, pain like the stabbing of an awl
872. 窜痛 *cuàn tòng*, scurrying pain
873. 胀痛 *zhàng tòng*, distending pain; distention and pain
874. 绕脐作痛 *rào qí zuò tòng*, pain around the umbilicus
875. 绕脐痛 *rào qí tòng*, pain around the umbilicus

876. 脐腹痛 *qí fù tòng*, pain in the umbilical region

877. 小腹痛 *xiǎo fù tòng*, smaller-abdominal pain

878. 少腹痛 *shào fù tòng*, lesser-abdominal pain

879. 腹满 *fù mǎn*, abdominal fullness

880. 腹冷 *fù lěng*, cold in the abdomen

881. 肠鸣 *cháng míng*, rumbling intestines

882. 肠鸣作痛 *cháng míng zuò tòng*, rumbling intestines and abdominal pain

883. 肠鸣腹痛 *cháng míng fù tòng*, rumbling intestines and abdominal pain

第二节　第二十七组				SECTION 2: SET 27

问饮食、口味 / Inquiry About Food, Drink & Taste in the Mouth

807	* 饮 亻	飲 食	*yǐn*	drink /drɪŋk/
808	* 食 食	食 食	*shí*	eat /it/
809	* 口 口	口 口	*kǒu*	mouth /maʊθ/
810	* 味 口	味 口	*wèi*	taste /test/
811-n629	* 渴 氵	渴 水	*kě*	thirst /θɝˑst/
812	多 夕	多 夕	*duō*	*much, many, copious*
813	少 小	少 小	*shǎo*	*little, scant*
814-n630	* 欲 谷	欲 欠	*yù*	desire /dɪˈzaɪr/
815-n631	* 欲 谷	慾 心	*yù*	desire /dɪˈzaɪr/
816	* 纳 纟	納 糸	*nà*	intake /ɪntek/
817-n632	* 呆 口	呆 口	*dāi*	torpid /ˈtɔrpɪd/ *adj.* torpor /ˈtɔrpɚ/ *n.*
818-n633	* 厌 厂	厭 厂	*yàn*	aversion to /əˈvɚʒn̩ tu/
819-n634	易 日	易 日	*yì*	*easy, easily*
820-n635	* 饥 亻	饑 食	*jī*	hunger /ˈhʌŋgɚ/
821	* 思 田	思 心	*sī*	think /θɪŋk/ thought /θɔt/
822	偏 亻	偏 人	*piān*	*bias*
823-n636	嗜 口	嗜 口	*shì*	*like, fond of*
824-n637	* 异 已	異 田	*yì*	strange /strendʒ/
825	* 淡 氵	淡 水	*dàn*	bland /blænd/
826	* 甜 舌	甜 甘	*tián*	sweet /swit/
827	* 黏 和	黏 黍	*nián*	sticky /ˈstɪkɪ/
828	* 腻 月	膩 肉	*nì*	slimy /ˈslaɪmɪ/
829	* 酸 酉	酸 酉	*suān*	sour /saʊr/

830	* 咸 戊　鹹 鹵	*xián*	salty /ˈsɔltɪ/
831	* 苦 艹　苦 艸	*kǔ*	bitter /ˈbɪtɚ/

注 Notes:

1. The Chinese for thirst is 渴 *kě* or 口渴 *kǒu kě*. Very often, there is also an indication of whether the thirst causes increased fluid intake or not, since thirst with no desire for fluids is a sign of water-damp or static blood.

2. Chinese has a variety of expressions meaning 'poor appetite'. The most common expression in the ordinary language, 胃口不好 *wèi kǒu bù hǎo*, does not normally appear in Chinese medical texts. 食欲不振 *shí yù bú zhèn*, the term used in Western medicine, is commonly seen in modern texts. The terms traditionally used in Chinese medicine include 不思饮食 *bù sī yǐn shí*, no thought of food and drink, 饮食少思 *yǐn shí shǎo sī*, little thought of food and drink, and 纳谷不香 *nà gǔ bù xiāng*, no pleasure in eating. The last of these is of interest because the literal meaning is 'food taken in is not fragrant', describing a subjective feeling as an objective fact (compare also 'generalized heaviness').

3. The term 纳呆 *nà dāi* denotes indigestion and loss of appetite, sometimes with a sensation of bloating attributed to impairment of the stomach's governing of intake. This term is commonly seen in Chinese medical texts and since Western literature on Chinese medicine does not contain any terms that can be matched to the Chinese, we must suppose that translators render it loosely as 'indigestion' or 'loss of appetite'. In actual fact, no existing English term covers the range of symptoms included in the definition, or reflects etiology of the condition. For this reason, we render it as 'torpid intake'.

4. Inquiry about taste in the mouth is a feature of Chinese medicine. It apparently has its origins in the correspondences between the flavors and the five phases. In the diagnostic context, sweet taste in the mouth is 口甜 *kǒu tián*, rather than 口甘 *kǒu gān*. A bland taste in the mouth is 口淡 *kǒu dàn* or 口淡无味 *kǒu dàn wú wèi*. The character 淡, bland, has previously been encountered in the sense of 'pale'.

复合词 Compounds:

884. 口渴 *kǒu kě*, thirst
885. 口大渴 *kǒu dà kě*, great thirst
886. 大渴 *dà kě*, thirst
887. 口渴引饮 *kǒu kě yǐn yǐn*, thirst with taking of fluids
888. 大渴引饮 *dà kě yǐn yǐn*, great thirst with taking of fluids

889. 口渴喜饮 *kǒu kě xǐ yǐn*, thirst with a liking of fluids
890. 口渴多饮 *kǒu kě duō yǐn*, thirst with large fluid intake
891. 口渴不欲饮 *kǒu kě bú yù yǐn*, thirst with no desire for fluids
892. 口渴不多饮 *kǒu kě bù duō yǐn*, thirst without great intake of fluids
893. 渴喜凉饮 *kě xǐ liáng yǐn*, thirst with a liking for cool drinks
894. 食欲 *shí yù*, appetite
895. 纳谷 *nà gǔ*, food intake (lit. 'take in grain')
896. 纳呆 *nà dāi*, torpid intake
897. 食欲不振 *shí yù bú zhèn*, poor appetite
898. 不思饮食 *bù sī yǐn shí*, no thought of food and drink
899. 饮食少思 *yǐn shí shǎo sī*, little thought of food and drink
900. 纳谷不香 *nà gǔ bù xiāng*, no pleasure in eating (lit. 'food taken in not fragrant')
901. 饮食不喜 *yǐn shí bù xǐ*, no pleasure in eating and drinking
902. 纳谷减少 *nà gǔ jiǎn shǎo*, reduced food intake
903. 厌食 *yàn shí*, aversion to food
904. 食不下 *shí bú xià*, inability to get food down
905. 善食易饥 *shàn shí yì jī*, large appetite with rapid hungering
906. 喜食异物 *xǐ shí yì wù*, predilection for strange foods
907. 偏食异物 *piān shí yì wù*, predilection for strange foods
908. 偏嗜 *piān shì*, predilection for strange foods; predilection for certain foods
909. 嗜食甘 *shì shí gān*, predilection for sweet foods
910. 异嗜 *yì shì*, predilection for strange foods
911. 口甜 *kǒu tián*, sweet taste in the mouth
912. 口苦 *kǒu kǔ*, bitter taste in the mouth
913. 口酸 *kǒu suān*, sour taste in the mouth
914. 口咸 *kǒu xián*, salty taste in the mouth
915. 口淡 *kǒu dàn*, bland taste in the mouth
916. 口淡无味 *kǒu dàn wú wèi*, bland taste in the mouth
917. 口腻 *kǒu nì*, slimy sensation in the mouth
918. 口黏腻 *kǒu nián nì*, sticky slimy sensation in the mouth

第二节　第二十八组   **SECTION 2: SET 28**

问大便   **Inquiry About Stool**

832   * 便 亻 便 人   *biàn*   stool /stul/

833-n638	* 屎 尸	屎 尸	*shǐ*	stool /stul/
834	矢 丿	矢 矢	*shǐ*	*stool*
835	* 溏 氵	溏 水	*táng*	sloppy /ˈslɑpɪ/
836	* 薄 竹	薄 竹	*bó*	thin /θɪn/
837	* 鸭 鸟	鴨 鳥	*yā*	duck /ˈdʌk/
838-n639	* 泄 氵	泄 水	*xiè*	diarrhea /ˌdaɪəˈrɪə/
839-n640	* 泻 氵	瀉 水	*xiè*	diarrhea /ˌdaɪəˈrɪə/
840	失 丿	失 大	*shī*	*loss*
841-n641	禁 示	禁 示	*jìn*	*confinement*
842-n642	* 秘 禾	秘 禾	*bì*	constipation /ˌkɑnstɪˈpeʃən/
843	* 干 干	乾 乙	*gān*	dry /draɪ/
844	* 结 纟	結 糸	*jié*	bound /baʊnd/
845	* 秽 禾	穢 禾	*huì*	foul /faʊl/
846	* 脓 月	膿 肉	*nóng*	pus /pʌs/
847-n643	* 频 页	頻 頁	*pín*	frequent /ˈfrikwənt/
848	* 裂 衣	裂 衣	*liè*	splitting /ˈsplɪtɪŋ/

注 Notes:

1. Constipation: Chinese has a number of terms that approximate the English 'constipation'. The standard term, which is also the colloquial term, is 便秘 *biàn bì*. It seems to be agreed that 秘, meaning closed, tight, or secret, is pronounced as *bì*, but some people say the term with the pronunciation *mì*, which the character has in other contexts (e.g., 秘密 *mì mì*, secret). An expanded form of this term is 大便秘结 *dà biàn mì jié*, 'bound stool'. Other terms include 大便干结 *dà biàn gān jié*, 'dry bound stool', 大便不通 *dà biàn bù tōng*, 'fecal stoppage', and 腑气不通 *fù qì bù tōng*, 'stoppage of bowel qi'.

2. Diarrhea: The modern colloquial term is 拉肚子 *lā dù zi*, which interestingly has the literal meaning of 'drawing belly', but this is not normally seen in medical texts. The Western medical term 腹泻 *fù xiè* now commonly appears. The traditional standard term is 泄泻 *xiè xiè*, a combination of two close synonyms. 泄 *xiè* means pour, flow, discharge, and is explained in this context to mean remittent sloppy stool; 泻 *xiè* means flow, drain, and is explained in this context as meaning defecation like the pouring down of water. In compound terms expressing etiology such as 'cold diarrhea' and 'heat diarrhea', the two characters are reduced to one, the choice apparently being arbitrary (e.g., 寒泻 *hán xiè* or 寒泄 *hán xiè*).

复合词 Compounds:

919. 大便 *dà biàn*, stool

920. 粪便 *fèn biàn*, stool
921. 便秘 *biàn bì*, constipation
922. 大便不通 *dà biàn bù tōng*, fecal stoppage; constipation
923. 腑气不通 *fǔ qì bù tōng*, stoppage of bowel qi
924. 大便秘结 *dà biàn bì jié*, bound stool
925. 大便干结 *dà biàn gān jié*, dry bound stool
926. 大便艰难 *dà biàn jiān nán*, difficult defecation
927. 便难 *biàn nán*, difficult defecation
928. 排便不爽 *pái biàn bù shuǎng*, ungratifying defecation
929. 里急后重 *lǐ jí hòu zhòng*, tenesmus; abdominal urgency and rectal heaviness
930. 上吐下泻 *shàng tù xià xiè*, simultaneous vomiting and diarrhea
931. 大便失禁 *dà biàn shī jìn*, fecal incontinence
932. 腹痛则泄，泄后痛减 *fù tòng zé xiè, xiè hòu tòng jiǎn*, abdominal pain followed and relieved by diarrhea
933. 泄泻 *xiè xiè*, diarrhea
934. 久泄 *jiǔ xiè*, enduring diarrhea
935. 腹泻 *fù xiè*, diarrhea
936. 水泻 *shuǐ xiè*, water diarrhea
937. 大便脓血 *dà biàn nóng xuè*, stool containing pus and blood
938. 大便下血 *dà biàn xià xuè*, precipitation of blood with the stool
939. 便血 *biàn xuè*, bloody stool
940. 先便后血 *xiān biàn hòu xuè*, blood following stool
941. 先血后便 *xiān xuè hòu biàn*, stool following blood
942. 矢气多 *shǐ qì duō*, passing of flatus
943. 矢气频频 *shǐ qì pín pín*, frequent passing of flatus
944. 肛门灼热 *gāng mén zhuó rè*, scorching heat in the anus
945. 肛裂 *gāng liè*, splitting of the anus

第二节　第二十九组			**SECTION 2: SET 29**
问小便			**Inquiry About Urine**
849	* 尿 尸　尿 尸	*niào*	urine /ˈjurɪn/ urination /ˌjurɪˈneʃən/ voiding /ˈvɔɪdɪŋ/
850-n644	溺 氵　溺 水	*niào*	*urine, same as* 尿
851	便 亻　便 人	*biàn*	*urine, usually with* 小
852	* 长 丿　長 長	*cháng*	long /lɔŋ/

853	* 短 矢	短 矢	*duǎn*	short /ʃɔrt/
854	* 多 夕	多 夕	*duō*	copious /ˈkopɪəs/
855	* 少 小	少 小	*shǎo*	scant /skænt/
856	* 清 氵	清 水	*qīng*	clear /klɪr/
857-n645	* 夜 宀	夜 夕	*yè*	night /naɪt/
858	* 浊 氵	濁 水	*zhuó*	turbid /ˈtɜ·bɪd/
859	* 涩 氵	澀 水	*sè*	rough /rʌf/
				inhibited /ɪnˈhɪbɪtɪd/
860	* 频 页	頻 頁	*pín*	frequent /ˈfrikwənt/
861-n646	* 数 攵	數 攴	*shuò*	frequent /ˈfrikwənt/
862	* 刺 刂	刺 刀	*cì*	sting /stɪŋ/
863-n647	* 利 禾	利 刀	*lì*	uninhibited /ˌʌnɪnˈhɪbɪtɪd/
864-n648	* 畅 申	暢 日	*chàng*	uninhibited /ˌʌnɪnˈhɪbɪtɪd/
865	* 闭 门	閉 門	*bì*	block /blɑk/
866-n649	* 淋 氵	淋 水	*lín*	dribble /ˈdrɪbl̩/
867-n650	* 漓 氵	漓 水	*lí*	dribble /ˈdrɪbl̩/
868-n651	* 沥 氵	瀝 水	*lì*	dribble /ˈdrɪbl̩/
869-n652	遗 辶	遺 辵	*yí*	*loss, leak*

注 Notes:

1. The expression 小便 *xiǎo biàn* literally means 'lesser convenience', and stands in contrast to 大便 *dà biàn* 'greater convenience' (stool). Note that 便 standing alone most often refers to stool rather than urine, e.g., 便难 *biàn nán*, 'difficult defecation'.

2. Of interest among the terms describing urination are 小便清长 *xiǎo biàn qīng cháng*, 'long voidings of clear urine', and 小便短赤 *xiǎo biàn duǎn chì*, 'short voidings of reddish urine'. Traditionally, urine is not described in quantitative terms as in Western medicine (polyuria, oliguria), but in terms of the length of the urinary voiding. In general, this matter is neglected by translators who let themselves be guided by Western medical conceptions of urination rather than by the meaning of the Chinese terms. The point may be of trivial clinical significance.

复合词 Compounds:

946. 小便 *xiǎo biàn*, urine
947. 小便清长 *xiǎo biàn qīng cháng*, long voidings of clear urine
948. 小便短赤 *xiǎo biàn duǎn chì*, short voidings of reddish urine
949. 小便失禁 *xiǎo biàn shī jìn*, urinary incontinence

950. 小便淋赤刺痛 *xiǎo biàn lín chì cì tòng*, dribbling urination with reddish urine and stinging pain

951. 夜间多尿 *yè jiān duō niào*, profuse urination at night

952. 遗尿 *yí niào*, enuresis

953. 小便频数 *xiǎo biàn pín shuò*, frequent urination

954. 小便疼痛 *xiǎo biàn téng tòng*, painful urination

955. 小便热痛 *xiǎo biàn rè tòng*, painful voidings of hot urine

956. 小便涩痛 *xiǎo biàn sè tòng*, rough (inhibited) painful voidings

957. 尿后馀沥 *niào hòu yú lì*, dribble after voiding

958. 小便不利 *xiǎo biàn bú lì*, inhibited urination

959. 小便不畅 *xiǎo biàn bú chàng*, inhibited urination

960. 小便不通 *xiǎo biàn bù tōng*, urinary stoppage

961. 尿闭 *niào bì*, urinary block

962. 小便淋漓不禁 *xiǎo biàn lín lí bú jìn*, dribbling urinary incontinence

---

第二节　第组				**SECTION 2: SET 30**

问睡眠   **Inquiry About Sleep**

870-n653	* 睡目	睡目	*shuì*	sleep /slip/
871-n654	* 眠目	眠目	*mián*	sleep /slip/
872-n655	* 寐宀	寐宀	*mèi*	sleep /slip/
873	嗜口	嗜口	*shì*	*like, fond of*
874-n656	* 梦夕	夢夕	*mèng*	dreaming /ˈdrimɪŋ/

注 Notes:

1. The terms 不寐 *bú mèi* and 失眠 *shī mián* are the same in meaning. The former is the classical term, while the latter is used in Western medicine and in the modern spoken language.

2. The character 昏 *hūn* appears in a number of expressions: 昏厥 *hūn jué*, clouding reversal (loss of consciousness), 目昏 *mù hūn*, clouded vision, and, in the present set of terms, 昏睡 *hūn shuì*, clouding sleep. The latter term is equivalent to hypersomnia in Western medicine.

复合词 Compounds:

963. 嗜睡 *shì shuì*, somnolence

964. 昏睡 *hūn shuì*, clouding sleep

965. 多梦 *duō mèng*, profuse dreaming

966. 易醒 *yì xǐng*, tendency to wake up easily

967. 梦游 *mèng yóu*, dream walking, sleep walking

968. 不寐 *bú mèi*, sleeplessness

969. 失眠 *shī mián*, insomnia

第二节　第组				**SECTION 2: SET 31**

问神与情志				**Inquiry About the Spirit & Affect-Mind**
875	* 情 忄	情 心	*qíng*	affect /ˈæfɛkt/
876	* 志 士	志 心	*zhì*	mind /maɪnd/
877-n657	健 亻	健 人	*jiàn*	*constantly; fortify*
878-n658	* 忘 亡	忘 心	*wàng*	forget /fɚˈgɛt/
879	* 烦 火	煩 火	*fán*	vexation /vɛksˈeʃən/
880-n659	善 羊	善 口	*shàn*	*good at, tend to*
881	易 日	易 日	*yì*	*easy, easily, tend to*
882	* 喜 士	喜 口	*xǐ*	joy /dʒɔɪ/
883	* 忧 忄	憂 心	*yōu*	anxiety /æŋˈzaɪətɪ/
884	* 思 田	思 心	*sī*	thought /θɔt/
885	* 悲 非	悲 心	*bēi*	sorrow /ˈsɑro/
886	* 恐 心	恐 心	*kǒng*	fear /fɪr/
887	* 惊 忄	驚 馬	*jīng*	fright /fraɪt/
888-n660	* 郁 阝	鬱 鬯	*yù*	depression /dɪˈprɛʃən/
889	* 闷 门	悶 門	*mèn*	oppression /əˈprɛʃən/

注 Notes:

1. The 五志 *wǔ zhì*, the five minds, and 七情 *qī qíng*, the seven affects have already been discussed. Unnatural tendencies towards these are often expressed with the character 善, meaning 'good (at)', 'to tend to'.

2. Forgetfulness in Chinese is 健忘 *jiàn wàng*. The character 健 *jiàn* normally means healthy or strong. Further ahead, we will also encounter it in a related sense in the term 健脾 *jiàn pí*, to fortify the spleen, but here it means constantly or continually.

复合词 Compounds:

970. 健忘 *jiàn wàng*, forgetfulness

971. 心烦 *xīn fán*, vexation
972. 易惊 *yì jīng*, susceptibility to fright
973. 善惊 *shàn jīng*, susceptibility to fright
974. 善喜 *shàn xǐ*, tendency to joy
975. 善悲 *shàn bēi*, tendency to sorrow
976. 善恐 *shàn kǒng*, susceptibility to fear
977. 善怒 *shàn nù*, irascibility
978. 善忧思 *shàn yōu sī*, anxiety and preoccupation
979. 郁闷 *yù mèn*, depression

第二节　第组					**SECTION 2: SET 32**

问月经　　　　　　　　Inquiry About Menstruation

890-n661	* 月 月	月 肉	*yuè*	month /mʌnθ/
891	* 经 纟	經 糸	*jīng*	menstruation /ˌmɛnstruˈeʃən/ *n.*
				menstrual /ˈmɛnstruəl/ *adj.*
				menstrual flow /ˈmɛnstruəl ˈdɪflo/
892-n662	* 浅 氵	淺 水	*qiǎn*	light(-colored) /ˈlaɪtˌkʌləˈd/
893-n663	* 黯 黑	黯 黑	*àn*	dull /dʌl/
894	* 稠 禾	稠 禾	*chóu*	thick /θɪk/
895	* 黏 禾	黏 黍	*nián*	sticky /ˈstɪkɪ/
896-n664	期 月	期 肉	*qī*	*period*
897	定 宀	定 宀	*dìng*	*set, fixed*
898	行 彳	行 彳	*xíng*	*move, be in progress*
899	* 闭 门	閉 門	*bì*	block /blɑk/
900	* 淋 氵	淋 水	*lín*	dribble /ˈdrɪbl̩/
901	* 漓 氵	漓 水	*lí*	dribble /ˈdrɪbl̩/
902-n665	断 斤	斷 斤	*duàn*	*break, interrupt*

注 Notes:

1. In Chinese, menstruation is expressed as 月经 *yuè jīng*; 月 means 'month' (as does 'mens' in Latin); 经 means 'warp', and has extended meanings of 'constant', 'regular', 'pass along', 'undergo', 'channel', etc. It is also used alone in the specific sense of menstruation, as many of the examples below reveal. See also Channels and Network Vessels.

2. The expressions 过多 *guò duō* and 过少 *guò shǎo*, literally 'over much' and 'over little', are rendered here as 'profuse' and 'scant'.

复合词 Compounds:

980. 经色浅淡 *jīng sè qiǎn dàn*, light-colored menstrual flow
981. 经色深红 *jīng sè shēn hóng*, deep red menstrual flow
982. 经色紫黑 *jīng sè zǐ hēi*, purple-black menstrual flow
983. 经色紫黯 *jīng sè zǐ àn*, dark purple menstrual flow
984. 经血夹块 *jīng xuè jiā kuài*, clots in the menstrual flow; clotted menstrual flow
985. 经质黏稠 *jīng zhì nián chóu*, thick sticky menstrual flow
986. 经质清稀 *jīng zhì qīng xī*, thin clear menstrual flow
987. 经行先期 *jīng xíng xiān qí*, advanced menstruation
988. 经行后期 *jīng xíng hòu qí*, delayed menstruation
989. 经行先后无定期 *jīng xíng xiān hòu wú dìng qí*, menstruation at irregular intervals
990. 经痛 *jīng tòng*, menstrual pain
991. 经来小腹胀痛 *jīng lái xiǎo fù zhàng tòng*, smaller-abdominal distention and pain during menstruation
992. 月经过多 *yuè jīng guò duō*, profuse menstruation
993. 月经过少 *yuè jīng guò shǎo*, scant menstruation
994. 月经大下不止 *yuè jīng dà xià bù zhǐ*, continual heavy menstrual flow
995. 月经淋漓不断 *yuè jīng lín lí bú duàn*, continual dribbling menstrual flow

---

第二节　第组	**SECTION 2: SET 33**

问带下	**Inquiry About Vaginal Discharge**

903	* 带 巾　带 巾　*dài*	vaginal discharge /ˈvædʒɪnl̩ (vəˈdʒaɪnl̩) ˈdɪstʃɑrdʒ/

注 Note:

In Chinese, 白带 *bái dài* is used in Western medicine as the equivalent of leukorrhea, and is used in the modern common language to denote vaginal discharge in general. Chinese medicine distinguishes vaginal discharges of different colors. The term leukorrhea, whose literal meaning is 'white flow', is therefore an unsuitable equivalent for any other than white vaginal discharge.

复合词 Compounds:

996. 白带 *bái dài*, white vaginal discharge; vaginal discharge
997. 带下色白 *dài xià sè bái*, white vaginal discharge
998. 带下色黄 *dài xià sè huáng*, yellow vaginal discharge
999. 带下色青 *dài xià sè qīng*, green-blue vaginal discharge
1000. 带下色赤白 *dài xià sè chì bái*, red and white vaginal discharge
1001. 带下清稀 *dài xià qīng xī*, clear thin vaginal discharge
1002. 带下黏稠 *dà xià nián chóu*, thick sticky vaginal discharge
1003. 带下量多 *dài xià liàng duō*, copious vaginal discharge
1004. 带下味腥 *dài xià wèi xīng*, fishy-smelling vaginal discharge
1005. 带下臭秽 *dài xià chòu huì*, foul-smelling vaginal discharge

---

第二节　第组					**SECTION 2: SET 34**

问男人　　　　　　　　　　**Inquiry for Men**

904-n666	* 男 田	男 田	*nán*	man /mæn/ *n.*
				male /mel/ *adj.*
905	* 精 米	精 米	*jīng*	semen /ˈsimən/ *n.*
				seminal /ˈsɛmɪnl̩/ *adj.*
906-n667	* 射 身	射 寸	*shè*	shoot /ʃut/
907	* 失 丿	失 大	*shī*	loss /lɔs/
908-n668	* 泄 氵	洩 水	*xiè*	ejaculate /ɪˈdʒækjuˌlet/ *vi.*
				ejaculation /ɪˌdʒækjuˈleʃən/ *n.*
909	* 遗 辶	遺 辶	*yí*	emission /ɪˈmɪʃən/
910	* 交 亠	交 亠	*jiāo*	intercourse /ˈɪntɚkors/
911-n669	挟 扌	挾 手	*jiā*	*clasp, contain*
912	* 萎 艹	萎 艸	*wěi*	wilt /wɪlt/
913	* 痿 疒	痿 疒	*wěi*	wilt /wɪlt/
914	* 缩 纟	縮 糸	*suō*	retracted /rɪˈtræktɪd/
915-n670	* 瘙 疒	瘙 疒	*sào*	itch /ɪtʃ/
916	* 痒 疒	癢 疒	*yǎng*	itch /ɪtʃ/
917	* 茎 艹	莖 艸	*jīng*	penis /ˈpinɪs/
918	* 睾 丿	睾 目	*gāo*	testicle /ˈtɛstɪkl̩/
919	* 囊 亠	囊 口	*náng*	scrotum /ˈskrotəm/
920-n671	* 事 一	事 亅	*shì*	matter /ˈmætɚ/
921	举 丶	舉 臼	*jǔ*	*rise*

注 Notes:

1. The term 阳痿, 'yáng wilt', i.e., impotence, can also be written as 阳萎. Further synonyms include 阴痿 *yīn wěi* and 阳事不举 *yáng shì bù jǔ* the 'male matter failing to rise'. In the last term, the 'yáng matter' (事 is affair, matter, business) refers to the penis. All of these terms, including the English impotence, are euphemistic in the sense that they do not spell out the problem completely.

2. Chinese medicine makes a distinction between seminal emission while dreaming, and seminal emission without dreaming. The English 'wet dreams', despite its literal meaning, loosely refers to any form of seminal emission during sleep, and is therefore imprecise in the Chinese medical context.

复合词 Compounds:

1006. 阳萎 *yáng wěi*, 'yáng wilt'; impotence

1007. 阳痿 *yáng wěi*, 'yáng wilt'; impotence

1008. 阴痿 *yīn wěi*, 'yīn wilt'; impotence

1009. 阳事不举 *yáng shì bù jǔ*, the 'male matter failing to rise'; impotence

1010. 阳事易举 *yáng shì yì jǔ*, 'frequent rising of the male matter'; frequent erections

1011. 早泄 *zǎo xiè*, premature ejaculation

1012. 遗精 *yí jīng*, seminal emission

1013. 小便挟精 *xiǎo biàn jiá jīng*, semen in the urine

1014. 血精 *xuè jīng*, bloody semen

1015. 精液清冷 *jīng yè qīng lěng*, clear cold semen

1016. 不射精 *bú shè jīng*, inability to ejaculate

1017. 阴举不衰 *yīn jǔ bù shuāi*, persistent erection

1018. 阴冷 *yīn lěng*, genital cold

1019. 阴缩 *yīn suō*, retracted genitals

1020. 茎中痛痒 *jīng zhōng tòng yǎng*, pain and itching in the penis

1021. 睾丸胀痛 *gāo wán zhàng tòng*, distention and pain of the testicles

1022. 阴囊瘙痒 *yīn náng sāo yǎng*, scrotal itch

1023. 梦遗 *mèng yí*, dream emission

1024. 不梦而遗 *bú mèng ér yí*, seminal emission without dreaming

1025. 无梦而遗 *wú mèng ér yí*, seminal emission without dreaming

1026. 梦交失精 *mèng jiāo shī jīng*, seminal loss while dreaming of intercourse

1027. 梦失精 *mèng shī jīng*, seminal loss while dreaming

习题 Exercise:

248. *pà lěng* ....

249. abhorrence of cold ....

250. 憎寒壮热 ....

251. *wèi wù fēng hán* ....

252. physical cold and cold limbs ....

253. 寒热往来 ....

254. *cháo rè* ....

255. late afternoon tidal heat [effusion] ....

256. 无汗 ....

257. *hàn duō* ....

258. shiver sweating ....

259. 自汗 ....

260. *dào hàn* ....

261. dizzy head ....

262. 目眩 ....

263. *tóu zhòng* ....

264. head heavy as if swathed ....

265. 头摇 ....

266. *mù tòng* ....

267. dizzy vision ....

268. 目涩 ....

269. *shì yī wéi èr* ....

270. tearing ....

271. 耳痛 ....

272. *bí tòng* ....

273. sore throat ....

274. 倦怠 ....

275. *pí láo* ....

276. fatigued body and lack of strength ....

277. 食后困顿 ....

278. *zhōu shēn suān chǔ* ....

279. fatigued limbs and lack of strength ....

280. 背痛 ....

281. *yāo xī wú lì* ....

282. limp aching lumbus and knees ....

283. 胸痛 ....

284. *xiōng mèn* ....

285. chest and rib-side fullness ....

286. 胸胁胀满 ....

287. *xié lè yǐn tòng* ....

288. hypertonicity of both rib-sides ....

289. 心下悸 ....

290. *è nì* ....

291. nausea ....

292. 吐衄 ....

293. *tòng yǒu dìng chù* ....

294. scurrying pain ....

295. 绕脐痛 ....

296. *shào fù tòng* ....

297. rumbling intestines ....

298. 口渴 ....

299. *kǒu kě yǐn yǐn* ....

300. thirst with a liking of fluids ....

301. 口渴不多饮 ....

302. *shí yù bú zhèn* ....

303. no thought of food and drink ....

304. 喜食异物 ....

305. *piān shì* ....

306. sour taste in the mouth ....

307. 口腻 ....

308. What are the two English equivalents of 淡 that have been encountered so far? ....

309. *dà biàn* ....

310. stool ....

311. 大便不通 ....

312. *biàn nán* ....

313. simultaneous vomiting and diarrhea ....

314. 大便失禁 ....

315. *xiè xiè* ....

316. water diarrhea ....

317. 便血 ....

318. *shǐ qì pín pín* ....

319. urine ....

320. 小便短赤 ....

321. *xiǎo biàn lín chì cì tòng* ....

322. frequent urination ....

323. 尿后馀沥 ....

324. *xiǎo biàn bù tōng* ....

325. dribbling urinary incontinence ....

326. 易醒 ....

327. *shī mián* ....

328. forgetfulness ....

329. 心烦 ....

330. *shàn yōu sī* ....

331. depression ....

332. 经血挟块 ....

333. *yuè jīng guò duō* ....

334. scant menstruation ....

335. 经行先期 ....

336. *jīng xíng xiān hòu wú dìng qí* ....

337. aversion to wind ....

338. 带下色黄 ....

339. *dài xià sè qīng* ....

340. thick sticky vaginal discharge ....

341. 带下味腥 ....

342. *yáng wěi* ....

343. premature ejaculation ....

344. 遗精 ....

切诊
Palpation

切脉 **Pulse-Taking**

第二节　第组	**SECTION 2: SET 35**

切脉 | **Pulse-Taking**

922		切 刀	切 刀	*qiē*	*take*
923	*	脉 月	脈 肉	*mài*	pulse /pʌls/
924-n672	*	按 扌	按 手	*àn*	press /prɛs/
925-n673	*	把 扌	把 手	*bǎ*	take /tek/
926	*	诊 讠	診 言	*zhěn*	examine /ɪgzˈæmɪn/
927-n674	*	持 扌	持 手	*chí*	take /tek/
928-n675	*	跗 扌	跗 足	*fū*	instep /ˈɪnstɛp/
929-n676	*	候 亻	候 人	*hòu*	indicator /ˈɪndɪketɚ/
930-n677		迎 辶	迎 辵	*yíng*	*predict*
931	*	寸 寸	寸 寸	*cùn*	inch /ɪntʃ/
					cun /tswʊn/
932	*	口 口	口 口	*kǒu*	opening /ˈopənɪŋ/
933	*	关 丷	關 門	*guān*	bar /bɑr/
934	*	尺 尺	尺 尸	*chǐ*	cubit /ˈkjubɪt/
935-n678	*	左 𠂇	左 工	*zuǒ*	left /lɛft/
936-n679	*	右 𠂇	右 口	*yòu*	right /raɪt/

注 Notes:

1. The term 脉 *mài* is translated in the present context as 'pulse'. In the context of the channels and network vessels, it is translated as 'vessel'.

2. In ancient times, the pulse was not only felt at the wrist but also at 'man's prognosis', the pulsating vessel at the sides of the neck, and the 'instep yáng' on the dorsum of the foot. In the term 人迎 *rén yíng*, man's prognosis, the character 迎 *yíng*, better known to most in the sense of ' to meet' or 'to welcome', is understood as the fate the patient is expected to 'meet'.

3. The term 三部九候 *sān bù jiǔ hòu*, three positions and nine indicators, has two definitions. In the context of the wrist pulse, the inch, bar, and cubit are the three positions, and the superficial level, midlevel, and deep level of each of these are the nine indicators. According to an older theory that is now rarely applied, the head, upper limbs, and lower limbs are the three positions, each area having three pulse points (indicators), which in most cases can be located by the acupuncture point found at the site.

Head
 Greater Yáng (*tài yáng*)
 TB-21 (*ěr mén*, Ear Gate)
 ST-4 (*dì cāng*, Earth Granary)
 ST-5 (*dà yíng*, Great Reception)

Upper limbs
 wrist pulse
 HT-7 (*shén mén*, Spirit Gate)
 LI-4 (*hé gǔ*, Union Valley)

Lower limbs
 LV-10 (*zú wǔ lǐ*, Foot Five Li) in men
 LV-3 (*tài chōng*, Supreme Surge) in women
 SP-11 (*jī mén*, Winnower Gate)
 ST-42 (*chōng yáng*, Surging Yáng)
 KI-3 (*tài xī*, Great Ravine)

4. 寸 *cùn*, inch, 关 *guān*, bar, and 尺 *chǐ*, cubit, are three positions of the pulse. 寸 *cùn*, inch and 尺 *chǐ*, cubit, are two units of length, the 尺 being equal to ten 寸. The inch position is so called because it is located close to the high bone (高骨 *gāo gǔ*, i.e., the styloid process of the radius), which is one Chinese inch behind (proximal to) fish margin (鱼际 *yú jì*, i.e., the thenar eminance). Another suggestion, from the *Nàn Jīng*, is that it is 9 tenths of an inch (9 fēn) in length. The Chinese 尺 *chǐ* is usually associated with the English 'foot', however, it does not derive, as the English 'foot', from the lower extremity of the body, and some scholars think that it originally meant the distance from the elbow to the wrist. The use of the word in Chinese medicine provides a little confirmation of this view. The 尺 *chǐ* pulse position is so called because it is one 尺 from the point 尺泽 on the transverse crease of the elbow. Furthermore, the area surface of the flesh between the wrist pulse and the elbow is called the 尺肤 *chǐ fū*, cubit skin. The English word 'cubit' denotes an old unit of length based on the length of the forearm, usually from the elbow to the tip of the middle finger. It is derived from the Latin *cubitum*, elbow. 'Cubit' therefore appears to be a more appropriate translation for 尺

than 'foot'. Finally, the bar position is so called because it separates the inch from the cubit.

5. 斜飞脉 *xié fēi mài*, oblique-running pulse, and 反关脉 *fǎn guān mài*, pulse on the back of the wrist, refer to anomalies in the pathway of the blood vessel at which the wrist pulse is felt.

复合词 Compounds:

1028. 把脉 *bǎ mài*, take the pulse, pulse-taking
1029. 持脉 *chí mài*, hold the pulse
1030. 按脉 *àn mài*, press the pulse
1031. 诊脉 *zhěn mài*, examine the pulse
1032. 脉诊 *mài zhěn*, pulse examination
1033. 候脉 *hòu mài*, examine the pulse; pulse examination
1034. 气口 *qì kǒu*, wrist pulse
1035. 寸口 *cùn kǒu*, inch opening; wrist pulse
1036. 寸脉 *cùn mài*, inch pulse, cun pulse
1037. 关脉 *guān mài*, bar pulse
1038. 尺脉 *chǐ mài*, cubit pulse
1039. 三部九候 *sān bù jiǔ hòu*, three positions and nine indicators
1040. 跌阳脉 *fū yáng mài*, instep yáng pulse
1041. 人迎 *rén yíng*, man's prognosis
1042. 人迎脉 *rén yíng mài*, man's prognosis pulse
1043. 斜飞脉 *xié fēi mài*, oblique-running pulse
1044. 反关脉 *fǎn guān mài*, pulse on the back of the wrist

第二节　第组				**SECTION 2: SET 36**

脉象　　　　　　　　　　　　　　　Pulses

937-n680	象 刀	象 豕	*xiàng*	*appearance, sign*
938	* 浮 氵	浮 水	*fú*	floating /ˈfloʊtɪŋ/
939-n681	* 沉 氵	沉 水	*chén*	sunken /ˈsʌŋkən/ deep /dip/
940-n682	* 迟 辶	遲 辵	*chí*	slow /sloʊ/
941	* 数 攵	數 攴	*shuò*	rapid /ˈræpɪd/
942-n683	* 虚 虍	虛 虍	*xū*	vacuous /ˈvækjuəs/
943-n684	* 实 宀	實 宀	*shí*	replete /rɪˈplit/
944	* 滑 氵	滑 水	*huá*	slippery /ˈslɪpərɪ/
945	* 涩 氵	澀 水	*sè*	rough /rʌf/

946	* 弦 弓	弦 弓	*xián*	stringlike /ˈstrɪŋlaɪk/
947	* 濡 氵	濡 水	*rú*	soggy /ˈsɒgɪ/
948-n685	* 洪 氵	洪 水	*hóng*	surging /ˈsɝdʒɪŋ/
949	* 微 彳	微 彳	*wēi*	faint /feɪnt/
950	* 细 纟	細 糸	*xì*	fine /faɪn/
951	* 弱 弓	弱 弓	*ruò*	weak /wik/
952	* 大 大	大 大	*dà*	large /lɑrdʒ/
953-n686	* 散 夂	散 攴	*sàn*	dissipated /ˈdɪsɪpetɪd/ scattered /ˈskætɚd/
954-n687	* 紧 纟	緊 糸	*jǐn*	tight /taɪt/
955-n688	* 芤 艹	芤 艸	*kōu*	scallion-stalk /ˈskæljən,stɔk/
956-n689	* 革 革	革 革	*gé*	drumskin /ˈdrʌmskɪn/
957-n690	* 牢 宀	牢 牛	*láo*	confined /kənˈfaɪnd/
958-n691	* 疾 疒	疾 疒	*jí*	racing /ˈresɪŋ/
959	* 动 力	動 力	*dòng*	stirred /stɝd/
960-n692	* 伏 亻	伏 人	*fú*	hidden /ˈhɪdn̩/
961-n693	* 缓 纟	緩 糸	*huǎn*	moderate /ˈmɑdərət/
962	* 促 亻	促 人	*cù*	skipping /ˈskɪpɪŋ/
963	* 结 纟	結 糸	*jié*	bound /baʊnd/
964-n694	* 代 亻	代 人	*dài*	intermittent /ˌɪntɚˈmɪtənt/
965	* 长 丿	長 長	*cháng*	long /lɔŋ/
966	* 短 矢	短 矢	*duǎn*	short /ʃɔrt/
967	* 力 力	力 力	*lì*	force /fɔrs, fors/
968	* 软 车	軟 車	*ruǎn*	soft /sɔft/
969-n695	* 钩 钅	鉤 金	*gōu*	hook /hʊk/
970	* 毛 毛	毛 毛	*máo*	down /daʊn/
971	* 石 石	石 石	*shí*	stone /ston/
972	* 合 人一口	合 口	*hé*	combine /kəmˈbaɪn/ *vt, vi.* combination /ˌkɑmbɪˈneʃən/ *n.*

注 Notes:

1. The term 脉象 *mài xiàng* literally means 'pulse manifestation'. It refers to any pulse (type) such as 'floating pulse' or 'large pulse'.

2. The term 数脉 *shuò mài* is here translated as 'rapid pulse'. In the term 小便频数 *xiǎo biàn pín shuò*, it was translated as 'frequent'. Its opposite, the 迟脉 *chí mài*, is the slow pulse, 迟 *chí* literally meaning delayed or tardy.

3. 洪脉 *hóng mài* is here translated as 'surging pulse'. In English texts, it is often called a 'flooding pulse'. In Chinese, 洪水 *hóng shuǐ* means 'flood'.

However, the English word flood implies an excessive amount of water expanding over land; its literal meaning is closer to the Chinese 泛 *fàn*. The Chinese 洪 implies a great swell of water along the pathway of a river, and in the context of the pulse this image is more accurately captured by 'surging'.

4. English pulse terminology varies considerably. The 迟脉 *chí mài* is called 'slow' by some and 'retarded' by others; 数脉 *shuò mài* is called 'rapid' by some and 'frequent' by others. 沉脉 *chén mài* is called 'deep' by some and 'sunken' by others; 洪脉 *hóng mài* is called 'flooding' by some and 'surging' by others; 涩脉 *sè mài* is called 'rough' by some and 'choppy' by others.

Distinctions between terms are easily lost. The terms 弱 *ruò* and 无力 *wú lì* in pulse descriptions are here rendered as 'weak' and 'forceless', respectively. These English terms, as indeed the Chinese terms, are not as synonymous as they would appear. A forceless pulse is one lacking in strength, whereas a weak pulse is one that not only lacks in strength, but is also sunken, and according to some definitions, is also fine. The stringlike pulse (弦脉 *xián mài*) should not be confused with the fine pulse (细脉 *xì mài*). The stringlike pulse is one that is long and taut and feels like a zither string to the touch, and that is associated with diseases of the liver and gallbladder, and in particular with ascendant liver yáng. The fine pulse is one that feels like a well-defined thread under the fingers, and that indicates dual vacuity of qi and blood, or of yīn and yáng, and in particular points to blood and yīn vacuity. The term 'thready pulse' commonly used by Western students and practitioners could theoretically be applied to both.

5. Pulse descriptions take two forms. Standard pulses are usually described in qualifier-qualified construction (e.g., 浮脉, floating pulse). Descriptions of combined pulses usually take the form of qualified-qualifier (e.g., 脉浮紧有力 *mài fú jǐn yǒu lì*). See Part I.

6. The term 小脉 *xiǎo mài*, which normally appears only in older literature, is synonymous with 细脉 *xì mài*, fine pulse, and is the opposite of the 大脉 *dà mài*, large pulse.

复合词 Compounds:

1045. 脉象 *mài xiàng*, pulse manifestation, pulse
1046. 正常脉 *zhèng cháng mài*, normal pulse
1047. 常脉 *cháng mài*, normal pulse
1048. 病脉 *bìng mài*, morbid pulse
1049. 浮脉 *fú mài*, floating pulse
1050. 沉脉 *chén mài*, sunken pulse, deep pulse
1051. 迟脉 *chí mài*, slow pulse
1052. 数脉 *shuò mài*, rapid pulse

1053. 虚脉 *xū mài*, vacuous pulse

1054. 实脉 *shí mài*, replete pulse

1055. 滑脉 *huá mài*, slippery pulse

1056. 涩脉 *sè mài*, rough pulse

1057. 弦脉 *xián mài*, stringlike pulse

1058. 濡脉 *rú mài*, soggy pulse

1059. 洪脉 *hóng mài*, surging pulse

1060. 微脉 *wēi mài*, faint pulse

1061. 细脉 *xì mài*, fine pulse

1062. 小脉 *xiǎo mài*, small pulse

1063. 弱脉 *ruò mài*, weak pulse

1064. 大脉 *dà mài*, large pulse

1065. 散脉 *sàn mài*, dissipated pulse

1066. 紧脉 *jǐn mài*, tight pulse

1067. 芤脉 *kōu mài*, scallion-stalk pulse

1068. 革脉 *gé mài*, drumskin pulse

1069. 牢脉 *láo mài*, confined pulse

1070. 疾脉 *jí mài*, racing pulse

1071. 动脉 *dòng mài*, stirred pulse

1072. 伏脉 *fú mài*, hidden pulse

1073. 缓脉 *huǎn mài*, moderate pulse

1074. 促脉 *cù mài*, skipping pulse, rapid irregularly interrupted pulse

1075. 结脉 *jié mài*, bound pulse

1076. 代脉 *dài mài*, regularly interrupted pulse

1077. 长脉 *cháng mài*, long pulse

1078. 短脉 *duǎn mài*, short pulse

1079. 相兼脉象 *xiāng jiān mài xiàng*, combined pulses

1080. 躁疾脉 *zào jí mài*, agitated racing pulse

1081. 脉微欲绝 *mài wēi yù jué*, a faint pulse verging on expiration

1082. 脉豁大无力 *mài huò dà wú lì*, a forceless large gaping pulse

1083. 脉细软无力 *mài xì ruǎn wú lì*, a forceless soft fine pulse

1084. 脉细 *mài xì*, a fine pulse

1085. 脉数 *mài shuò*, a rapid pulse

1086. 脉软 *mài ruǎn*, a soft pulse

1087. 脉濡软 *mài rú ruǎn*, a soft soggy pulse

1088. 脉细数 *mài xì shuò*, a fine rapid pulse

1089. 脉弦紧 *mài xián jǐn*, a tight stringlike pulse

1090. 脉弦滑 *mài xián huá*, a slippery stringlike pulse

1091. 脉弦细 *mài xián xì*, a fine stringlike pulse

1092. 脉滑数 *mài huá shuò*, a slippery rapid pulse
1093. 脉浮数 *mài fú shuò*, a rapid floating pulse
1094. 脉迟而紧 *mài chí ér jǐn*, a tight slow pulse
1095. 脉弦紧迟沉 *mài xián jǐn chén chí*, a sunken slow tight stringlike pulse
1096. 脉洪数有力 *mài hóng shuò yǒu lì*, a forceful rapid surging pulse
1097. 脉细数无力 *mài xì shuò wú lì*, a forceless rapid fine pulse
1098. 脉洪大而数 *mài hóng dà ér shuō*, a rapid large surging pulse
1099. 脉沉滑 *mài chén huá*, a slippery sunken pulse
1100. 脉沉弦 *mài chén xián*, a stringlike sunken pulse
1101. 脉沉实有力 *mài chén shí yǒu lì*, a forceful replete sunken pulse
1102. 脉濡数 *mài rú shuò*, a rapid soggy pulse
1103. 脉细而数 *mài xì ér shuò*, a fine rapid pulse
1104. 春脉弦 *chūn mài xián*, the spring pulse is stringlike
1105. 夏脉钩 *xià mài gōu*, the summer pulse is hooklike (surging)
1106. 秋脉毛 *qiū mài máo*, the autumn pulse is downy (floating)
1107. 冬脉石 *dōng mài shí*, the winter pulse is stonelike (sunken)
1108. 肝脉弦 *gān mài xián*, the liver pulse is stringlike
1109. 心脉洪 *xīn mài hóng*, the heart pulse is surging
1110. 两尺脉沉 *liǎng chǐ mài chén*, a sunken pulse at both cubits; a pulse that is sunken at both cubits
1111. 右关脉弱 *yòu guān mài ruò*, a weak right bar pulse; a pulse that is weak at the right bar
1112. 左寸脉沉而无力 *zuǒ cùn mài chén ér wú lì*, a forceless sunken left inch pulse; a pulse that is sunken and forceless at the left inch
1113. 重按无力 *zhòng àn wú lì*, forceless under heavy pressure
1114. 脾脉缓 *pí mài huǎn*, the spleen pulse is moderate
1115. 肺脉浮 *fèi mài fú*, the lung pulse is floating
1116. 肾脉沉 *shèn mài chén*, the kidney pulse is sunken

按诊　**Body Palpation**

第二节　第组	**SECTION 2: SET 37**

按诊				**Body Palpation**
973	* 按 扌　按 手	*àn*	palpate /pæl'pet/ press /prɛs/ *vt.* pressure /'prɛʃər/ *n.*
974	久 丿　久 丿	*jiǔ*	*for a long time, enduring, prolonged*

975-n696	*	甚 一	甚 甘	*shèn*	pronounced /prə'naʊnst/
976-n697	*	柔 矛	柔 木	*róu*	soft /sɔft/
977		甲 田	甲 田	*jiǎ*	*scale*
978		错 钅	錯 金	*cuò*	*wrong, deranged*
979		近 辶	近 辵	*jìn*	*near; approach, get near*
980		即 艮	即 卩	*jí*	*then, immediately*
981		清 氵	清 水	*qīng*	*cool*
982	*	欠 欠	欠 欠	*qiàn*	lack /læk/
983	*	逆 辶	逆 辵	*nì*	counterflow /ˈkaʊntəˌflo/
984	*	厥 厂	厥 厂	*jué*	reversal /rɪˈvɝsl̩/
985	*	痞 疒	痞 疒	*pǐ*	glomus /ˈgloməs/
986	*	块 土	塊 土	*kuài*	lump /lʌmp/
987	*	喜 士	喜 口	*xǐ*	like /laɪk/
988-n698	*	拒 扌	拒 手	*jù*	reject /rɪˈdʒɛkt/
989-n699	*	坚 土	堅 土	*jiān*	hard /hɑrd/
990-n700	*	硬 石	硬 石	*yìng*	hard /hɑrd/
991-n701	*	窅 穴	窅 穴	*yǎo*	pit /pɪt/
992-n702	*	没 氵	沒 水	*mò*	engulf /ɪnˈgʌlf/
993-n703		举 丶	舉 臼	*jǔ*	*lift*
994-n704		起 走	起 走	*qǐ*	*rise*
995	*	凹 丨	凹 凵	*āo*	pit /pɪt/
996		陷 阝	陷 阜	*xiàn*	*fall, collapse, sink*

注 Notes:

1. The Chinese 按 usually means to press or to apply pressure. In the context of the four examinations, it includes the idea of light touch (such as to detect warmth or cold).

2. Note the construction exemplified by 按之柔软 *àn zhī róu ruǎn*, literally, 'press it and it is soft', i.e., it feels soft under pressure. A similar construction is seen in 轻按即痛 *qīng àn jí tòng*, literally 'press (it) lightly, then (it) immediately hurts', i.e., painful at the slightest pressure. Again, 按之凹陷，举手即起 *àn zhī āo xiàn, jǔ shǒu jí qǐ* literally means 'press it and it pits, lift it and it comes straight up', i.e., pitting that disappears as soon as pressure is released.

3. The Chinese 窅 *yǎo* corresponds to the English 'pitting' in the examination of swelling. It is also expressed with the compound 凹陷 *āo xiàn*, previously rendered as 'hollow' in inspection of the abdomen.

4. The character 欠 *qiàn* means to lack. It has previously appeared in this text in the less common sense of to yawn (呵欠 *hē qiàn*).

5. The terms 四肢厥冷 *sì zhī jué lěng*, reversal cold of the limbs, and 四肢逆冷 *sì zhī nì lěng*, counterflow cold of the limbs, are identical in meaning. 厥 *jué* and 逆 *nì* both mean an ebbing of the normal outward flow of qì to the extremities.

复合词 Compounds:

1117. 按肌肤 *àn jī fū*, palpation of the skin
1118. 肌肤干燥 *jī fū gān zào*, dry skin
1119. 肌肤甲错 *jī fū jiǎ cuò*, encrusted skin
1120. 初按甚热，久按热反转轻 *chū àn shèn rè, jiǔ àn rè fǎn zhuǎn qīng*, pronounced heat on initial palpation that becomes less pronounced on prolonged palpation
1121. 按手足 *àn shǒu zú*, palpation of the limbs
1122. 手背热 *shǒu bèi rè*, heat in the backs of the hands
1123. 手足心烦热 *shǒu zú xīn fán rè*, vexing heat in the heart of the palms and soles
1124. 手足心热 *shǒu zú xīn rè*, heat in the (heart of the) palms and soles
1125. 四肢不温 *sì zhī bù wēn*, lack of warmth in the limbs
1126. 手足不温 *shǒu zú bù wēn*, lack of warmth in the extremities
1127. 四肢欠温 *sì zhī qiàn wēn*, lack of warmth in the limbs
1128. 手足寒 *shǒu zú hán*, cold extremities
1129. 四肢清冷 *sì zhī qīng lěng*, cold limbs
1130. 手足清冷 *shǒu zú qīng lěng*, cold extremities
1131. 四肢厥冷 *sì zhī jué lěng*, reversal cold of the limbs
1132. 手足厥寒 *shǒu zú jué hán*, reversal cold of the extremities
1133. 手足寒厥 *shǒu zú hán jué*, cold reversal in the extremities
1134. 手足厥冷 *shǒu zú jué lěng*, reversal cold of the extremities
1135. 手足厥 *shǒu zú jué*, reversal of the extremities
1136. 四肢逆冷 *sì zhī nì lěng*, counterflow cold of the limbs
1137. 手足逆冷 *shǒu zú nì lěng*, counterflow cold of the extremities
1138. 手足逆寒 *shǒu zú nì hán*, counterflow cold of the extremities
1139. 按之窅而不起 *àn zhī yǎo ér bù qǐ*, pitting when pressure is applied
1140. 按之没指 *àn zhī mò zhǐ*, engulfs the fingers when pressure is applied
1141. 按之凹陷，举手即起 *àn zhī āo xiàn, jǔ shǒu jí qǐ*, pitting that disappears as soon as pressure is released
1142. 按胸腹 *àn xiōng fù*, palpation of the chest and abdomen
1143. 腹中痞块 *fù zhōng pǐ kuài*, abdominal lump glomus
1144. 腹痛拒按 *fù tòng jù àn*, abdominal pain that rejects pressure
1145. 腹痛喜按 *fù tòng xǐ àn*, abdominal pain that likes pressure

1146. 按之柔软 *àn zhī róu ruǎn*, (feels) soft under pressure
1147. 按之坚硬 *àn zhī jiān yìng*, (feels) hard under pressure
1148. 按之疼痛 *àn zhī téng tòng*, (feels) painful under pressure
1149. 按之有痞块 *àn zhī yǒu pǐ kuài*, lump glomus that can be felt under pressure
1150. 痛不可近 *tòng bù kě jìn*, pain exacerbated by the slightest pressure (lit. '[so] painful [that one] cannot get near [it]')
1151. 轻按即痛 *qīng àn jí tòng*, painful at the slightest pressure

习题 Exercise:

347. 寸、关、尺 ....
348. *yòu chǐ* ....
349. left inch ....
350. 把脉 ....
351. *fǎn guān mài* ....
352. wrist pulse ....
353. 动脉 ....
354. *fú mài* ....
355. normal pulse ....
356. 大脉 ....
357. *sàn mài* ....
358. floating pulse ....
359. 迟脉 ....
360. *shuò mài* ....
361. faint pulse ....
362. 濡脉 ....
363. *gān mài xián* ....
364. heart pulse is surging ....
365. 脾脉缓 ....
366. *cù mài* ....
367. vacuous pulse ....
368. 实脉 ....
369. *huá mài* ....
370. rough pulse ....

371. 弦脉 ....

372. *hóng mài* ....

373. sunken pulse, deep pulse ....

374. 细脉 ....

375. *mài xiǎo* ....

376. weak pulse ....

377. 紧脉 ....

378. *kōu mài* ....

379. calm pulse ....

380. 长脉 ....

381. *bìng mài* ....

382. drumskin pulse ....

383. 牢脉 ....

384. *jí mài* ....

385. moderate pulse ....

386. 结脉 ....

387. *dài mài* ....

388. short pulse ....

389. 脉洪大而数 ....

390. *mài chén huá* ....

391. a stringlike sunken pulse ....

392. 脉数 ....

393. *mài chén huá* ....

394. a forceful replete sunken pulse ....

395. 脉濡数 ....

396. *mài fú* ....

397. a forceless fine rapid pulse ....

398. 寸微，关滑，尺带数 ....

399. *zuǒ guān mài xián* ....

400. a slippery floating right inch pulse; a pulse that is floating and slippery at the right inch ....

401. What are the two meanings of 欠 *qiàn* so far encountered? ....

402. 按肌肤 ....

403. *jī fū jiǎ cuò* ....

404. palpation of the limbs ....

405. 手足心烦热 ....

406. *sì zhī qiàn wēn* ....

407. cold limbs ....

408. 四肢逆冷 ....

409. *fù tòng jù àn* ....

410. (feels) soft under pressure ....

411. 按之有痞块 ....

412. *àn zhī mò zhǐ* ....

第三节：疾病用字
Section 3: Diseases

The term 病 *bìng* means 'illness', 'sickness', or 'disease', i.e., any morbid condition of the body. The term 疾病 *jí bìng* or 疾 *jí* disease (entity), denotes a morbid condition manifesting in the same basic signs or course of development wherever it occurs and whomever it affects.

Many diseases such as jaundice, dysentery, goiter, cholera, consumption, epilepsy, mumps, measles, malaria, and lockjaw are marked by such specific signs (jaundice by yellowing of the skin, dysentery by pus [mucus] and blood in the stool, etc.) that they have been identified by Westerners and Chinese alike. Modern medicine too recognizes most of these as disease entities.

Disease categories are by no means universal, though. The Chinese medical concepts of 痿 *wěi*, 'wilting', 痹 *bì*, 'impediment', and 疝 *shàn*, 'mounting', for example, have no natural equivalents in English. English names have to be devised for these concepts. In these three cases, we have chosen literal translations of the Chinese terms.

Furthermore, the same objective disease identified by both Chinese and Westerners are often conceived and explained in different ways, and the name given to the disease reflects something of the technical understanding. For example, the condition called 风火眼 *fēng huǒ yǎn* is also called 'acute conjunctivitis' in Western medicine, each term reflecting the respective understanding of the condition. We have adopted the principle that if a term reflects Western medical knowledge that is alien to Chinese medicine, it should not be used to represent a Chinese medical disease entity. Instead, a term that reflects the Chinese medical concept should be devised. Here, neither 'conjunctiva' nor 'inflammation', as such, are Chinese medical concepts, and hence 风火眼 *fēng huǒ yǎn* is rendered literally as 'wind-fire eye'. The term 中风 *zhòng fēng*, literally meaning 'wind stroke', could be rendered by the layman's term 'stroke' or the now little used medical term 'apoplexy' (from the Greek *plessein*, to strike), but to call it 'cerebrovascular accident' would imply an understanding of the condition that Chinese medicine does not have.

It is sometimes difficult to decide whether an existing term can be used or a new term should be created. 霍乱 *huò luàn*, 'cholera', is a good example. The literal meaning of the Chinese term is reflected in the term coined by Bensky et al., 'sudden turmoil', since cholera is a sudden major disruption of the digestive tract that takes the form of violent vomiting and diarrhea of sudden onset. The word 'cholera' came into use in English in the 14th century. Its literal meaning is ambiguous, since *kholē* in Greek meant 'bile' (one of the four humors of humoral pathology) or 'anger', and might even be derived from *cholades*, intestines. Whichever meaning is operant, the term is premodern and reflects no modern medical knowledge of the disease. It was originally used to denote a condition of violent vomiting and diarrhea, and it was not until much later that the term was redefined to denote a disease characterized by violent vomiting and diarrhea and caused by the bacterium *Vibrio cholera*. Western medicine has appropriated the word and redefined it. In theory, however, we can argue that 'cholera' can still be thought of in its wider meaning (any violent vomiting and diarrhea), which is precisely what the Chinese *huò luàn* denotes.

The literal translation *sudden turmoil* is very acceptable. However, in view of the fact that the Chinese *huò luàn* may actually have been borrowed from the Greek word *cholera*,[29] there is just as much reasons for retaining the familiar disease name.

Many conditions that Chinese medicine classes as 'diseases' might appear to us to be like symptom names.

第三节　第一组				SECTION 3: SET 1

内科疾病   Diseases of Internal Medicine

997	* 病 疒	病 疒	bìng	illness /ˈɪlnɪs/ disease /dɪˈziz/
998	* 疾 疒	疾 疒	jí	disease /dɪˈziz/
999-n705	* 症 疒	症 疒	zhèng	pathocondition /ˈpæθokənˌdɪʃən/
1000-n706	* 证 讠	證 言	zhèng	pattern /ˈpætən/
1001	* 候 亻	候 人	hòu	indicator /ˈɪndɪˌketə/
1002-n707	* 感 心	感 心	gǎn	contract /kənˈtrækt/ vt., contraction* /kənˈtræktʃən/ n.
1003	* 伤 亻	傷 人	shāng	damage /ˈdæmɪdʒ/
1004	* 中 中	中 丨	zhòng	strike /straɪk/ vt, vi. stroke /strok/ n.
1005	* 温 氵	溫 水	wēn	warm /wɔrm/ adj. warmth /wɔrmθ/ n.
1006-n708	* 疫 疒	疫 疒	yì	epidemic /ˌɛpɪˈdɛmɪk/ n., adj.
1007-n709	* 瘟 疒	瘟 疒	wēn	scourge /skɝdʒ/
1008	* 天 天	天 大	tiān	heaven /ˈhɛvən/
1009	* 行 彳	行 彳	xíng	current /ˈkɝənt/
1010-n710	* 虾 虫	蝦 虫	há	toad /tod/

---

[29] See Unschuld, *Chinese Medicine*, Brookline MA, Paradigm Publications, 1998, Chapter 1.

1011-n711	*	蟆 虫	蟆 虫	*má*	toad /tod/
1012-n712	*	痧 疒	痧 疒	*shā*	sand /sænd/
1013	*	雷 雨	雷 雨	*léi*	thunder /ˈθʌndɚ/
1014-n713	*	癆 疒	癆 疒	*láo*	consumption /kənˈsʌmpʃən/
1015-n714	*	尸 尸	尸 尸	*shī*	corpse /kɔrps/
1016	*	劳 艹	勞 力	*láo*	taxation /tæksˈeʃən/
1017-n715	*	疟 疒	瘧 疒	*nüè*	malaria /məˈlɛrɪə/
1018	*	悬 心	懸 心	*xuán*	suspend /səˈspɛnd/ *vt.*
					suspended /səˈspɛndɪd/ *adj.*
1019-n716	*	溢 氵	溢 水	*yì*	spill /spɪl/ *vt, vi.*
					spillage /ˈspɪlɪdʒ/ *n.*
1020	*	支 十	支 支	*zhī*	propping /ˈprɑpɪŋ/
1021-n717	*	怔 忄	怔 心	*zhēng*	fear /fɪr/
1022-n718	*	忡 忄	忡 心	*chōng*	fear /fɪr/
1023-n719	*	痹 疒	痹 疒	*bì*	impediment /ɪmˈpɛdɪmɛnt/
1024-n720	*	着 羊	着 艸	*zháo*	fixed /fɪkst/
1025	*	痿 疒	痿 疒	*wěi*	wilting /ˈwɪltɪŋ/
1026-n721	*	瘫 疒	癱 疒	*tān*	paralysis /pəˈræləsɪs/
1027-n722	*	痪 疒	瘓 疒	*huàn*	paralysis /pəˈræləsɪs/
1028-n723	*	痉 疒	痙 疒	*jìng*	tetany /ˈtɛtənɪ/
1029-n724		破 石	破 石	*pò*	*break*
1030-n725	*	痢 疒	痢 疒	*lì*	dysentery /ˈdɪsn̩ˌtɛrɪ/
1031-n726	*	疰 疒	疰 疒	*zhù*	infixation /ˌɪnfɪksˈeʃən/
1032-n727	*	注 氵	注 水	*zhù*	influx /ˈɪnflʌks/
1033-n728	*	噎 口	噎 口	*yē*	dysphagia /dɪsˈfædʒɪə/
1034	*	膈 月	膈 肉	*gé*	occlusion /əˈkluʒən/
1035-n729	*	疸 疒	疸 疒	*dǎn*	jaundice /ˈdʒɔndɪs/
1036	*	黄 土	黃 黃	*huáng*	jaundice /ˈdʒɔndɪs/
1037-n730	*	疝 疒	疝 疒	*shàn*	mounting /ˈmaʊntɪŋ/
1038-n731	*	癥 疒	癥 疒	*zhēng*	concretion /kənˈkriʃən/
1039-n732	*	瘕 疒	瘕 疒	*jiǎ*	conglomeration /kənˌglɑməˈreʃən/
1040-n733	*	积 禾	積 禾	*jī*	accumulation /əˌkjumuˈleʃən/
1041-n734	*	聚 耳	聚 耳	*jù*	gathering /ˈgæðərɪŋ/
1042-n735	*	痃 疒	痃 疒	*xián*	string /strɪŋ/
1043-n736	*	癖 疒	癖 疒	*pǐ*	aggregation /ˌægrɪˈgeʃən/
1044-n737	*	澼 氵	澼 水	*pǐ*	afflux /ˈæflʌks/
1045	*	鼓 鼓	鼓 鼓	*gǔ*	drum /drʌm/
1046-n738	*	臌 月	臌 肉	*gǔ*	drum distention /ˈdrʌm–dɪstɛnʃən/
1047-n739	*	飧 夕	飧 夕	*sūn*	swill /swɪl/
1048-n740	*	洞 氵	洞 水	*dòng*	throughflux /ˈθruflʌks/

1049-n741	* 濡 氵	濡 水	*rú*	soggy /ˈsɔgɪ/
1050	* 淋 氵	淋 水	*lín*	strangury /ˈstræŋgjurɪ/
1051	* 沙 氵	沙 水	*shā*	sand /sænd/
1052	* 石 石	石 石	*shí*	stone /ston/
1053-n742	* 膏 高	膏 肉	*gāo*	unctuous /ˈʌŋktjuəs/
1054-n743	* 癃 疒	癃 疒	*lóng*	dribbling block /ˈdrɪblɪŋ blɑk/
1055-n744	* 瘿 疒	癭 疒	*yǐng*	goiter /ˈgɔɪtɚ/
1056	* 脚 月	腳 肉	*jiǎo*	foot /fʊt/
				leg /lɛg/
1057	* 癫 疒	癲 疒	*diān*	withdrawal /wɪðˈdrɔəl/
1058	* 狂 犭	狂 犬	*kuáng*	mania /ˈmenɪə/
1059-n745	* 痫 疒	癇 疒	*xián*	epilepsy /ˈɛpɪˌlɛpsɪ/
1060-n746	* 痴 疒	癡 疒	*chī*	feeble-minded /ˌfibl̩ˈmaɪndɪd/ *adj.*
				feeble-mindedness /ˌfibl̩ˈmaɪndɪdnɪs/ *n.*
1061	* 呆 口	呆 口	*dāi*	torpor /ˈtɑrpɚ/
1062-n747	* 霍 雨	霍 雨	*huò*	sudden /ˈsʌdn̩/
1063	* 乱 舌	亂 乙	*luàn*	deranged /dɪˈrendʒd/

注 Notes:

1. The character 疾 *jí*, disesase, has already been encountered in the sense of racing. Here it means disease.

2. The term 天行 *tiān xíng*, literally translated here as 'heaven current', figures in names of diseases that move through the atmosphere. (天 *tiān* means heaven, sky, above the ground.) This is equivalent to 疫 *yì*, epidemic.

3. We often apply the practice of including parenthesized Pīnyīn for newly coined disease names, e.g., mounting, sand, wilting.

4. The character 痧 *shā*, translated as 'sand', is composed of the illness signific with the element 沙 *shā*, sand. It denotes diseases characterized by speckled rashes, and, curiously, some that are not.

5. The Chinese 噎膈 *yē gé* is a disease characterized by the sensation of blockage on swallowing, difficulty in getting food and drink down, and, in some cases, immediate vomiting of ingested food. The elements of the term are 噎, inability to swallow (dysphagia), and 膈, explained as meaning a blockage preventing food from going down (occlusion). Furthermore, 噎 can also denote the throat, while the primary meaning of 膈 (with the flesh signific 肉) is the diaphragm.

6. The term 黄疸 *huáng dǎn*, jaundice, is sometimes abbreviated to 黄, as in the term 退黄 *tuì huáng*, abate jaundice.

7. The character 痨, consumption, is homophonic with 劳 *láo*, taxation, and its differs in the written form only by the addition of the disease signific 疒; sometimes the two characters are wrongly interchanged. Consumption manifests as vacuity taxation (severe vacuity) pattern, but a now obsolete name, 传尸痨 *chuán shī láo*, shows that the Chinese have long been aware that it differs from vacuity taxation patterns by its transmissibility.

8. The term 中风 *zhòng fēng*, wind stroke, in the 伤寒论 *Shāng Hán Lùn* meant any disease caused by external wind. It now usually denotes what is referred to in lay English speech as stroke and in Western medicine as 'apoplexy'. In the Chinese term, the character 中 *zhòng* means strike, and is the same as 中, center. It derives from the representation of an arrow passing through the center of a round target; hence it conveys both the idea of 'center' and that of 'strike'.

9. The terms 心悸 *xīn jì*, palpitation, and 怔忡 *zhēng chōng*, fearful throbbing, denote two different kinds of throbbing of the heart. The former is a general term for throbbing of the heart, but is also used specifically in the sense of palpitation brought on by emotional stimulus. In this sense it is specifically referred to as 惊悸 *jīng jì*, fright palpitation. The term 怔忡 *zhēng chōng*, which literally means fear or apprehension and which is rendered here as fearful throbbing, refers to throbbing of the heart that arises spontaneously.

10. The Chinese 痉 *jìng* means severe spasm such as rigidity in the neck, clenched jaw, convulsion of the limbs, and arched-back rigidity. As used in Western medicine, the term tetany is narrower in meaning than 痉 *jìng*; however, in origin, it means nothing more than spasm (from the Greek *teinein*, cognate with English words such as tend, tension, distention), i.e., 'lockjaw', which is the classic but not the only form of 痉 *jìng*.

11. The term 癥假积聚 *zhēng jiǎ jī jù*, which is rendered in the present text as 'concretions, conglomerations, accumulations, and gatherings', denotes four kinds of abdominal masses associated with pain and distention. Very often this term is loosely translated as 'abdominal masses'. However, there are theoretical differences between the four kinds. Concretions and accumulations are masses of definite form and fixed location, associated with pain of fixed location. They stem from disease in the viscera and in the blood aspect. Conglomerations and gatherings are masses of indefinite form, which gather and dissipate at irregular intervals and are attended by pain of unfixed location. They are attributed to disease in the bowels and in the qì aspect. Accumulations and gatherings chiefly occur in the middle burner. Concretions and conglomerations chiefly occur in the lower burner and in many cases are the result of gynecological diseases. In general, concretions, conglomerations, concretions, and gatherings (which can be referred to by the short form

'concretions and gatherings') arise when emotional depression or dietary intemperance causes damage to the liver and spleen.

As to the translation of 癥瘕積聚 *zhēng jiǎ jī jù*, we have given each character its own rendering. 積 *jī* and 聚 *jù* are everyday words meaning to 'accumulate' and to 'gather', respectively, and we have rendered them as such in the technical context. The other two characters, 癥 *zhēng* and 瘕 *jiǎ*, both have the disease signific; in other words, they were created to specifically denote disease conditions. The word *zhēng* has a phonetic component *zhēng*, which could be taken as a semantic component if we accept 'contraction' as one of its less common meanings. Since this character's denotative meaning is a definite lump of fixed location, we have rendered it as 'concretion', which is suggestive of hard lump. The word 瘕 *jiǎ* contains the phonetic 假 *jiǎ*, which, again, could also be taken as a semantic component since it means 'false' or 'spurious'. This is quite likely since the *jiǎ* type of lump comes and goes, and is of unfixed location; it is therefore a 'false' or 'phantom' lump. We have rendered this term as 'conglomeration', which suggests a looser type of lump than 'concretion'.

12. The term 疝 *shàn* refers to any of various diseases characterized by pain or swelling of the abdomen or scrotum. One of these, 疝气 *shàn qì*, is used in modern medicine as the equivalent of 'hernia', and this might induce translators to render 疝 *shàn* as 'hernia' in all contexts. In traditional Chinese medicine, however, 疝 *shàn* is broader in its denotation, including notably what modern doctors call 'hydrocele of the testis', a swelling of the testicle due to an accumulation of serous fluid. The disease conditions denoted by the term 疝 *shàn* are not bound by a common characteristic, since they do not all involve the scrotum, and do not necessarily involve abdominal pain. The Chinese term 疝 *shàn* is made of the illness signific with the character 山 *shān*, 'mountain', which may simply be a phonetic component, but it is highly probable that it is in fact a semantic component, implying accumulation expressed through a natural metaphor. Given the likelihood of this latter explanation, and given the difficulty of definition based on denotation, we have rendered this term as 'mounting' (a physical accumulation or an accumulation of evil).

13. The term 痿 *wěi*, translated in this text as 'wilting', denotes weakness and limpness of the sinews that in severe cases prevents the lifting of the arms and legs. English has no existing term for such a disease condition. Our translation, as with 疝, is based on the character composition. The composition of the character can be explained as the illness signific combined with a phonetic 委 *wěi*. However, a much more likely explanation appears to be that when another character 萎, which is composed of the the phonetic 委 topped with a grass signific and meaning 'wilt' or 'wither', came to be used to denote a

physical condition of wilting or withering of the limbs, the grass signific was replaced with the illness signific. The Chinese expression for 'impotence', 阳痿（阳萎）*yáng wěi*, literally 'yáng wilting' (yáng being a euphemism for the penis), can be written with either of the two characters. The term 委 *wěi* has been rendered by Bensky et al., as 'Atrophy' and previously by Wiseman as 'atony'. Both these terms are Western medical terms that do not reflect the original metaphor inherent in the Chinese term. Both terms are over-specific, and neither reflects the Chinese metaphor.

14. Another disease affecting the limbs is 痹 *bì*, which is defined as blockage of the channels arising when wind, cold, and/or dampness invade the fleshy exterior and the joints, and manifesting in signs such as joint pain, sinew and bone pain, and heaviness or numbness of the limbs. The character 痹 *bì* is generally understood to mean 'paralyzed' or 'crippled'. However, in Chinese medical texts, it is usually explained as meaning 'blocked', and is often seen in this meaning (in 喉痹 *hóu bì*, 'throat impediment', usually denoting severe soreness and swelling of the throat; no notion of crippling is implied). Our English rendering, 'impediment', primarily reflects the medical meaning (Latin *im* + *ped*, foot, originally meant fettering of the feet).

15. The term 淋 *lín* denotes any condition characterized by dribbling and painful urination. The character represents an ordinary everyday word meaning to drip, dribble, or sprinkle. We have rendered it in the medical context as 'strangury', a now little used Western medical term that comes from the Greek *stragx-*, *stragg*, drop, drip, and *ouron*, urine. 'Strangury' denotes the same clinical reality, and its literal meaning matches the literal meaning of the Chinese term.

复合词 Compounds:

1152. 外感热病 *wài gǎn rè bìng*, externally contracted febrile disease; externally contracted heat disease
1153. 外感 *wài gǎn*, external contraction
1154. 伤寒 *shāng hán*, cold damage
1155. 伤暑 *shāng shǔ*, summerheat damage
1156. 中风 *zhòng fēng*, wind stroke
1157. 时疫 *shí yì*, seasonal epidemic
1158. 天行时疫 *tiān xíng shí yì*, heaven-current seasonal epidemic
1159. 虾蟆瘟 *há má wēn*, toad-head scourge
1160. 大头瘟 *dà tóu wēn*, massive-head scourge
1161. 痧气 *shā qì*, sand qì
1162. 疟疾 *nüè jí*, malaria
1163. 痉病 *jìng bìng*, tetanic disease

1164. 刚痉 *gāng jìng*, hard tetany

1165. 柔痉 *róu jìng*, soft tetany

1166. 破伤风 *pò shāng fēng*, lockjaw

1167. 瘫痪 *tān huàn*, paralysis

1168. 痿 *wěi*, wilting

1169. 肺痿 *fèi wěi*, lung wilting

1170. 肺痈 *fèi yōng*, welling-abscess of the lung

1171. 肺胀 *fèi zhàng*, distention of the lung; pulmonary distention

1172. 咳嗽 *ké sòu*, cough

1173. 痰咳 *tán ké*, phlegm cough

1174. 干咳 *gān ké*, dry cough

1175. 劳嗽 *láo sòu*, taxation cough

1176. 哮 *xiāo*, wheezing

1177. 喘 *chuǎn*, panting

1178. 痨瘵 *láo zhài*, consumption

1179. 传尸痨 *chuán shī láo*, corpse-transmitted consumption

1180. 痰饮 *tán yǐn*, phlegm-rheum

1181. 悬饮 *xuán yǐn*, suspended rheum

1182. 溢饮 *yì yǐn*, spillage rheum

1183. 支饮 *zhī yǐn*, propping rheum

1184. 咳血 *ké xuè*, coughing of blood

1185. 吐血 *tù xuè*, blood ejection

1186. 便血 *biàn xuè*, bloody stool

1187. 尿血 *niào xuè*, bloody urine

1188. 心悸 *xīn jì*, palpitation

1189. 惊悸 *jīng jì*, fright palpitation

1190. 怔忡 *zhēng chōng*, fearful throbbing

1191. 不寐 *bú mèi*, sleeplessness

1192. 尸厥 *shī jué*, deathlike reversal (lit. 'corpse reversal')

1193. 注夏 *zhù xià*, summer influx

1194. 夏痓 *xià zhù*, summer infixation

1195. 头痛 *tóu tòng*, headache

1196. 眩晕 *xuàn yūn*, dizziness

1197. 雷头风 *léi tóu fēng*, thunder head wind

1198. 痹 *bì*, impediment

1199. 五痹 *wǔ bì*, five impediments

1200. 风痹 *fēng bì*, wind impediment

1201. 行痹 *xíng bì*, moving impediment

1202. 寒痹 *hán bì*, cold impediment

1203. 痛痹 *tòng bì*, painful impediment

1204. 湿痹 *shī bì*, damp impediment

1205. 着痹 *zháo (zhuó) bì*, fixed impediment

1206. 热痹 *rè bì*, heat impediment

1207. 胸痹 *xiōng bì*, chest impediment

1208. 筋痹 *jīn bì*, sinew impediment

1209. 痿 *wěi*, wilting

1210. 脚气 *jiǎo qì*, leg qì (beriberi)

1211. 噎膈 *yē gé*, dysphagia-occlusion

1212. 气膈 *qì gé*, qì occlusion

1213. 呕吐 *ǒu tù*, vomiting (and retching)

1214. 反胃 *fǎn wèi*, stomach reflux

1215. 呃逆 *è nì*, hiccup

1216. 胃脘痛 *wèi wǎn tòng*, stomach duct pain

1217. 腹痛 *fù tòng*, abdominal pain

1218. 黄疸 *huáng dǎn*, jaundice

1219. 阴黄 *yīn huáng*, yīn jaundice

1220. 阳黄 *yáng huáng*, yáng jaundice

1221. 酒疸 *jiǔ dǎn*, liquor jaundice

1222. 黑疸 *hēi dǎn*, black jaundice

1223. 癥瘕积聚 *zhēng jiǎ jī jù*, concretions, conglomerations, accumulations, and gatherings

1224. 鼓胀 *gǔ zhàng*, drum distention

1225. 臌胀 *gǔ zhàng*, drum distention

1226. 泄泻 *xiè xiè*, diarrhea

1227. 湿泄 *shī xiè*, damp diarrhea

1228. 脾泄 *pí xiè*, spleen diarrhea

1229. 肾泄 *shèn xiè*, kidney diarrhea

1230. 五更泄 *wǔ gēng (jīng) xiè*, fifth-watch diarrhea

1231. 晨泄 *chén xiè*, early morning diarrhea

1232. 食泄 *shí xiè*, food diarrhea

1233. 火泄 *huǒ xiè*, fire diarrhea

1234. 飧泄 *sūn xiè*, swill diarrhea

1235. 洞泄 *dòng xiè*, throughflux diarrhea

1236. 濡泄 *rú xiè*, soggy diarrhea

1237. 痢疾 *lì jí*, dysentery

1238. 霍乱 *huò luàn*, cholera, sudden turmoil

1239. 便秘 *biàn bì*, constipation

1240. 癃闭 *lóng bì*, dribbling urinary block

1241. 水肿 *shuǐ zhǒng*, water swelling
1242. 阳水 *yáng shuǐ*, yáng water
1243. 阴水 *yīn shuǐ*, yīn water
1244. 风水 *fēng shuǐ*, wind swelling
1245. 皮水 *pí shuǐ*, skin water
1246. 正水 *zhèng shuǐ*, regular water
1247. 石水 *shí shuǐ*, stone water
1248. 五淋 *wǔ lín*, five stranguries
1249. 石淋 *shí lín*, stone strangury
1250. 沙淋 *shā lín*, sand strangury
1251. 血淋 *xuè lín*, blood strangury
1252. 气淋 *qì lín*, qi strangury
1253. 膏淋 *gāo lín*, unctuous strangury
1254. 热淋 *rè lín*, heat strangury
1255. 劳淋 *láo lín*, taxation strangury
1256. 冷淋 *lěng lín*, cold strangury
1257. 腰痛 *yāo tòng*, lumbar pain
1258. 胁痛 *xié tòng*, rib-side pain
1259. 消渴 *xiāo kě*, dispersion-thirst
1260. 疝气 *shàn qì*, mounting qi
1261. 肉瘿 *ròu yǐng*, flesh goiter
1262. 石瘿 *shí yǐng*, stone goiter
1263. 痴呆 *chī dāi*, feeble-mindedness
1264. 癫狂 *diān kuáng*, mania and withdrawal
1265. 痫 *xián*, epilepsy
1266. 虚劳 *xū láo*, vacuity taxation
1267. 内伤发热 *nèi shāng fā rè*, internal damage heat effusion

习题 Exercise:

413. 伤寒 ....
414. *shāng shǔ* ....
415. seasonal epidemic ....
416. 天行赤眼 ....
417. *dà tóu wēn* ....
418. malaria ....
419. 痢疾 ....
420. *huò luàn* ....

421. tetanic disease ....

422. 刚痉 ....

423. *pò shāng fēng* ....

424. wilting ....

425. 瘵瘵 ....

426. *xià zhù* ....

427. chest impediment ....

428. 噎膈 ....

429. *huáng dǎn* ....

430. concretions, conglomerations, accumulations, and gatherings ....

431. 哮 ....

432. *chuǎn* ....

433. phlegm-rheum ....

434. 悬饮 ....

435. *yì yǐn* ....

436. propping rheum ....

437. 便血 ....

438. *xīn jì* ....

439. fright palpitation ....

440. 怔忡 ....

441. *xíng bì* ....

442. cold impediment ....

443. 着痹 ....

444. *jiǔ dǎn* ....

445. drum distention ....

446. 湿泄 ....

447. *pí xiè* ....

448. fifth-watch diarrhea ....

449. 晨泄 ....

450. *yáng shuǐ* ....

451. wind swelling ....

452. 正水 ....

453. *ròu yǐng* ....

454. stone goiter ....

455. 虚劳 ....

456. *dòng xiè* ....

457. soggy diarrhea ....

458. 癃闭 ....

459. *wǔ lín* ....

460. sand strangury ....

461. 膏淋 ....

462. *shàn qì* ....

463. feeble-mindedness ....

464. 痫 ....

第三节　第二组　　　　　　　　SECTION 3: SET 2

外科疾病　　　　　　　　　　External Medicine Diseases

1064-n748	科 禾　科 禾	*kē*	*department, branch*
1065-n749	* 疮 疒　瘡 疒	*chuāng*	sore /sɔr, sor/
1066-n750	* 疡 疒　瘍 疒	*yáng*	sore /sɔr, sor/
1067-n751	* 疖 疒　癤 疒	*jiē*	boil /bɔil/
1068-n752	* 癞 疒　癩 疒	*lài*	lai /laɪ/
1069-n753	* 疔 疒　疔 疒	*dīng*	clove sore /ˈklov–sɔr (sor)/
1070-n754	* 丝 纟　絲 糸	*sī*	thread /θrɛd/
1071	* 走 走　走 走	*zǒu*	running /ˈrʌnɪŋ/
1072-n755	* 痈 疒　癰 疒	*yōng*	welling-abscess /ˈwɛlɪŋæbsɪs/
1073-n756	* 疽 疒　疽 疒	*jū*	flat-abscess /ˈflatæbsɪs/
1074-n757	* 瘤 疒　瘤 疒	*liú*	tumor /ˈtjumɚ/
1075-n758	* 岩 山　岩 山	*yán*	rock /rɑk/
1076	* 发 又　發 癶	*fā*	effusion /ɪˈfjuʒən/
1077-n759	搭 扌　搭 手	*dā*	*reach, touch*
1078-n760	* 荣 艹　榮 火	*róng*	glory /ˈɡlɔrɪ, ˈɡlorɪ/
1079	* 疳 疒　疳 疒	*gān*	gan /ɡæn, ɡɑn/
1080-n761	* 癣 疒　癬 疒	*xiǎn*	lichen /ˈlaɪkən/
1081-n762	* 牛 牛　牛 牛	*niú*	ox /ɔks/
1082-n763	* 松 木　松 木	*sōng*	pine /paɪn/
1083-n764	* 翻 羽　翻 羽	*fān*	evert /ɪˈvɝt/

1084	* 花 ⁺⁺	花 艸	*huā*	flower /ˈflaʊɚ/
1085-n765	* 圆 口	圓 口	*yuán*	coin /kɔɪn/
1086-n766	* 疕 疒	疕 疒	*bǐ*	crust /krʌst/
1087-n767	* 秃 禾	禿 禾	*tū*	bald /bɔld/
1088-n768	* 鹅 鸟	鵝 鳥	*é*	goose /gus/
1089	* 灰 ナ	灰 火	*huī*	ashen /ˈæʃən/
1090-n769	* 痘 疒	痘 疒	*dòu*	pox /pɑks/
1091-n770	* 丹 丿	丹 丶	*dān*	cinnabar /ˈsɪnəˌbɑr/
1092	* 毒 ㇐	毒 毋	*dú*	toxin /ˈtɑksɪn/
1093-n771	缠 纟	纏 糸	*chán*	tie
1094	* 蛇 虫	蛇 虫	*shé*	snake /snek/
1095-n772	* 疥 疒	疥 疒	*jiè*	scab /skæb/
1096	* 痦 疒	痦 疒	*péi*	miliaria /ˌmɪlɪˈɛrɪə/
1097-n773	* 瘰 疒	瘰 疒	*luǒ*	scrofula /ˈskrɔfjələ/ (small)
1098-n774	* 疬 疒	癧 疒	*lì*	scrofula /ˈskrɔfjələ/ (large)
1099-n775	* 核 木	核 木	*hé*	node /nod/
1100-n776	* 痤 疒	痤 疒	*cuó*	pimple /ˈpɪmpl̩/
1101-n777	* 痱 疒	痱 疒	*fèi*	prickly heat /ˌprɪklɪ hit/
1102-n778	* 痔 疒	痔 疒	*zhì*	hemorrhoid /ˈhɛməˌrɔɪd/
1103-n779	* 漏 氵	漏 水	*lòu*	fistula /ˈfɪstjulə/
1104-n780	* 瘘 疒	瘻 疒	*lòu*	fistula /ˈfɪstjulə/
1105	* 脱 月	脫 肉	*tuō*	prolapse /ˈprolæps/
1106-n781	* 折 扌	折 手	*zhé*	fracture /ˈfræktʃɚ/
1107-n782	落 ⁺⁺	落 艸	*lào*	*fall, drop*
1108	枕 木	枕 木	*zhěn*	*pillow*

注 Notes:

1. The term 疔 *dīng* denotes a small, hard sore with a deep root, appearing most commonly on the face and ends of the fingers. The character 疔 *dīng* contains the character 丁 *dīng*, which has numerous disparate meanings but which because of its shape came to be used to denote a carpenter's nail (usually written as 钉). This meaning of the character probably explains its appearance in 疔 *dīng*, a sore that penetrates deep into the flesh like a nail. In translation, we render the term as *clove*, denoting an object similar in shape to a nail and derived from the Latin *clavus*, meaning a carpenter's nail. This choice avoids the confusion arising through the ambiguity of the word *nail* in English.

2. 癣 *xiǎn* is a skin disease characterized by elevation of the skin, serous discharge, scaling, and itching. The character 癣 *xiǎn* contains 鲜, apparently

in the meaning of 蘚, moss or lichen. It describes skin diseases that take the form of slightly raised patches on the skin having the appearance of lichen on a stone or tree bark. The compound 圓癬 *yuán xiǎn*, coin lichen, describes lichen taking the form of patches that spread outward and then begin to heal in the center, giving the appearance of an old Chinese coin that is pierced with a hole.

3. The term 翻花痔 *fān huā zhì*, everted flower hemorrhoids, describes hemorrhoids having the appearance of a flower that is past its prime, with petals fully opened and turned back.

4. The language of sores includes a couple of terms that are virtually impossible to translate owing to the absence of a single clear definition and the absence of any literal meaning in the character. The term 疳 *gān* means child malnutrition and could be rendered as such without hesitation were it not for that fact that it also denotes certain kinds of ulceration sometimes related and sometimes unrelated to malnutrition. No English word unites these two definitions. The term 癩 *lài* denotes various diseases of the head characterized by hair loss or leprosy. Paul U. Unschuld has pointed out that the character is composed of the illness signific combined with a character 癩 *lài*, which, if not functioning merely as phonetic element, may be taken to mean 'repudiation', thus indicating that the essential characteristic of diseases called 癩 *lài* was originally the social rejection of its victims.

复合词 Compounds:

1268. 疔疮 *dīng chuāng*, clove sore
1269. 红丝疔 *hóng sī dīng*, red-thread clove sore
1270. 疔疮走黄 *dīng chuāng zǒu huáng*, clove sore running yellow
1271. 红丝走窜 *hóng sī zǒu cuàn*, running red threads
1272. 疖肿 *jié zhǒng*, swollen boil
1273. 痈疽 *yōng jū*, welling and flat-abscesses
1274. 发背 *fā bèi*, effusion
1275. 搭手 *dā shǒu*, reachable sore
1276. 圆癣 *yuán xiǎn*, coin lichen
1277. 牛皮癣 *niú pí xiǎn*, oxhide lichen
1278. 松皮癣 *sōng pí xiǎn*, pine bark lichen
1279. 脚湿气 *jiǎo shī qì*, damp foot qi
1280. 鹅爪风 *é zhǎo fēng*, goose-foot wind
1281. 灰指甲 *huī zhǐ jiǎ*, ashen nail
1282. 白秃疮 *bái tū chuāng*, bald white scalp sore
1283. 白疕 *bái bǐ*, white crust

1284. 癞疮 *lài chuāng*, lai sore
1285. 癞大风 *lài dà fēng*, lai great wind; leprosy
1286. 肉瘤 *ròu liú*, flesh tumor
1287. 肾岩 *shèn yán*, kidney rock
1288. 翻花下疳 *fān huā xià gān*, everted-flower lower body gan
1289. 失荣 *shī róng*, loss-of-glory
1290. 丹毒 *dān dú*, cinnabar toxin [sore]
1291. 缠腰火丹 *chán yāo huǒ dān*, fire-girdle cinnabar
1292. 缠腰蛇丹 *chán yāo shé dān*, snake-girdle cinnabar
1293. 无名肿毒 *wú míng zhǒng dú*, innominate toxin swelling
1294. 痔漏 *zhì lòu*, hemorrhoids and fistula
1295. 翻花痔 *fān huā zhì*, everted-flower hemorrhoids
1296. 脱肛 *tuō gāng*, prolapse of the rectum
1297. 肛裂 *gāng liè*, splitting of the anus
1298. 肛漏 *gāng lòu*, anal fistula
1299. 瘰疬 *luǒ lì*, scrofula
1300. 痰核 *tán hé*, phlegm node
1301. 乳头破裂 *rǔ tóu pò liè*, cracked nipple
1302. 痱子 *fèi zǐ*, prickly heat
1303. 粉刺 *fěn cì*, acne
1304. 痤疮 *cuó chuāng*, pimples; acne
1305. 痤痱 *cuó fèi*, pock pimples
1306. 骨折 *gǔ zhé*, bone fracture
1307. 落枕 *lào zhěn*, crick in the neck

习题 Exercise:

465. *dīng chuāng* ....
466. clove sore running yellow ....
467. 疖肿 ....
468. *fā bèi* ....
469. coin lichen ....
470. 松皮癣 ....
471. *bái tū chuāng* ....
472. lai great wind; leprosy ....
473. 失荣 ....
474. *chán yāo shé dān* ....
475. prolapse of the rectum ....

476. 瘰疬 ....
477. *fěn cì* ....

第三节　第三组				SECTION 3: SET 3

耳鼻喉科　　　　　　　　　　　Ear, Nose, & Throat Diseases

1109	* 耳 耳	耳 耳	*ěr*	ear /ɪr/
1110	* 鼻 鼻	鼻 鼻	*bí*	nose /noz/
1111	* 喉 口	喉 口	*hóu*	larynx /ˈlærɪŋks/
				throat /θrot/
1112	悬 心	懸 心	*xuán*	suspend, hang
1113-n783	* 旗 方	旗 方	*qí*	flag /flæg/
1114-n784	旗 广	旗 广	*qí*	disease name, apparently after 旗
1115	* 聋 士	聾 耳	*lóng*	deafness /ˈdɛfnɪs/
1116	* 鸣 口	鳴 口	*míng*	ringing /ˈrɪŋɪŋ/
				tinnitus /təˈnaɪtəs/
1117-n785	* 聤 耳	聤 耳	*tíng*	purulent ear /ˈpjʊrələnt ˈɪr/
1118-n786	* 鼽 鼻	鼽 鼻	*qiú*	sniveling /ˈsnɪvl̩ɪŋ/
1119-n787	* 齇 鼻	齇 鼻	*zhā*	drinker's nose /ˈdrɪŋkɚz noz/
1120	* 嗅 口	嗅 口	*xiù*	smell (sense of) /smɛl/
1121	* 鱼 鱼	魚 魚	*yú*	fish /fɪʃ/
1122-n788	* 鲠 鱼	鯁 魚	*gěng*	stuck /stʌk/ (of fish bones)
1123	* 衄 血	衄 血	*nü*	spontaneous external
				bleeding /spɑnˈteniəs ɪksˈtɝnl̩ ˈblidɪŋ/
1124-n789	* 梅 木	梅 木	*méi*	plum /plʌm/
1125	* 核 木	核 木	*hé*	pit /pɪt/

注 Notes:

1. The term 悬旗风 *xuán qí fēng*, flying flag wind, is a disease of the uvula characterized by redness and swelling. An alternate name is 悬旗风 *xuán qí fēng*, which is the same except that 旗 *qí*, flag, is replaced by 旗. This character is given only one definition by the 中文大辞典 *Zhōng Wén Dà Cí Diǎn*, a person's name. The alternate name is given the same English rendering, 'flying flag wind', for want of information.

2. The term 乳蛾 *rǔ é*, in this text translated as 'baby moth', denotes a red, sore swelling on either or both sides of the pharynx. The word 乳 *rǔ* means breast (or nipple) or milk; it is also used as a qualifier to mean 'suckling'

(e.g., 乳猪 *rǔ zhū*, suckling pig). In this latter sense, it is sometimes even applied to the young of non-mammals. The combination 乳蛾 *rǔ é* refers to what modern medicine calls tonsillitis, which appears as lumps at the sides of the throat. The term describes the resemblance of these lumps to 'nipples or moths' or to 'baby moths', depending on how 乳 *rǔ* is interpreted.

复合词 Compounds:

1308. 耳聋 *ěr lóng*, deafness
1309. 暴聋 *bào lóng*, fulminant deafness
1310. 耳鸣 *ěr míng*, ringing in the ears
1311. 耳衄 *ěr nü*, spontaneous bleeding of the ear
1312. 耳聤 *ěr tíng*, purulent ear
1313. 耳内长肉 *ěr nèi zhǎng ròu*, growth in the ear
1314. 耳痔 *ěr zhì*, ear pile
1315. 鼻渊 *bí yuān*, deep-source nasal congestion
1316. 鼻鼽 *bí qiú*, sniveling
1317. 鼻齄 *bí zhā*, drinker's nose
1318. 酒齄鼻 *jiǔ zhā bí*, drinker's nose
1319. 红鼻子 *hóng bí zǐ*, red nose
1320. 鼻衄 *bí nü*, nosebleed
1321. 失嗅 *shī xiù*, loss of smell
1322. 梅核气 *méi hé qì*, plum-pit qi
1323. 乳蛾 *rǔ é*, baby moth; nipple moth
1324. 喉蛾 *hóu é*, throat moth
1325. 石蛾 *shí é*, stone moth
1326. 白喉 *bái hóu*, diphtheria
1327. 悬雍下垂 *xuán yōng xià chuí*, pendulous uvula
1328. 悬旗风 *xuán qí fēng*, flying flag wind
1329. 悬旗风 *xuán qí fēng*, flying flag wind
1330. 鱼骨鲠喉 *yú gǔ gěng hóu*, fish bones stuck in the throat
1331. 鱼刺鲠喉 *yú cì gěng hóu*, fish bones stuck in the throat (long, fine fish bones are usually called 刺 rather than 骨)

习题 Exercise:

478. deafness ....
479. 耳衄 ....
480. *bí yuān* ....
481. sniveling ....

482. 酒齄鼻 ....

483. *méi hé qì* ....

484. flying flag wind ....

485. 鱼骨鲠喉 ....

第三节　第四组　　　　　　　　　SECTION 3: SET 4

眼科疾病　　　　　　　　　　　　Eye Diseases

1126	* 睑 目	瞼 目	*jiǎn*	eyelid /ˈaɪlɪd/
1127	* 胞 月	胞 肉	*bāo*	eyelid /ˈaɪlɪd/
1128-n790	偷 亻	偷 人	*tōu*	*steal*
1129	针 钅	針 金	*zhēn*	*needle*
1130-n791	跳 足	跳 足	*tiào*	*jump*
1131-n792	* 垂 丿	垂 土	*chuí*	droop /drup/
1132	漏 氵	漏 水	*lòu*	*leak*
1133	* 烂 火	爛 火	*làn*	ulceration /ˌʌlsəˈreʃən/
1134	* 涩 氵	澀 水	*sè*	dry /draɪ/
1135	* 干 疒	乾 疒	*gān*	dry /draɪ/
1136-n793	* 椒 木	椒 木	*jiāo*	peppercorn /ˈpɛpəˌkɔrn/
1137-n794	* 粟 西	粟 木	*sù*	millet /ˈmɪlɪt/
1138-n795	拳	拳 手	*quán*	*curled*
1139-n796	* 睫 目	睫 目	*jié*	eyelash /ˈaɪlæʃ/
1140-n797	倒 亻	倒 人	*dào*	*inverted*
1141	* 漏 氵	漏 水	*lòu*	leak /lik/
1142	* 溢 氵	溢 水	*yì*	spill /spɪl/ *vt, vi.*
				spillage /ˈspɪlɪdʒ/ *n.*
1143-n798	* 膜 月	膜 肉	*mò*	membrane /ˈmɛmbren/
1144-n799	* 胬 疒	胬 疒	*nǔ*	excrescence /ɪkskrˈɛsəns/
1145-n800	攀 手	攀 手	*pān*	*climb*
1146-n801	抱 扌	抱 手	*bào*	*embrace*
1147	* 轮 车	輪 車	*lún*	wheel /wil, hwil/
1148-n802	* 星 日	星 日	*xīng*	star /stɑr/
1149-n803	* 翳 羽	翳 羽	*yì*	screen /skrin/
1150-n804	* 蟹 虫	蟹 虫	*xiè*	crab /kræb/
1151	* 冲 冫	衝 行	*chōng*	surge /sɝdʒ/
1152	* 昏 氏	昏 日	*hūn*	clouding /ˈklaʊdɪŋ/
1153	偏 亻	偏 人	*piān*	*biased, skew*
1154	* 近 辶	近 辵	*jìn*	near /nɪr/

1155	*	远 辶	遠 辵	*yuǎn*	far /fɑr/
1156	*	视 礻	視 見	*shì*	sight /saɪt/ *n.*
					see /si/ *vt, vi.*
1157	*	瞳 目	瞳 目	*tóng*	pupil /ˈpjupl̩/
1158-n805	*	灌 氵	灌 水	*guàn*	pour /pɔr, por/
1159	*	丝 纟	絲 糸	*sī*	thread /θrɛd/
1160-n806	*	虬 虫	虬 虫	*qiú*	tangled /ˈtæŋgl̩d/
1161-n807	*	睆 白	睆 白	*huāng*	dim /dɪm/
1162	*	乱 舌	亂 乙	*luàn*	chaotic /keˈɑtɪk/
1163-n808	*	盲 亡	盲 目	*máng*	blindness /ˈblaɪndnɪs/
1164	*	暴 日	暴 日	*bào*	sudden /ˈsʌdən/
					fulminant /ˈfʌlmɪnənt/
1165	*	夜 亠	夜 夕	*yè*	night /naɪt/
1166-n809	*	雀 小	雀 隹	*què*	sparrow /ˈspæro/
1167-n810	*	障 阝	障 阜	*zhàng*	obstruction /əbˈstrʌkʃən/

注 Note:

1. Many of the terms for eye diseases are descriptive of the clinical features. Many of them will make some sense to students unfamiliar with them. Below, we discuss just a few of the terms.

2. The Chinese 拳毛倒睫 *quán máo dào jié*, ingrown eyelash, literally means 'curled-hair inverted eyelash'. The character 拳 *quán* normally means a fist, but is here used in the sense of curled, an idea that is more commonly expressed as 卷 *juǎn* in the common language.

3. 青盲 *qīng máng* refers to gradual loss of vision unaccompanied by any change in the eye itself. The word 青 means green-blue, and may mean black in this context, if the term refers, as it appears to do, to the absence of any change in the color of the pupil. Clear-eye blindness is equivalent to optic atrophy in Western medicine. It is attributed to insufficiency of the liver and kidney with depletion of essence blood, combined with spleen-stomach vacuity that prevents essential qì from reaching up to the eyes. 暴盲 *bào máng*, sudden blindness, is sudden loss of sight, attributable to liver qì ascending counterflow, qì stagnation and blood stasis, or major vacuity of original qì.

4. 胬肉攀睛 *nǔ ròu pān jīng*, excrescence creeping over the eye, is a gray-white fleshy growth at the canthus that progressively grows over the eye, in severe cases partially affecting vision. It arises when heat congesting in the heart and lung channels causes qì stagnation and blood stasis. It may also result from effulgent yin vacuity fire. It corresponds to pterygium in Western medicine.

5. 蟹睛 *xiè jīng*, crab's-eye, is a condition characterized by an erosive screen on the dark of the eye (iris and cornea) from which a bead-like formation resembling the eye of a crab emerges. It is caused by accumulated heat in the liver surging up into the eyes or by external injury. The bead-like formation is surrounded by a white screen and is associated with acute eye pain, aversion to light, and tearing. It leaves a scar on healing, and if the "spirit jelly" (vitreous humor) of the eye escapes, blindness usually ensues. It corresponds to iridoptosis in Western medicine.

6. 内障 *nèi zhàng*, internal obstruction, refers to any of a number of diseases of the spirit pupil and inner eye manifesting in poor vision. It stands in contrast to 外障 *wài zhàng*, external obstruction, which refers to any disease of the eyelids, canthi, white of the eye, or the black of the eye. External obstructions include red sore swollen eyes (e.g., fire eye), erosion, tearing, eye discharge, or dryness of the eyes, eye screens and membranes, and excrescences of the canthi.

7. Several of the terms denoting eye conditions listed below include the word 生 *shēng*, meaning to arise, grow (and which we have already encountered in the sense of 'engender'). For example, 眼生痰核 *yǎn shēng tán hé* is a phlegm node growing on the eye. Note that the word *growing* is deleted from the formal rendering.

复合词 Compounds:

1332. 天行赤眼 *tiān xíng chì yǎn*, heaven-current red eye
1333. 星翳 *xīng yì*, starry screen
1334. 胞睑肿胀 *bāo jiǎn zhǒng zhàng*, swelling of the eyelid
1335. 眼胞瘀痛 *yǎn bāo yū tòng*, stasis pain in the eyelids
1336. 眼睑丹毒 *yǎn jiǎn dān dú*, cinnabar toxin of the eyelid
1337. 眼生偷针 *yǎn shēng tōu zhēn*, sty of the eye
1338. 眼皮跳 *yǎn pí tiào*, twitching of the eyelids
1339. 上胞下垂 *shàng bāo xià chuí*, drooping of the upper eyelid
1340. 眼生痰核 *yǎn shēng tán hé*, phlegm node of the eye
1341. 目生粟疮 *mù shēng sù chuāng*, millet sore of the eye
1342. 目生椒疮 *mù shēng jiāo chuāng*, peppercorn sore of the eye
1343. 目生椒粟 *mù shēng jiāo sù*, peppercorn or millet sore of the eye
1344. 胞内生肉 *bāo nèi shēng ròu*, growth inside the eyelid
1345. 拳毛倒睫 *quán máo dào jié*, ingrown eyelash
1346. 漏睛 *lòu jīng*, weeping canthus
1347. 眼弦赤烂 *yǎn xián chì làn*, ulceration of the eyelid rim
1348. 白睛生疳 *bái jīng shēng gān*, gan of the white of the eye

1349. 白睛鱼胞 *bái jīng yú bāo*, fish-belly eye white

1350. 白睛溢血 *bái jīng yì xuè*, blood spillage in the white of the eye

1351. 赤脉传睛 *chì mài chuán jīng*, red vessels crossing the eye

1352. 赤膜下垂 *chì mó xià chuí*, hanging red membrane

1353. 胬肉攀睛 *nǔ ròu pān jīng*, excrescence creeping over the eye

1354. 赤丝虬脉 *chì sī qiú mài*, tangled red-thread vessels

1355. 赤丝乱脉 *chì sī luàn mài*, chaotic red-thread vessels

1356. 抱轮红 *bào lún hóng*, red areola surrounding the dark of the eye

1357. 目生星翳 *mù shēng xīng yì*, starry eye screen

1358. 疳翳 *gān yì*, gan screen

1359. 蟹睛 *xiè jīng*, crab's-eye

1360. 黄液上冲 *huáng yè shàng chōng*, upsurging yellow humor

1361. 目昏 *mù hūn*, clouded vision

1362. 目珠自胀 *mù zhū zì zhàng*, feeling of distention in the eyes (the character 自 *zì*, self, here implies that the distention is felt only by the patient himself and is not objectively apparent to the observer)

1363. 目视无神 *mù shì wú shén*, spiritless eyes

1364. 目偏视 *mù piān shì*, squint

1365. 瞳神散大 *tóng shén sàn dà*, dilated pupils

1366. 血灌瞳神 *xuè guàn tóng shén*, blood pouring into the pupil spirit

1367. 雀目 *què mù*, sparrow's vision

1368. 近视 *jìn shì*, nearsightedness

1369. 远视眈眈 *yuǎn shì huāng huāng*, seeing dimly afar

1370. 远视 *yuǎn shì*, farsightedness

1371. 暴盲 *bào máng*, sudden blindness

1372. 内障 *nèi zhàng*, internal obstruction

1373. 夜盲 *yè máng*, night blindness

1374. 青盲 *qīng máng*, clear-eye blindness

习题 Exercise:

486. *xīng yì* ....

487. cinnabar toxin of the eyelid ....

488. 眼生痰核 ....

489. *quán máo dào jié* ....

490. 眼弦赤烂 ....

491. *nǔ ròu pān jīng* ....

492. crab's-eye ....

493. 雀目 ....

494. *nèi zhàng* ....

495. clear-eye blindness ....

第三节　第五组   SECTION 3: SET 5

男科疾病   Men's Diseases

1168	* 男 田	男 田	*nán*	man /mæn/ male /mel/
1169	* 泄 氵	洩 水	*xiè*	ejaculate /ɪ'dʒækjuˌlet/ *vi.* ejaculation /ɪˌdʒækju'leʃən/ *n.*
1170	* 遗 辶	遺 辵	*yí*	emission /ɪ'mɪʃən/
1171	* 淫 氵	淫 水	*yín*	ooze /uz/
1172	* 强 弓	強 弓	*jiàng*	rigid /'rɪdʒɪd/ *adj.* rigidity* /rɪ'dʒɪdətɪ/ *n.*
1173	* 子 子	子 子	*zǐ*	testicle /'tɛstɪkl/
1174-n811	绣 纟	繡 糸	*xiù*	*brocade*
1175-n812	球 王	球 玉	*qiú*	*ball*
1176-n813	* 癞 疒	癩 疒	*tuí*	prominence /'pramɪnəns/ *n.* prominent /'pramɪnənt/ *adj.*
1177-n814	* 狐 犭	狐 犬	*hú*	fox /faks/ *n.* foxy /'faksɪ/ *adj.*
1178	* 浊 氵	濁 水	*zhuó*	turbid /'tɝbɪd/ *adj.* turbidity /tɝ'bɪdɪtɪ/ *n.*

复合词 Compounds:

1375. 阳痿 *yáng wěi*, 'yáng wilt', impotence

1376. 早泄 *zǎo xiè*, premature ejaculation

1377. 遗精 *yí jīng*, seminal emission

1378. 梦遗 *mèng yí*, dream emission

1379. 阳强 *yáng jiàng*, 'rigid yáng', persistent erection

1380. 强中 *jiàng zhōng*, 'rigid center,' persistent erection with seminal loss

1381. 血精 *xuè jīng*, bloody semen

1382. 子痈 *zǐ yōng*, testicular welling-abscess

1383. 囊痈 *náng yōng*, scrotal welling-abscess

1384. 绣球风 *xiù qiú fēng*, bobble wind

1385. 子痰 *zǐ tán*, testicular phlegm

1386. 寒疝 *hán shàn*, cold mounting

1387. 癩疝 *tuí shàn*, prominent mounting

1388. 狐疝 *hú shàn*, foxy mounting

1389. 白淫 *bái yín*, white ooze

1390. 白浊 *bái zhuó*, white turbidity

1391. 赤浊 *chì zhuó*, red turbidity

496. 阳痿 ....

497. *zǎo xiè* ....

498. 'rigid *yáng*,' persistent erection ....

499. 子痈 ....

500. *zǐ tán* ....

501. white ooze ....

502. 赤浊 ....

第三节　第六组				**SECTION 3: SET 6**

小儿疾病				**Children's Diseases**
1179-n815	* 儿 儿	兒 儿	*ér*	child /tʃaɪld/ infant /ˈɪnfənt/ *n.* infantile /ˈɪnfəntaɪl/ *adj.*
1180	* 胎 月	胎 肉	*tāi*	fetus /ˈfitəs/ *n.* fetal /ˈfitl̩/ *adj.*
1181	* 弱 弓	弱 弓	*ruò*	feebleness /ˈfibl̩nɪs/
1182	* 囟 丿	囟 口	*xìn*	fontanels /ˌfɑntəˈnɛlz/
1183-n816	填 土	塡 土	*tián*	*fill up, stuff*
1184	凸 丨	凸 凵	*tú*	*stick out, protrude*
1185-n817	解 角	解 角	*jiě*	*untie, detach*
1186	* 颅 页	顱 頁	*lú*	skull /skʌl/
1187	合 人入	合 口	*hé*	*unite, together*
1188-n818	* 痄 疒	痄 疒	*zhà*	mumps /mʌmps/
1189	* 腮 月	腮 肉	*sāi*	cheek /tʃik/
1190	* 麻 麻	麻 麻	*má*	measles /ˈmizl̩z/
1191	* 疹 疒	疹 疒	*zhěn*	papules /ˈpæpjulz/
1192	* 顿 页	頓 頁	*dùn*	bout /baʊt/
1193	* 惊 忄	驚 馬	*jīng*	fright /fraɪt/
1194	* 积 禾	積 禾	*jī*	accumulation /əˌkjumuˈleʃən/

1195-n819	* 滞 氵	滯 水	zhì	stagnation /stæg'neʃən/
1196	* 急 心	急 心	jí	acute /ə'kjut/
1197	* 迟 辶	遲 辵	chí	slowness /'slonɪs/
1198-n820	* 立 立	立 立	lì	stand /stænd/
1199	* 语 讠	語 言	yǔ	speak /spik/ vi.
1200	* 齿 齿	齒 齒	chǐ	teethe /tiθ/
1201	* 发 又	髮 髟	fà	hair /hɛr/
1202	行 彳	行 彳	xíng	walk
1203-n821	鸡 又	雞 隹	jī	chicken, hen, cock
1204	* 丹 丿	丹 丶	dān	cinnabar /'sɪnəˌbɑr/
1205	* 痧 疒	痧 疒	shā	sand /sænd/
1206	* 疳 疒	疳 疒	gān	gan /gæn/

注 Notes:

1. The Chinese term for 'measles', 麻疹 *má zhěn*, derives from 麻子, literally 'sesame seeds', an expression first used by Páng Ān-Shí (庞安时) to describe the spots of measles or the pits left by it in severe cases. Note that 麻 also means 'hemp' or 'linen', and describes numbness and tingling (such as is produced by linen on the skin).

2. The term 鸡胸 *jī xiōng*, 'chicken breast', denotes a deformity in infants in which the chest protrudes at the center, giving it the appearance of a chicken's breast. In Western medicine, the condition is often referred to by the Latin name 'pectus gallinatum', whose literal meaning is identical with the Chinese (from *gallus*, a cock). In lay speech, people with the condition are more commonly described as 'pigeon-chested'.

3. The Chinese 水痘 *shuǐ dòu* literally means 'water pox'. The natural equivalent in English is 'chicken pox'.

复合词 Compounds:

1392. 胎毒 *tāi dú*, fetal toxin
1393. 胎弱 *tāi ruò*, fetal feebleness
1394. 胎赤 *tāi chì*, fetal redness
1395. 解颅 *jiě lú*, ununited skull
1396. 囟门不合 *xìn mén bù hé*, non-closure of the fontanels
1397. 囟陷 *xìn xiàn*, depressed fontanels
1398. 囟门下陷 *xìn mén xià xiàn*, depressed fontanels
1399. 囟填 *xìn tián*, bulging fontanels
1400. 囟门凸起 *xìn mén tú qǐ*, bulging fontanels

1401. 鸡胸 *jī xiōng*, chicken breast; pigeon chest

1402. 龟背 *guī bèi*, turtle's back

1403. 五迟 *wǔ chí*, five slownesses

1404. 发迟 *fà chí*, slowness to grow hair

1405. 齿迟 *chǐ chí*, slowness to teethe

1406. 立迟 *lì chí*, slowness to stand

1407. 行迟 *xíng chí*, slowness to walk

1408. 语迟 *yǔ chí*, slowness to speak

1409. 百日咳 *bǎi rì ké*, whooping cough (lit. 'hundred-day cough')

1410. 鸡咳 *jī ké*, hen cough, whooping cough

1411. 顿咳 *dùn ké*, long-bout cough (whooping cough)

1412. 痄腮 *zhà sāi*, mumps

1413. 急惊风 *jí jīng fēng*, acute fright wind

1414. 慢惊风 *màn jīng fēng*, chronic fright wind

1415. 麻疹 *má zhěn*, measles

1416. 疳积 *gān jī*, gan accumulation

1417. 小儿啼哭 *xiǎo ér tí kū*, crying in children

1418. 积滞 *jī zhì*, accumulation and stagnation

1419. 小儿麻疹 *xiǎo ér má zhěn*, measles in children

1420. 水痘 *shuǐ dòu*, chicken pox

1421. 小儿水痘 *xiǎo ér shuǐ dòu*, chicken pox in children

1422. 小儿丹痧 *xiǎo ér dān shā*, cinnabar sand in children

1423. 小儿丹毒 *xiǎo ér dān dú*, cinnabar toxin in children

1424. 小儿发热 *xiǎo ér fā rè*, heat effusion in children

1425. 小儿发黄 *xiǎo ér fā huáng*, yellowing of the complexion in children

1426. 小儿呕吐 *xiǎo ér ǒu tù*, vomiting in children

1427. 小儿腹泻 *xiǎo ér fù xiè*, diarrhea in children

1428. 小儿大便不通 *xiǎo ér dà biàn bù tōng*, constipation in children

1429. 小儿痞块 *xiǎo ér pǐ kuài*, lump glomus in children

1430. 小儿蛔虫 *xiǎo ér huí chóng*, roundworm in children

1431. 小儿浮肿 *xiǎo ér fú zhǒng*, puffy swelling in children

1432. 小儿遗尿 *xiǎo ér yí niào*, child enuresis

1433. 小儿鹅口 *xiǎo ér é kǒu*, goose mouth sore in children

1434. 小儿痿证 *xiǎo ér wěi zhèng*, infantile wilting pattern

1435. 小儿疳眼 *xiǎo ér gān yǎn*, child eye gan

习题 Exercise:

503. *tāi dú* ....

504. ununited skull ....

505. 鸡胸 ....

506. *chǐ chí* ....

507. whooping cough ....

508. 痄腮 ....

509. *má zhěn* ....

510. chicken pox ....

第三节　第七组   SECTION 3: SET 7

妇科疾病   Women's Diseases

1207-n822	* 妇 女	婦 女	*fù*	woman /ˈwʊmən/
1208	* 乱 舌	亂 乙	*luàn*	chaotic /keˈɑtɪk/
1209-n823	* 崩 山	崩 山	*bēng*	flooding /ˈflʌdɪŋ/
1210	* 漏 氵	漏 水	*lòu*	spotting /ˈspɑtɪŋ/
1211	* 带 巾	帶 巾	*dài*	vaginal discharge /ˈvædʒɪnl̩ (vəˈdʒɑɪnl̩) ˈdɪstʃɑrdʒ/
1212-n824	前 ˅	前 八	*qián*	*before, earlier, pre-*

注 Notes:

1. The term 崩漏 *bēng lòu* refers to profuse or minor discharge of blood through the vagina that is not attributable to normal menstrual bleeding or to damage during coitus. Within the compound, 崩 *bēng* literally means collapse or burst, and 漏 *lòu* literally means to leak or trickle. While many translators use the Western medical terms 'uterine bleeding' or 'metrorrhagia', the colloquial expressions 'flooding' and 'spotting' come much closer to the literal meaning of the Chinese terms. In Chinese, the two characters combined together are a generic term (flooding and spotting), but both 崩 *bēng* and 漏 *lòu* may be used singly or in combination with other characters: 崩中 *bēng zhòng*, flooding; 漏下 *lòu xià*, spotting.

2. In Chinese, amenorrhea is referred to as 经闭 *jīng bì*, 'menstrual block'.

复合词 Compounds:

1436. 月经不调 *yuè jīng bù tiáo*, menstrual irregularities

1437. 经乱 *jīng luàn*, chaotic menstruation

1438. 痛经 *tòng jīng*, menstrual pain

1439. 经行腹痛 *jīng xíng fù tòng*, menstrual abdominal pain

1440. 经行头痛 *jīng xíng tóu tòng*, menstrual headache

1441. 经行身痛 *jīng xíng shēn tòng*, menstrual body pain

1442. 经行腰痛 *jīng xíng yāo tòng*, menstrual lumbar pain

1443. 经行发热 *jīng xíng fā rè*, menstrual heat effusion

1444. 经行呕吐 *jīng xíng ǒu tù*, menstrual vomiting

1445. 经行泄泻 *jīng xíng xiè xiè*, menstrual diarrhea

1446. 经行吐衄 *jīng xíng tù nǜ*, menstrual blood ejection and spontaneous external bleeding

1447. 经行便血 *jīng xíng biàn xuè*, menstrual bloody stool

1448. 经行浮肿 *jīng xíng fú zhǒng*, menstrual puffy swelling

1449. 经行抽搐 *jīng xíng chōu chù*, menstrual convulsion

1450. 经前不寐 *jīng qián bú mèi*, premenstrual sleeplessness

1451. 经前乳胀 *jīng qián rǔ zhàng*, premenstrual distention of the breasts

1452. 经前腹痛 *jīng qián fù tòng*, premenstrual abdominal pain

1453. 经後腹痛 *jīng hòu fù tòng*, postmenstrual abdominal pain

1454. 经断复行 *jīng duàn fù xíng*, postmenopausal recommencement of periods

1455. 崩漏 *bēng lòu*, flooding and spotting

1456. 崩中 *bēng zhōng*, flooding

1457. 血崩 *xuè bēng*, flooding

1458. 暴崩 *bào bēng*, fulminant flooding

1459. 崩中暴下 *bēng zhōng bào xià*, fulminant flooding

1460. 漏下 *lòu xià*, spotting

1461. 经漏 *jīng lòu*, postmenstrual spotting

1462. 经闭 *jīng bì*, menstrual block

1463. 白带 *bái dài*, white vaginal discharge

1464. 黄带 *huáng dài*, yellow vaginal discharge

1465. 赤带 *chì dài*, red vaginal discharge

1466. 五色带 *wǔ sè dài*, five-colored vaginal discharge

第三节　第八组	**SECTION 3: SET 8**

妊娠疾病	**Pregnancy Diseases**

1213	* 胎 月	胎 肉	*tāi*	fetus /ˈfitəs/
1214-n825	* 妊 女	妊 女	*rèn*	pregnant /ˈprɛgnənt/ *adj.*
				pregnancy /ˈprɛgnənsɪ/ *n.*

1215-n826	* 娠 女	娠 女	*shēn*	pregnant /ˈprɛgnənt/ *adj.*
				pregnancy /ˈprɛgnənsɪ/ *n.*
1216-n827	* 孕 子	孕 子	*yùn*	pregnant /ˈprɛgnənt/ *adj.*
				pregnancy /ˈprɛgnənsɪ/ *n.*
1217	滑 氵	滑 水	*huá*	slip, slide

注 Note:

The Chinese 子痫 *zǐ xián* corresponds to eclampsia in Western medicine. In Chinese medicine, it was considered a form of epilepsy as is reflected in its name, literally translated as 'epilepsy of pregnancy'.

复合词 Compounds:

1467. 妊娠呕吐 *rèn shēn ǒu tù*, vomiting in pregnancy
1468. 妊娠腹痛 *rèn shēn fù tòng*, abdominal pain in pregnancy
1469. 妊娠心烦 *rèn shēn xīn fán*, vexation in pregnancy
1470. 妊娠咳嗽 *rèn shēn ké sòu*, cough in pregnancy
1471. 妊娠喑哑 *rèn shēn yīn yǎ*, loss of voice in pregnancy
1472. 妊娠肿胀 *rèn shēn zhǒng zhàng*, swelling and distention in pregnancy
1473. 妊娠眩晕 *rèn shēn xuàn yūn*, dizziness in pregnancy
1474. 妊娠下肢抽筋 *rèn shēn xià zhī chōu jīn*, lower limb cramp in pregnancy
1475. 妊娠心腹胀满 *rèn shēn xīn fù zhàng mǎn*, distention and fullness in the heart [region] and abdomen in pregnancy
1476. 妊娠腹痛 *rèn shēn fù tòng*, abdominal pain in pregnancy
1477. 妊娠小便不通 *rèn shēn xiǎo biàn bù tōng*, urinary stoppage in pregnancy
1478. 妊娠尿血 *rèn shēn niào xuè*, bloody urine in pregnancy
1479. 胎动不安 *tāi dòng bù ān*, stirring fetus
1480. 滑胎 *huá tāi*, habitual miscarriage
1481. 子痫 *zǐ xián*, epilepsy of pregnancy
1482. 胎水 *tāi shuǐ*, fetal water
1483. 胎漏 *tāi lòu*, fetal spotting
1484. 胎位不正 *tāi wèi bú zhèng*, malposition of the fetus
1485. 流产后闭经 *liú chǎn hòu bì jīng*, post-miscarriage menstrual block

第三节　第九组   **SECTION 3: SET 9**

产后疾病   **Postpartum Diseases**

1218	* 产 立	產 生	*chǎn*	delivery /dɪˈlɪvərɪ/
				childbirth /ˈtʃaɪldbɜ˞θ/
				partum /ˈpɑrtəm/
1219	* 乳 ⺇	乳 乙	*rǔ*	breast /brɛst/
				milk /mɪlk/
1220-n828	汁 氵	汁 水	*zhī*	*juice, sap*
1221	* 胞 月	胞 肉	*bāo*	placenta /pləˈsɛntə/
1222	衣 衣	衣 衣	*yī*	*clothing, wrapping*
1223	恶 亞	惡 心	*è*	*malign, evil*
1224	露 雨	露 雨	*lù*	*dew*
1225	* 枕 木	枕 木	*zhěn*	pillow /ˈpɪlo/
1226	* 败 貝	敗 貝	*bài*	vanquished /ˈvænkwɪʃt/

注 Notes:

1. The Chinese 乳 *rǔ* means both 'breast' and 'milk'.

2. The term 恶露 *è lù* denotes a liquid discharge from the uterus after childbirth. In English, this is known as lochia, which is derived from the Greek *lokhos*, childbirth (and related to *lechnos*, bed, and the English 'lie'). The Chinese term literally means 'malign dew'. Note that the word 恶 is pronounced in three different ways. In the sense of malign, it is pronounced as *è*; in the sense of aversion to or fear of it is pronounced as *wǔ*; and in the sense of nausea, it is pronounced as *ě*.

3. The term 儿枕痛 *ér zhěn tòng*, infant's-pillow pain, denotes postpartum lower abdominal pain caused by static blood. The condition probably gets its name from the association of the pain with an abdominal mass imagined to be the pillow on which the infant's head lay.

复合词 Compounds:

1486. 乳汁不行 *rǔ zhī bù xíng*, breast milk stoppage
1487. 乳汁自漏 *rǔ zhī zì lòu*, postpartum leakage of breast milk
1488. 胞衣不下 *bāo yī bú xià*, retention of the placenta
1489. 恶露 *è lù*, lochia (lit. 'malign dew')
1490. 恶露不下 *è lù bú xià*, retention of the lochia
1491. 恶露不断 *è lù bú duàn*, persistent flow of lochia
1492. 儿枕痛 *ér zhěn tòng*, infant's-pillow pain

1493. 败血冲肺 *bài xuè chōng fèi*, vanquished blood surging into the lung

1494. 败血冲胃 *bài xuè chōng wèi*, vanquished blood surging into the stomach

1495. 败血冲心 *bài xuè chōng xīn*, vanquished blood surging into the heart

1496. 产后血崩 *chǎn hòu xuè bēng*, postpartum flooding

1497. 产后腹痛 *chǎn hòu fù tòng*, postpartum abdominal pain

1498. 产后眩晕 *chǎn hòu xuàn yūn*, postpartum dizziness

1499. 产后发热 *chǎn hòu fā rè*, postpartum heat effusion

1500. 产后多汗 *chǎn hòu duō hàn*, postpartum profuse sweating

1501. 产后大便难 *chǎn hòu dà biàn nán*, postpartum defecation difficulty

1502. 产后小便不通 *chǎn hòu xiǎo biàn bù tōng*, postpartum urinary stoppage

1503. 产后小便频数 *chǎn hòu xiǎo biàn pín shuò*, postpartum urinary frequency

1504. 产后小便失禁 *chǎn hòu xiǎo biàn shī jìn*, postpartum urinary incontinence

1505. 产后浮肿 *chǎn hòu fú zhǒng*, postpartum puffy swelling

1506. 产后胁痛 *chǎn hòu xié tòng*, postpartum rib-side pain

1507. 产后腰痛 *chǎn hòu yāo tòng*, postpartum lumbar pain

1508. 产后身痛 *chǎn hòu shēn tòng*, postpartum body pain

1509. 产门不闭 *chǎn mén bú bì*, non-closure of the birth gate

1510. 产后阴户肿痛 *chǎn hòu yīn hù zhǒng tòng*, postpartum painful swelling of the yīn door

---

第三节　第十组　　　　　　　　　　SECTION 3: SET 10

妇人杂病　　　　　　　　　　**Miscellaneous Women's Diseases**

1227	* 脏 月	臟 肉	*zàng*	visceral /ˈvɪsərəl/
1228	* 躁 足	躁 足	*zào*	agitation /ˌædʒɪˈteʃən/
1229-n829	* 挺 扌	挺 手	*tǐng*	protrude /proˈtrud/
1230	* 交 亠	交 亠	*jiāo*	intercourse /ˈɪntɚˌkɔrs, -kors/
1231-n830	* 接 扌	接 手	*jiē*	*join, connect, receive*

注 **Note:**

阴挺 *yīn tǐng*, vaginal protrusion, is a women's disease characterized by heaviness, sagging, and swelling of the anterior yīn, or the protrusion of the

the internal organs outside the body. It is usually the result of center qì fall or insufficiency of kidney qì, if not due to holding breath and straining in childbirth.

复合词 Compounds:

1511. 妇人 *fù rén*, woman
1512. 不孕 *bú yùn*, infertility
1513. 癥瘕 *zhēng jiǎ*, concretions and conglomerations
1514. 妇人脏躁 *fù rén zàng zào*, visceral agitation in women
1515. 交接出血 *jiāo jiē chū xuè*, coital bleeding
1516. 阴痒 *yīn yǎng*, pudendal itch
1517. 阴挺 *yīn tǐng*, vaginal protrusion
1518. 外阴痈肿 *wài yīn yōng zhǒng*, genital welling-abscess
1519. 阴疮 *yīn chuāng*, genital sore

习题 Exercise:

511. 月经不调 ....
512. *jīng luàn* ....
513. menstrual headache ....
514. 经行腰痛 ....
515. *bēng lòu* ....
516. red vaginal discharge ....
517. 妊娠呕吐 ....
518. *rèn shēn fù tòng* ....
519. loss of voice in pregnancy ....
520. 妊娠心腹胀满 ....
521. *tāi dòng bù ān* ....
522. fetal water ....
523. 胎位不正 ....
524. *liú chǎn hòu bì jīng* ....
525. breast milk stoppage ....
526. 乳汁自漏 ....
527. *bāo yī bú xià* ....
528. lochia ....
529. 儿枕痛 ....

第四节：病机、辨证
Section 4: Pathomechanisms and Pattern Identification

The term 证 *zhèng*, which literally means 'testimony' or 'evidence', in the medical context means either a sign of disease (i.e., a symptom) or a pattern (a configuration of signs). Through pattern identification the nature and location of an illness can be established. The most general form of pattern identification is 八纲辨证 *bā gāng biàn zhèng*, eight-principle pattern identification, which determines whether an illness is in the exterior or interior and whether it is ascribed to cold or heat, vacuity or repletion, and to yīn or yáng. Through 脏腑辨证 *zàng fǔ biàn zhèng*, bowel and viscera pattern identification, 六经辨证 *liù jīng biàn zhèng*, six-channel pattern identification, and other procedures, a more detailed description of the condition can be established.

A pattern differs from a 疾病 *jí bìng* or 疾 *jí*, disease. A disease is a morbid condition that is characterized by a similar set of symptoms and similar course in all that it effects; one and the same disease may present different patterns at different stages of its development.

The concept of 病机 *bìng jī*, pathomechanism, is equivalent to the notions of etiology and pathogenesis in Western medicine. The distinction between terms describing pathomechanisms and terms describing patterns is blurred since many patterns are labelled by a pathomechanical term. Some consider 肝气郁结 *gān qì yù jié*, binding depression of liver qi, to be a pathomechanism and 肝郁 *gān yù*, liver depression, to be a pattern name, while others consider the former as a pattern name too.

In addition to names of organs, names of elements (qì, blood, etc.), and names of disease evils, which have already been introduced, the vocabulary of pathomechanisms and disease patterns notably comprises a large number of descriptive characters. These characters are the focus of the present section. These are first introduced in five sets, grouped according to similarity of meaning: 'vacuity', 'insecurity', 'repletion', 'heat and fire', and 'stagnation'. The categories 'heat and fire' and 'stagnation' are effectively subsets of 'vacuity' and 'repletion', while 'insecurity' is a subset of 'vacuity'. Together, these categories actually represent the main vectors in the dynamics of pathogenesis in the Chinese medical understanding. These lists are followed by a systematic presentation of terminology relating to pathomechanisms and the various forms of pattern identification.

第四节　第一组　　　　　　　　　　　**SECTION 4: SET 1**

「虚」类字词　　　　　　　　　　　'Vacuity' Terms

1232	*	虚 庀	虚 庀	xū	vacuity /vəˈkjuɪtɪ/
1233	*	足 足	足 足	xū	sufficiency /səˈfɪʃənsɪ/
1234-n831	*	衰 一	衰 衣	shuāi	debilitation /dəˌbɪlɪˈteʃən/
1235-n832	*	耗 耒	耗 耒	hào	wearing /ˈwɛrɪŋ/
1236-n833	*	亏 二	虧 庀	kuī	depletion /dɪˈpliʃən/
1237-n834	*	竭 立	竭 立	jié	exhaustion /ɪgzˈɔstʃən/
1238	*	劳 艹	勞 力	láo	taxation /tæksˈeʃən/
1239-n835	*	损 扌	損 手	sǔn	detriment /ˈdɛtrɪmənt/
1240-n836	*	亡 亡	亡 一	wáng	collapse /kəˈlæps/
1241	*	脱 月	脱 肉	tuō	desert /dɪˈzɜ·t/ vi.
					desertion /dɪˈzɜ·ʃən/ n.
1242	*	浮 氵	浮 水	fú	floating /ˈflotɪŋ/
1243	*	绝 纟	絕 糸	jué	expiration /ˌɛkspəˈreʃən/
1244-n837	*	夺 大	奪 大	duó	despoliate /dɪˈspolɪˌet/ vt.
					despoliation /dɪˌspolɪˈeʃən/ n.
1245	*	干 二	乾 乙	gān	dryness /ˈdraɪnɪs/ n.
1246	*	枯 木	枯 木	kū	desiccation /ˌdɛsɪˈkeʃən/
1247-n838	*	涸 氵	涸 水	hé	desiccation /ˌdɛsɪˈkeʃən/
1248	*	空 穴	空 穴	kōng	emptiness /ˈɛmptɪnɪs/
1249	*	振 扌	振 手	zhèn	vitalize /ˈvaɪtəlaɪz/
1250-n839	*	养 丷	養 食	yǎng	nourish /ˈnɜ·ɪʃ/
1251	*	涵 氵	涵 水	hán	moisten /ˈmɔɪsn̩/
1252	*	陷 阝	陷 阜	xiàn	fall /fɔl/

注 Notes:

1. The terms listed in this section denote various forms of vacuity. The Chinese 虚 xū is the opposite of 实 shí (which is the theme of the next set). Their meanings are empty/full, or insubstantial/substantial. In medicine, 虚 xū denotes a condition of the body arising from an insufficiency (不足 bù zú) of internal resources (blood, qì, essence, etc.). Repletion is a condition of the body created by a superabundance (有余 yǒu yú) of evil and the body's reaction to it.

The character 足 zú, sufficiency, is usually only used in the negative form 不足 bù zú, insufficiency, in contrast to 有余 yǒu yú, superabundance. Notice that the primary meaning of 足, 'foot', is extended to mean sufficiency by being the necessary 'basis' for activity. Interestingly, the English word 'sufficiency' derives from the Latin *suf* (*sub*) + *ficere* (*facere*), 'under make', which expresses the notion in a similar way.

2. Both insufficiency and vacuity are generic terms. The other words listed above are more specific. The word 亏 *kuī*, 'depletion', and 衰 *shuāi*, 'debilitation', mean severe forms of vacuity; 劳 *láo*, 'taxation', means severe chronic vacuity; 绝 *jué*, 'expiration', and 亡 *wáng*, 'collapse', are used in compound terms describing critical conditions; 损 *sǔn*, 'detriment', means loss or damage (to blood, fluids, organs, etc.), and specifically severe chronic damage; 夺 *duó*, 'despoliation' (previously translated as 'retrenchment'), describes a sudden loss as if by an act of plundering. Many translators ignore these distinctions and use generic terms instead.

3. In terms describing vacuity conditions, the characters 振 *zhèn*, 养 *yǎng*, and 函 *hán* are used in negative constructions such as 脾阳不振 *pí yáng bú zhèn*, devitalized spleen yáng, and 筋脉失养 *jīn mài shī yǎng*, sinews deprived of nourishment.

复合词 Compounds:

1520. 心气虚 *xīn qì xū*, heart qì vacuity
1521. 肾精不足 *shèn jīng bù zú*, insufficiency of kidney essence
1522. 夺精 *duó jīng*, despoliation of essence
1523. 热耗真阴 *rè hào zhēn yīn*, heat wearing true yīn
1524. 上厥下竭 *shàng jué xià jié*, upper body reversal and lower body exhaustion
1525. 肠液亏耗 *cháng yè kuī hào*, intestinal humor depletion
1526. 五劳所伤 *wǔ láo suǒ shāng*, damage by the five taxations
1527. 津液亏损 *jīn yè kuī sǔn*, fluid depletion
1528. 亡阴 *wáng yīn*, yīn collapse
1529. 气脱 *qì tuō*, qì desertion
1530. 阳强不能密，阴气乃绝 *yáng jiàng bù néng mì, yīn qì nǎi jué*, when yáng is overstrong and does not constrain itself, yīn qì expires
1531. 阴虚阳浮 *yīn xū yáng fú*, yīn vacuity and floating yáng
1532. 精气夺则虚 *jīng qì duó zé xū*, when essential qì is despoliated, there is vacuity
1533. 干血 *gān xuè*, dry blood
1534. 干血劳 *gān xuè láo*, dry blood taxation
1535. 津枯血燥 *jīn kū xuè zào*, desiccation of liquid and blood dryness
1536. 肾阴枯涸 *shèn yīn kū hé*, desiccation of kidney yīn
1537. 髓海空虚 *suǐ hǎi kōng xū*, emptiness of the sea of marrow
1538. 脾阳不振 *pí yáng bú zhèn*, devitalized spleen yáng

1539. 血不养筋 *xuè bù yǎng jīn*, blood failing to nourish the sinews

1540. 水不涵木 *shuǐ bù hán mù*, water failing to moisten wood

1541. 土不生金 *tǔ bù shēng jīn*, earth failing to engender metal

1542. 土不制水 *tǔ bù zhì shuǐ*, earth failing to dam water

第四节　第二组	**SECTION 4: SET 2**

「实」类字词   'Repletion' Terms

1253	* 实 宀	實 宀	*shí*	repletion /rɪˈpliʃən/
1254-n840	* 胜 月	勝 力	*shèng*	prevail /prɪˈvel/ *vi.* prevalence /ˈprɛvələns/
1255-n841	* 盛 皿	盛 皿	*shèng*	exuberance /ɪgzˈjubərəns/
1256-n842	* 余 人	餘 食	*yú*	superabundance /ˌsupərəˈbʌndəns/
1257-n843	* 犯 犭	犯 犬	*fàn*	invade /ɪnˈved/
1258-n844	* 侵 亻	侵 人	*qīn*	invade /ɪnˈved/
1259-n845	* 袭 龍	襲 衣	*xí*	assail /əˈsel/
1260	* 入 入	入 入	*rù*	enter /ɛntər/
1261	* 束 束	束 木	*shù*	fetter /ˈfɛtər/
1262	* 困 口	困 口	*kùn*	encumber /ɪnˈkʌmbər/
1263-n846	* 伏 亻	伏 人	*fú*	latent /ˈletənt/ deep-lying /ˈdipˌlaɪŋ/
1264-n847	* 客 宀	客 宀	*kè*	settle /ˈsɛtl̩/
1265-n848	* 留 田	留 田	*liú*	lodged /lɑdʒd/
1266-n849	恋 心	戀 心	*liàn*	*feel attachment to; reluctant to leave*
1267	* 蒙 艹	蒙 艸	*méng*	cloud /klaʊd/
1268-n850	* 蔽 艹	蔽 艸	*bì*	cloud /klaʊd/
1269-n851	* 迷 辶	迷 辵	*mí*	confound /kənˈfaʊnd/
1270-n852	* 扰 扌	擾 手	*rǎo*	harass /həˈræs, ˈhærəs/
1271	* 泛 氵	泛 水	*fàn*	flood /flʌd/
1272-n853	滥 氵	濫 水	*làn*	*flood, overflow, excessive*
1273	* 注 氵	注 水	*zhù*	pour /pɔr, por/
1274	* 射 身	射 寸	*shè*	shoot /ʃut/
1275-n854	* 凌 冫	凌 冫	*líng*	intimidate /ɪnˈtɪmɪdet/
1276-n855	* 蕴 艹	蘊 艸	*yùn*	brew /bru/
1277	* 冲 冫	衝 行	*chōng*	surge /sɝdʒ/
1278	* 动 力	動 力	*dòng*	stir /stɝ/
1279-n856	* 亢 亠	亢 亠	*kàng*	hyperactivity /ˌhaɪpərækˈtɪvɪtɪ/
1280-n857	* 迫 辶	迫 辵	*pò*	distress /dɪˈstrɛs/
1281	* 陷 阝	陷 阜	*xiàn*	fall /fɔl/

1282-n858　＊搏 扌　搏 手　*bó*　contend /kən'tɛnd/ *vi.*
1283　＊煽 火　煽 火　*shàn*　fan /fæn/ *vt.*

注 Note:

The vocabulary describing the entry of evils into the body and imbalances within the body are often described in an aggressive or militaristic tone: 'wind-heat assailing the lung', 'water-cold shooting into the heart', 'water qì intimidating the heart', 'wind and damp contending with each other', etc.

复合词 Compounds:

1543. 实热 *shí rè*, repletion heat
1544. 邪气盛 *xié qì shèng*, exuberant evil qì
1545. 邪气有馀 *xié qì yǒu yú*, superabundance of evil qì
1546. 风热袭肺 *fēng rè xí fèi*, wind-heat assailing the lung
1547. 风热犯肺 *fēng rè fàn fèi*, wind-heat invading the lung
1548. 风邪入侵经络 *fēng xié rù qīn jīng luò*, wind evil invading the channels and network vessels
1549. 热入气分 *rè rù qì fèn*, heat entering the qì aspect
1550. 风寒束肺 *fēng hán shù fèi*, wind-cold fettering the lung
1551. 寒湿困脾 *hán shī kùn pí*, cold-damp encumbering the spleen
1552. 湿遏热伏 *shī è rè fú*, dampness trapping hidden (deep-lying) heat
1553. 寒邪客于肺 *hán xié kè yú fèi*, cold evil settling in the lung
1554. 邪气客于内 *xié qì kè yú nèi*, evil qì settling in the inner body
1555. 痰留胸胁 *tán liú xiōng xié*, phlegm lodged in the chest and rib-side
1556. 温热留恋气分 *wēn rè liú liàn qì fèn*, warm-heat lodged in the qì aspect
1557. 痰蒙蔽心包 *tán zhuó méng bì xīn bāo*, phlegm clouding the pericardium
1558. 痰迷心窍 *tán mí xīn qiào*, phlegm confounding the orifices of the heart
1559. 痰火上扰 *tán huǒ shàng rǎo*, phlegm-fire harassing the upper body
1560. 肾虚水泛 *shèn xū shuǐ fàn*, kidney vacuity water flood
1561. 水湿泛滥 *shuǐ shī fàn làn*, water-damp flood
1562. 湿热下注大肠 *shī rè xià zhù dà cháng*, damp-heat pouring down into the large intestine
1563. 水寒射肺 *shuǐ hán shè fèi*, water-cold shooting into the lung
1564. 水气凌心 *shuǐ qì líng xīn*, water qì intimidating the heart
1565. 湿热蕴结肝胆 *shī rè yùn jié gān dǎn*, damp-heat brewing [and binding] in the liver and gallbladder

1566. 肝风内动 *gān fēng nèi dòng*, liver wind stirring internally

1567. 脚气冲心 *jiǎo qì chōng xīn*, leg qì surging into the heart

1568. 肝阳上亢 *gān yáng shàng kàng*, ascendant (hyperactivity of) liver yáng

1569. 肝风内动 *gān fēng nèi dòng*, liver wind stirring internally

1570. 太阳热邪迫肺 *tài yáng rè xié pò fèi*, greater yáng (*tài yáng*) heat evil distressing the lung

1571. 内陷 *nèi xiàn*, inward fall

1572. 风湿相搏 *fēng shī xiāng bó*, wind and dampness contending with each other; mutual contention of wind and dampness

---

第四节　第三组				**SECTION 4: SET 3**

「火」与「热」有关字词				**Fire & Heat Terms**
1284-n859	* 旺 日	旺 日	*wàng*	effulgent /ɪˈfʌldʒənt/
1285	* 盛 皿	盛 皿	*shèng*	exuberant /ɪgzˈjubərənt/
1286-n860	* 炎 火	炎 火	*yán*	flame /flem/
1287-n861	* 燔 火	燔 火	*fán*	blaze /blez/
1288-n862	* 焚 火	焚 火	*fén*	deflagrate /ˈdɛfləˌgret/
1289	* 灼 火	灼 火	*zhuó*	scorch /skɔrtʃ/
1290-n863	* 炼 火	煉 火	*liàn*	condense /kənˈdɛns/
1291	* 焦 隹	焦 火	*jiāo*	scorch /ˈskɔrtʃ/
1292-n864	* 炽 火	熾 火	*chì*	intense /ɪnˈtɛns/
1293	* 蒸 艹	蒸 艸	*zhēng*	steam /stim/
1294-n865	* 薰 艹	薰 艸	*xūn*	fume /fjum/
1295	* 浮 氵	浮 水	*fú*	float /flot/
1296-n866	* 刑 刂	刑 刀	*xíng*	torment /tɔrˈmɛnt/

注 Notes:

1. Heat and fire are yáng phenomena. However, distinction is made between repletion heat (or fire) and vacuity heat (or fire). Vacuity heat and fire usually arise from yīn vacuity; rarely, vacuity heat is the result of qì vacuity.

2. Except for the terms that describe vacuity heat and vacuity fire, the vocabulary of heat and fire is a subset of repletion terms. At first sight, many of the words appear to be near synonyms; closer inspection reveals important nuances. 旺 *wàng*, 'effulgence', is a relatively generic term describing a strong, bright fire. 蒸 *zhēng*, 'steaming' and 薰 *xūn*, 'fuming', are the metaphors of

damp-heat; 炎 *yán*, 'flaming', used in the compound *shàng yán*, 'flaming upward', is the metaphor describing the pathomechanism by which internal fire causes upper body signs; 灼 *zhuó*, 'scorching', describes the intense local action of heat; 燔 *fán*, 'blazing' and 焚 *fén*, 'deflagrating', are part of the stock vocabulary of warm disease; 浮 *fú*, 'floating', often in the compound 浮越 *fú yuè*, 'floating astray', describe the gentle upward movement of vacuity fire in severe conditions.

复合词 Compounds:

1573. 阴虚火旺 *yīn xū huǒ wàng*, effulgent yīn vacuity fire
1574. 热盛 *rè shèng*, exuberant heat
1575. 心火亢盛 *xīn huǒ kàng shèng*, exuberant heart fire
1576. 肝火上炎 *gān huǒ shàng yán*, liver fire flaming upward
1577. 气营两燔 *qì yíng liǎng fán*, qì and construction both ablaze
1578. 心火内焚 *xīn huǒ nèi fén*, heart fire deflagrating internally
1579. 胃火炽盛 *wèi huǒ chì shèng*, intense stomach fire
1580. 暑湿郁蒸 *shǔ shī yù zhēng*, depressed steaming summerheat-damp
1581. 热灼肾阴 *rè zhuó shèn yīn*, heat scorching kidney yīn
1582. 炼液为痰 *liàn yè chéng tán*, condense humor into phlegm
1583. 肺热叶焦 *fèi rè yè jiāo*, lung heat scorching the lobes
1584. 火盛刑金 *huǒ shèng xíng jīn*, exuberant fire tormenting metal
1585. 痰火扰心 *tán huǒ rǎo xīn*, phlegm-fire harassing the heart
1586. 肝火犯肺 *gān huǒ fàn fèi*, liver fire invading the lung
1587. 湿热蕴脾 *shī rè yùn pí*, damp-heat brewing in the spleen
1588. 胃热亢盛 *wèi rè kàng shèng*, hyperactive stomach heat
1589. 胃火上升 *wèi huǒ shàng shēng*, stomach fire bearing upward; upbearing of stomach fire

---

第四节　第四组　　　　　　　　　　　　SECTION 4: SET 4

「滞」类字词　　　　　　　　　　'Stagnation' Terms

1297	*	滞 氵	滯 水	*zhì*	stagnation /stæg'neʃən/
1298	*	瘀 疒	瘀 疒	*yū*	stasis /'stesɪs/
1299	*	郁 阝	鬱 鬯	*yù*	depression /dɪ'preʃən/
1300-n867	*	壅 土	壅 土	*yōng*	congestion /kən'dʒestʃən/
1301	*	闭 门	閉 門	*bì*	block /blɑk/
1302-n868	*	阻 阝	阻 阜	*zǔ*	obstruction /əb'strʌkʃən/
1303-n869	*	遏 辶	遏 辵	*è*	obstruction /əb'strʌkʃən/

				trap /træp/
1304	* 塞宀	塞土	*sāi*	blockage /ˈblɑkɪdʒ/
1305-n870	* 蓄艹	蓄艸	*xù*	amassment /əˈmæsmənt/
1306-n871	* 停亻	停人	*tíng*	collection /kəˈlɛkʃən/
1307	* 积禾	積禾	*jī*	accumulation /əˌkjumjuˈleʃən/
1308	* 聚耳	聚耳	*jù*	gathering /ˈgæðərɪŋ/
1309	* 结纟	結糸	*jié*	bind /baɪnd/
1310	* 逆辶	逆辵	*nì*	counterflow /ˈkaʊntɚflo/
1311	* 厥厂	厥厂	*jué*	reversal /rɪˈvɝsl̩/

注 Notes:

1. The above list includes not only characters meaning stagnation or blockage, but also denoting conditions that result from stagnation or blockage, such as 聚 *jù*, gathering, and 蓄 *xù*, amass. The characters 逆 *nì*, counterflow, and 厥 *jué*, reversal, refer to backward flow or ebbing that may be due to repletion or to stagnation.

2. The characters 滞 *zhì*, stagnation, and 郁 *yù*, depression, are similar in meaning. The former is more commonly used to generally denote the impairment of qì dynamic (气机 *qì jī*), while the latter often specifically denotes qì stagnation associated with emotional disturbance, referred to as 肝气郁结 *gān qì yù jié*, binding depression of liver qì.

3. The word 结 *jié* has many different meanings, all related to the original meaning of to 'tie (in a knot)', which is reflected in the silk (or thread) signific. The wider meanings include: 'condense', 'coagulate', 'stick', 'freeze', 'solidify'. In the Chinese medical context, we translate the term in most contexts as 'bind', since this word not only shares with *jié* the core meaning of to 'tie', but also has a similar range of extended meanings: to 'thicken' (fluids), 'tangle', 'stick', etc. This term notably appears in 热结 *rè jié*, 'heat bind', which refers to constipation due to heat in the intestines, and which is so named because heat causes the waste in the digestive tract to bind together forming a hard mass. It also occurs in 肝气郁结 *gān qì yù jié*, 'binding depression of liver qì', where it emphasizes the clogging nature of the depression. It could be argued that 结 *jié* in this context is superfluous.

4. The term 不利 *bú lì* is here rendered as 'inhibit' because it implies partial obstruction or difficulty of action. It occurs in pathomechanism terms such as 肺气不利 *fèi qì bú lì*, inhibited lung qì, and 膀胱气化不利 *páng guāng qì huà bú lì*, inhibited bladder qì transformation, but it is more common in diagnostic terms: 四肢屈伸不利 *sì zhī qū shén bú lì*, 'inhibited bending

and stretching of the limbs', 小便不利 *xiǎo biàn bú lì*, 'inhibited urination', and 语言不利 *yǔ yán bú lì*, 'inhibited speech'.

5. The words 聚 *jù*, 'gathering' and 积 *jī*, 'accumulation', are used in general descriptions of evils (邪 *xié*), but both can also denote specific forms of abdominal masses. In addition, 积, 'accumulation', often specifically denotes accumulation of the food in the digestive tract. The word 壅 *yōng*, 'congestion', mostly describes the clogging effect of evils and phlegm in the lung. The term 蓄 *xù*, 'amassment', is used in specific compound terms from the *Shāng Hán Lùn* such as 'blood amassment patterns' and 'water amassment patterns'.

6. The two terms, 逆 *nì*, 'counterflow', and 厥 *jué*, 'reversal', are similar in meaning and usage. Both mean a disturbance of normal flow, and both can describe how movement of yáng qì to the periphery of the body ebbs or recedes (四肢逆冷 *sì zhī nì lěng*, 'counterflow cold of the limbs'; 四肢厥冷 *sì zhī jué lěng*, 'reversal cold of the limbs'). In addition, 'counterflow' describes the adverse movement of lung, liver, or stomach qì, while 'reversal', describes other disturbances of qì that give rise to temporary loss of consciousness (called 昏厥 *hūn jué*, 'clouding reversal', in traditional terminology).

复合词 Compounds:

1590. 气滞 *qì zhì*, qì stagnation
1591. 血瘀 *xuè yū*, blood stasis
1592. 气郁 *qì yù*, qì depression
1593. 痰热壅肺 *tán rè yōng fèi*, phlegm-heat congesting the lung
1594. 气闭 *qì bì*, qì block
1595. 寒湿中阻 *hán shī zhōng zǔ*, cold-damp obstructing the center
1596. 湿遏卫阳 *shī è wèi yáng*, dampness obstructing defense yáng
1597. 伤寒蓄血 *shāng hán xù xuè*, cold damage blood amassment
1598. 水饮内停 *shuǐ yǐn nèi tíng*, water-rheum collecting internally
1599. 食积 *shí jī*, food accumulation
1600. 热结 *rè jié*, heat bind
1601. 气逆 *qì nì*, qì counterflow
1602. 厥证 *jué zhèng*, reversal pattern
1603. 肺气不利 *fèi qì bú lì*, inhibited lung qì
1604. 膀胱气化不利 *páng guāng qì huà bú lì*, inhibited bladder qì transformation

第四节　第五组 SECTION 4: SET 5

「不固」类字词				'Insecurity' Terms
1312-n872	* 固 口	固 口	*gù*	security /sɪˈkjʊrɪtɪ/
1313	* 利 禾	利 刀	*lì*	uninhibited /ˌʌnɪnˈhɪbɪtɪd/ diarrhea /ˌdaɪəˈrɪə/
1314	* 滑 氵	滑 水	*huá*	efflux /ˈɛflʌks/
1315	* 脱 月	脱 肉	*tuō*	desertion /dɪˈzɝˈʃən/
1316	* 泄 氵	泄 水	*xiè*	discharge /ˈdɪstʃɑrdʒ/
1317	* 遗 辶	遗 辵	*yí*	emission /ɪˈmɪʃən/
1318	* 浮 氵	浮 水	*fú*	floating /ˈflotɪŋ/
1319-n873	* 越 走	越 走	*yuè*	astray /əˈstre/

注 Notes:

1. Most of the words in the above list are used in symptom names as well as in the terminology of pathomechanisms and patterns.

2. 遗尿 *yí niào* literally means 'emission of urine', while the English term is 'enuresis', which literally means 'urinating in [bed]'.

3. The term 滑 *huá*, which in the context of the pulse is translated as 'slippery', here denotes an uncontrolled discharge (lit. 'slipping out') of fluid substances from the body such as stool or semen, and is rendered as 'efflux'.

4. The word 脱 *tuō*, 'desertion', is similar to *huá* in denoting an uncontrollable outward flow, but applies most commonly to yīn, yáng, qì, and blood. The literal meaning of 脱 *tuō* is to 'shed', as a snake sheds its skin. We chose desertion since 'shed' has positive connotations in English that *tuō* does not have in the medical context. Note that 脱肛 *tuō gāng*, 'prolapse of the rectum', is not translated with the standard term 'desertion' even though 'prolapse of the rectum' forms part of a desertion pattern. 'Desertion of the anus' would be a more exact literal translation that would place this sign in its right contextual frame of reference. Reluctantly, we opted for 'prolapse of the rectum' only because it is familiar to all readers.

复合词 Compounds:

1605. 表气不固 *biǎo qì bú gù*, insecurity of exterior qi
1606. 下利清谷 *xià lì qīng gǔ*, clear-food diarrhea
1607. 气脱 *qì tuō*, qi desertion
1608. 滑脱 *huá tuō*, efflux desertion
1609. 气随血脱 *qì suí xuè tuō*, qi deserting with the blood

1610. 宗气外泄 *zōng qì wài xiè*, discharge of ancestral qì
1611. 心神浮越 *xīn shén fú yuè*, heart spirit floating astray
1612. 中气下陷 *zhōng qì xià xiàn*, center qì fall
1613. 久泻滑脱 *jiǔ xiè huá tuō*, enduring diarrhea efflux desertion
1614. 滑精 *huá jīng*, seminal emission
1615. 遗精 *yí jīng*, seminal emission
1616. 梦遗 *mèng yí*, dream emission
1617. 遗尿 *yí niào*, enuresis
1618. 精液大泄 *jīng yè dà xiè*, great discharge of semen

第四节　第六组 | **SECTION 4: SET 6**

病机 — Pathomechanisms

1320	* 机 木	機 木	*jī*	mechanism /ˈmɛkəˌnɪzəm/
1321	* 盛 皿	盛 皿	*shèng*	exuberance /ɪgzˈjubərəns/
1322	* 胜 月	勝 力	*shèng*	prevail /prɪˈvel/
1323	* 衰 亠	衰 衣	*shuāi*	debilitated /dəˈbɪlɪˌtetɪd/
1324-n874	则 贝	則 刀	*zé*	*then, so*
1325-n875	* 承 →	承 丿	*chéng*	bear /bɛr/

复合词 Compounds:

1619. 病机 *bìng jī*, pathomechanism
1620. 邪气盛则实 *xié qì shèng zé shí*, when evil qì is exuberant, there is repletion
1621. 精气夺则虚 *jīng qì duó zé xū*, when essential qì is despoliated, there is vacuity
1622. 阳胜则热 *yáng shèng zé rè*, when yáng prevails, there is heat
1623. 阴胜则寒 *yīn shèng zé hán*, when yīn prevails, there is cold
1624. 阳盛则外热 *yáng shèng zé wài rè*, when yáng is exuberant, there is external heat
1625. 阳胜则阴病 *yáng shèng zé yīn bìng*, when yáng prevails, yīn ails
1626. 阴胜则阳病 *yīn shèng zé yáng bìng*, when yīn prevails, yáng ails
1627. 热盛则肿 *rè shèng zé zhǒng*, when heat is exuberant, there is swelling
1628. 寒胜则浮 *hán shèng zé fú*, when cold prevails, there is swelling
1629. 湿胜则濡泻 *shī shèng zé rú xiè*, when dampness prevails, there is soft-stool diarrhea

1630. 湿胜则阳微 *shī shèng zé yáng wēi*, when dampness prevails, yáng is debilitated (the character 微 is here taken to mean 衰微 and is therefore translated as 'debilitated')

1631. 燥胜则干 *zào shèng zé gān*, when dryness prevails, there is aridity

1632. 风胜则动 *fēng shèng zé dòng*, when wind prevails, there is stirring

1633. 肝常有馀 *gān cháng yǒu yú*, liver is often in superabundance

1634. 阳虚则外寒 *yáng xū zé wài hán*, when yáng is vacuous, there is external cold

1635. 阴虚则内热 *yīn xū zé nèi rè*, when yīn is vacuous, there is internal heat

1636. 津不上承 *jīn bú shàng chéng*, liquid failing to bear upward

1637. 水饮内停 *shuǐ yǐn nèi tíng*, water-rheum collecting internally

1638. 水湿泛滥 *shuǐ shī fàn làn*, water-damp flood

1639. 清阳不升 *qīng yáng bù shēng*, clear yáng failing to bear upward; non-upbearing of clear yáng

1640. 浊阴不降 *zhuó yīn bú jiàng*, turbid yīn failing to bear downward; non-downbearing of turbid yīn

1641. 心神失守 *xīn shén shī shǒu*, heart spirit failing to contain itself

1642. 脾失健运 *pí shī jiàn yùn*, spleen failing to move and transform

1643. 气化不利 *qì huà bú lì*, inhibited qì transformation

1644. 肺气不宣 *fèi qì bù xuān*, lung qì failing to diffuse; non-diffusion of lung qì

1645. 肺失肃降 *fèi shī sù jiàng*, impaired depurative downbearing

1646. 肺津不布 *fèi jīn bú bù*, lung liquid failing to distribute; non-distribution of lung liquid

1647. 肝失疏泄 *gān shī shū xiè*, liver failing to course freely; impairment of the liver's free coursing

1648. 肾失固藏 *shèn shī gù cáng*, kidney failing to store securely

1649. 肝不藏血 *gān bù cáng xuè*, liver failing to store the blood

1650. 脾不统血 *pí bù tǒng xuè*, spleen failing to control (manage) the blood

---

第四节　第七组	SECTION 4: SET 7

八纲辨证	**Eight-Principle Pattern Identification**

1326-n876	* 八 八　八 八	*bā*	eight /et/
1327-n877	纲 纟　綱 糸	*gāng*	*headrope, guiding principle*
1328-n878	* 辨 辛　辨 辛	*biàn*	identify /aɪˈdɛntɪˌfaɪ/ *vi.*
			identification /aɪˌdɛntɪfɪˈkeʃən/ *n.*

1329	* 证 讠	證 言	*zhèng*	pattern /ˈpætən/
1330	* 表 主	表 衣	*biǎo*	exterior /ɪksˈtɪrɪəˈ/
1331	* 里 里	裡 衣	*lǐ*	interior /ɪnˈtɪrɪəˈ/
1332	* 寒 宀	寒 宀	*hán*	cold /kold/
1333	* 热 灬	熱 火	*rè*	heat /hit/
1334	* 虚 虍	虛 虍	*xū*	vacuity /vəˈkjuɪtɪ/
1335	* 实 宀	實 宀	*shí*	repletion /rɪˈpliʃən/
1336	* 阴 阝	陰 阜	*yīn*	yīn /jɪn/
1337	* 阳 阝	陽 阜	*yáng*	yáng /jɑŋ, jæŋ/
1338-n879	夹 大	夾 大	*jiā*	*mingled*
1339	错 钅	錯 金	*cuò*	*mingled*
1340	杂 木	雜 隹	*zá*	*miscellaneous, adulterated*
1341	* 半 丨	半 十	*bàn*	half /hæf/
1342	* 真 十	眞 目	*zhēn*	true
1343	* 假 亻	假 人	*jiǎ*	false /fɔls/
1344-n880	转 車	轉 車	*zhuǎn*	*turn, reverse*
1345	* 化 亻	化 匕	*huà*	transform /trænsˈfɔrm/

注 Notes:

1. Combinations of vacuity/repletion and of heat/cold are written without hyphens, e.g., vacuity cold, repletion heat, vacuity heat, since the meaning is 'cold arising through vacuity'. For the same reason, 'vacuous cold' should also be avoided.

2. Combinations are expressed as: 'vacuity heat', 'vacuity cold', 'repletion heat', but usually 'cold repletion' rather than 'repletion cold'.

3. Complexes of vacuity and repletion and of heat and cold are written with a hyphen, e.g., 'heat-cold complex', since heat and cold are a polarity complex.

复合词 Compounds:

1651. 表里 *biǎo lǐ*, exterior and interior, exterior-interior
1652. 寒热 *hán rè*, cold and heat, cold-heat
1653. 寒实 *hán shí*, cold repletion
1654. 实寒 *shí hán*, repletion cold
1655. 实热 *shí rè*, repletion heat
1656. 虚寒 *xū hán*, vacuity cold
1657. 虚热 *xū rè*, vacuity heat
1658. 虚实 *xū shí*, vacuity and repletion, vacuity-repletion

1659. 阴阳 *yīn yáng*, yīn and yáng, yīn-yáng

1660. 表虚 *biǎo xū*, exterior vacuity

1661. 里实 *lǐ shí*, interior repletion

1662. 虚热 *xū rè*, vacuity heat

1663. 相兼 *xiāng jiān*, combination

1664. 真假 *zhēn jiǎ*, truth and falsity

1665. 错杂 *cuò zá*, complex

1666. 夹杂 *jiā zá*, complex

1667. 转化 *zhuǎn huà*, conversion

1668. 半表半里 *bàn biǎo bàn lǐ*, half interior half exterior; midstage penetration

1669. 真寒假热 *zhēn hán jiǎ rè*, true cold and false heat

1670. 真虚假实 *zhēn xū jiǎ shí*, true vacuity and false repletion

1671. 寒热错杂 *hán rè cuò zá*, cold and heat complex

1672. 寒热夹杂 *hán rè jiā zá*, cold and heat complex

1673. 表里同病 *biǎo lǐ tóng bìng*, disease of both the exterior and interior

1674. 寒热的真假 *hán rè de zhēn jiǎ*, true or false heat or cold

1675. 虚实转化 *xū shí zhuǎn huà*, conversion between vacuity and repletion

1676. 阴虚 *yīn xū*, yīn vacuity

1677. 阳虚 *yáng xū*, yáng vacuity

1678. 阴阳两虚 *yīn yáng liǎng xū*, dual vacuity of yīn and yáng; yīn and yáng vacuity

1679. 气血两虚 *qì xuè liǎng xū*, dual vacuity of qì and blood; qì-blood vacuity

1680. 气阴两虚 *qì yīn liǎng xū*, dual vacuity of qì and yīn; qì and yīn vacuity

1681. 亡阴 *wáng yīn*, yīn collapse

1682. 亡阳 *wáng yáng*, yáng collapse

第四节　第八组　　　　　　　SECTION 4: SET 8

气血辨证　　　　　　　Qì-Blood Pattern Identification

1346	* 气 气	氣 气	*qì*	qì /tʃi/
1347	* 血 血	血 血	*xuè*	blood /blʌd/
1348	* 虚 虍	虛 虍	*xū*	vacuity /vəˈkjuɪtɪ/
1349	* 陷 阝	陷 阜	*xiàn*	fall /fɔl/
1350	* 脱 月	脱 肉	*tuō*	desertion /dɪˈzɝˌʃən/
1351	* 滞 氵	滯 水	*zhì*	stagnation /stægˈneʃən/
1352	* 逆 辶	逆 辵	*nì*	counterflow /ˈkɑʊntɚˌflo/

1353	* 闭门 閉門	*bì*	block /blɑk/
1354	* 瘀疒 瘀疒	*yū*	stasis /ˈstesɪs/
1355	* 妄亡 妄女	*wàng*	frenetic /frənˈɛtɪk/

复合词 Compounds:

1683. 气虚 *qì xū*, qì vacuity
1684. 气陷 *qì xiàn*, qì fall
1685. 气脱 *qì tuō*, qì desertion
1686. 气滞 *qì zhì*, qì stagnation
1687. 气逆 *qì nì*, qì counterflow
1688. 气闭 *qì bì*, qì block
1689. 血虚 *xuè xū*, blood vacuity
1690. 血脱 *xuè tuō*, blood desertion
1691. 气随血脱 *qì suí xuè tuō*, qì deserting with the blood
1692. 血瘀 *xuè yū*, blood stasis
1693. 血热 *xuè rè*, blood heat
1694. 血热妄行 *xuè rè wàng xíng*, frenetic movement of hot blood
1695. 血燥 *xuè zào*, blood dryness
1696. 血寒 *xuè hán*, blood cold
1697. 气滞血瘀 *qì zhì xuè yū*, qì stagnation and blood stasis
1698. 热极生风 *rè jí shēng fēng*, extreme heat engendering wind
1699. 血虚生风 *xuè xū shēng fēng*, blood vacuity engendering wind

---

| 第四节　第九组 | **SECTION 4: SET 9** |

| 脏腑辨证 | **Organ Pattern Identification** |

1356	* 脏月 臟肉	*zàng*	viscus /ˈvɪskəs/ *sing.* viscera /ˈvɪsərə/ *pl.*
1357	* 腑月 腑肉	*fǔ*	bowel /ˈbauəl/
1358	* 虚虍 虚虍	*xū*	vacuity /vəˈkjuɪtɪ/
1359	* 脱月 脫肉	*tuō*	desertion /dɪˈzɚʃən/
1360	* 亢亠 亢亠	*kàng*	hyperactivity /ˌhaɪpərækˈtɪvɪtɪ/
1361	* 扰扌 擾手	*rǎo*	harass /həˈræs, ˈhærəs/
1362	* 凌冫 凌冫	*líng*	intimidate /ɪnˈtɪmɪˌdet/
1363	* 亏二 虧虍	*kuī*	depletion /dɪˈpliʃən/
1364	* 郁阝 鬱鬯	*yù*	depression /dɪˈprɛʃən/
1365	* 动力 動力	*dòng*	stir /stɝ/

1366	* 炎火	炎火	*yán*	flame /flem/
1367	* 化亻	化匕	*huà*	transform /trænsˈfɔrm/
1368	* 生丿	生生	*shēng*	engender /ɪnˈgɛndɚ/
1369	* 陷阝	陷阜	*xiàn*	fall /fɔl/
1370	* 统纟	統糸	*tǒng*	manage /ˈmænɪdʒ/ control /kənˈtrol/
1371	* 困口	困口	*kùn*	encumber /ɪnˈkʌmbɚ/
1372	* 足足	足足	*zú*	sufficiency /səˈfɪʃənsɪ/
1373	* 纳纟	納糸	*nà*	absorb /əbˈsɔrb/
1374	* 泛氵	泛水	*fàn*	flood /flʌd/
1375	* 交一	交一	*jiāo*	interact /ˌɪntəˈrækt/
1376	* 犯犭	犯犬	*fàn*	invade /ɪnˈved/

复合词 Compounds:

1700. 心气虚 *xīn qì xū*, heart qì vacuity

1701. 心血虚 *xīn xuè xū*, heart blood vacuity

1702. 心阴虚 *xīn yīn xū*, heart yīn vacuity

1703. 心阳虚 *xīn yáng xū*, heart yáng vacuity

1704. 心阳暴脱 *xīn yàng bào tuō*, fulminant desertion of heart yáng

1705. 心气血两虚 *xīn qì xuè liǎng xū*, dual vacuity of heart qì and blood; heart qì and blood vacuity

1706. 心气阴两虚 *xīn qì yīn liǎng xū*, dual vacuity of heart qì and yīn; heart qì and yīn vacuity

1707. 心阴阳两虚 *xīn yīn yáng liǎng xū*, dual vacuity of heart yīn and heart yáng; heart yīn and yáng vacuity

1708. 心火亢盛 *xīn huǒ kàng shèng*, hyperactive heart fire

1709. 心脉痹阻 *xīn mài bì zǔ*, heart vessel obstruction

1710. 水气凌心 *shuǐ qì líng xīn*, water qì intimidating the heart

1711. 肝血虚 *gān xuè xū*, liver blood vacuity

1712. 肝血亏虚 *gān xuè kuī xū*, liver blood depletion

1713. 肝阴虚 *gān yīn xū*, liver yīn vacuity

1714. 肝气郁结 *gān qì yù jié*, binding depression of liver qì

1715. 肝火上炎 *gān huǒ shàng yán*, liver fire flaming upward

1716. 肝阳上亢 *gān yáng shàng kàng*, ascendant hyperactivity of liver yáng

1717. 肝风内动 *gān fēng nèi dòng*, liver wind stirring internally

1718. 肝阳化风 *gān yáng huà fēng*, liver yáng transforming into wind

1719. 肝经湿热犯耳 *gān jīng shī rè fàn ěr*, liver channel damp-heat invading the ear

1720. 脾气虚 *pí qì xū*, spleen qì vacuity

1721. 脾气下陷 *pí qì xià xiàn*, spleen qì fall

1722. 脾不统血 *pí bù tǒng xuè*, spleen failing to control the blood

1723. 脾阴虚 *pí yīn xū*, spleen yīn vacuity

1724. 脾阳虚 *pí yáng xū*, spleen yáng vacuity

1725. 脾虚湿困 *pí xū shī kùn*, spleen vacuity with damp encumbrance

1726. 脾虚生痰 *pí xū shēng tán*, spleen vacuity engendering phlegm

1727. 肺气虚 *fèi qì xū*, lung qì vacuity

1728. 肺阴虚 *fèi yīn xū*, lung yīn vacuity

1729. 肺阳虚 *fèi yáng xū*, lung yáng vacuity

1730. 肺气不利 *fèi qì bú lì*, inhibited lung qì

1731. 肺气不宣 *fèi qì bù xuān*, lung qì failing to diffuse; non-diffusion of lung qì

1732. 肺失肃降 *fèi shī sù jiàng*, impaired depurative downbearing of the lung

1733. 肺气阴两虚 *fèi qì yīn liǎng xū*, dual vacuity of lung qì and yīn; lung qì and yīn vacuity

1734. 肺气衰绝 *fèi qì shuāi jué*, expiration of lung qì

1735. 肾气虚气化无权 *shèn qì xū qì huà wú quán*, kidney vacuity and impaired qì transformation

1736. 肾精不足 *shèn jīng bù zú*, insufficiency of kidney essence

1737. 肾阴虚 *shèn yīn xū*, kidney yīn vacuity

1738. 肾阳虚 *shèn yáng xū*, kidney yáng vacuity

1739. 肾气不足 *shèn qì bù zú*, insufficiency of kidney qì

1740. 肾不纳气 *shèn bú nà qì*, kidney failing to absorb qì

1741. 肾阴阳两虚 *shèn yīn yáng liǎng xū*, dual vacuity of kidney yīn and yáng

1742. 肾阳虚水泛 *shèn yáng xū shuǐ fàn*, kidney yáng vacuity water flood

1743. 心肝血虚 *xīn gān xuè xū*, heart-liver blood vacuity

1744. 心肝火盛 *xīn gān huǒ shèng*, exuberant heart-liver fire

1745. 心肺气虚 *xīn fèi qì xū*, heart-lung qì vacuity

1746. 心肺阳虚 *xīn fèi yáng xū*, heart-lung yáng vacuity

1747. 心肺阴虚 *xīn fèi yīn xū*, heart-lung yīn vacuity

1748. 心脾两虚 *xīn pí liǎng xū*, dual vacuity of the heart and spleen; heart-spleen vacuity

1749. 心脾血虚 *xīn pí xuè xū*, heart-spleen blood vacuity

1750. 心脾阳虚 *xīn pí yáng xū*, heart-spleen yáng vacuity

1751. 心肾阳虚 *xīn shèn yáng xū*, heart-kidney yáng vacuity

1752. 心肾气虚 *xīn shèn qì xū*, heart-kidney qì vacuity

1753. 心肾血虚 *xīn shèn xuè xū*, heart-kidney blood vacuity

1754. 心肾阴虚 *xīn shèn yīn xū*, heart-kidney yīn vacuity

1755. 心肾不交 *xīn shèn bù jiāo*, non-interaction of the heart and kidney

1756. 心胃火盛 *xīn wèi huǒ shèng*, exuberant heart-stomach fire

1757. 心胆不宁 *xīn dǎn bù níng*, disquieting of the heart and gallbladder

1758. 肝脾不调 *gān pí bù tiáo*, liver-spleen disharmony

1759. 肝脾两虚 *gān pí liǎng xū*, dual vacuity of the liver and spleen; liver-spleen vacuity

1760. 脾湿肝郁 *pí shī gān yù*, spleen dampness and liver depression

1761. 肝气犯脾 *gān qì fàn pí*, liver qì invading the spleen

1762. 肝胃不和 *gān wèi bù hé*, liver-stomach disharmony

1763. 肝气犯胃 *gān qì fàn wèi*, liver qì invading the stomach

1764. 胃腑气滞 *wèi fǔ qì zhì*, stomach bowel qì stagnation

1765. 肝火犯肺 *gān huǒ fàn fèi*, liver fire invading the lung

1766. 肝肾阴虚 *gān shèn yīn xū*, liver-kidney yīn vacuity

1767. 肝肾欲绝 *gān shèn yù jué*, liver and kidney verging on expiration

1768. 脾肺气虚 *pí fèi qì xū*, spleen-lung qì vacuity

1769. 脾肾阳虚 *pí shèn yáng xū*, spleen-kidney yáng vacuity

1770. 脾胃湿热 *pí wèi shī rè*, spleen-stomach damp-heat

1771. 脾胃阳虚 *pí wèi yáng xū*, spleen-stomach yáng vacuity

1772. 脾胃气败 *pí wèi qì bài*, vanquished spleen and stomach qì

1773. 肺脾肾阳虚 *fèi pí shèn yáng xū*, lung-spleen-kidney yáng vacuity

1774. 肺肾阴虚 *fèi shèn yīn xū*, lung-kidney yīn vacuity

1775. 胆气虚 *dǎn qì xū*, gallbladder qì vacuity

1776. 胆热 *dǎn rè*, gallbladder heat

1777. 胆郁痰扰 *dǎn yù tán rǎo*, depressed gallbladder with harassing phlegm

1778. 胃气虚 *wèi qì xū*, stomach qì vacuity

1779. 胃阴虚 *wèi yīn xū*, stomach yīn vacuity

1780. 胃寒 *wèi hán*, stomach cold

1781. 胃气虚寒 *wèi qì xū hán*, stomach qì vacuity cold

1782. 胃虚寒 *wèi xū hán*, stomach vacuity cold

1783. 胃阳虚寒 *wèi yáng xū hán*, stomach yáng vacuity cold

1784. 胃实寒 *wèi shí hán*, stomach repletion cold

1785. 胃热 *wèi rè*, stomach heat

1786. 胃火 *wèi huǒ*, stomach fire

1787. 胃热亢盛 *wèi rè kàng shèng*, hyperactive stomach heat

1788. 胃实热 *wèi shí rè*, stomach repletion heat

1789. 胃火炽盛 *wèi huǒ chì shèng*, intense stomach fire

1790. 胃火上升 *wèi huǒ shàng shēng*, stomach fire bearing upward; upbearing of stomach fire

1791. 胃腑血瘀 *wèi fǔ xuè yū*, stomach bowel blood stasis

1792. 胃阴阳两虚 *wèi yīn yáng liǎng xū*, dual vacuity of stomach yīn and yáng; stomach yīn and yáng vacuity

1793. 大肠湿热 *dà cháng shī rè*, large intestinal damp-heat

1794. 大肠结热 *dà cháng jié rè*, large intestinal heat bind

1795. 大肠津亏 *dà cháng jīn kuī*, large intestinal liquid depletion

1796. 大肠液亏 *dà cháng yè kuī*, large intestinal humor depletion

1797. 大肠虚寒 *dà cháng xū hán*, large intestinal vacuity cold

1798. 湿阻大肠 *shī zǔ dà cháng*, dampness obstructing the large intestine

1799. 小肠虚寒 *xiǎo cháng xū hán*, small intestinal vacuity cold

1800. 小肠气滞 *xiǎo cháng qì zhì*, small intestinal qì stagnation

1801. 膀胱虚寒 *páng guāng xū hán*, bladder vacuity cold

1802. 膀胱湿热 *páng guāng shī rè*, bladder damp-heat

第四节　第十组				**SECTION 4: SET 10**

病邪辨证				**Disease-Evil Pattern Identification**

1377	* 胜 月	勝 力	*shèng*	prevail /prɪˈvel/
1378	* 犯 犭	犯 犬	*fàn*	invade /ɪnˈved/
1379	* 袭 龍	襲 衣	*xí*	assail /əˈsel/
1380	* 侵 亻	侵 人	*qīn*	invade /ɪnˈved/
1381	* 束 束	束 木	*shù*	fetter /ˈfɛtɚ/
1382	* 阻 阝	阻 阜	*zǔ*	obstruction /əbˈstrʌkʃən/
1383	* 滞 氵	滯 水	*zhì*	stagnation /stægˈneʃən/
1384	* 结 纟	結 糸	*jié*	bind /baɪnd/
1385	* 蕴 艹	蘊 艸	*yùn*	brew /bru/
1386	* 扰 扌	擾 手	*rǎo*	harass /həˈræs, ˈhærəs/
1387	* 蒙 艹	蒙 艸	*méng*	cloud /klaʊd/
1388	* 蔽 艹	蔽 艸	*bì*	cloud /klaʊd/
1389	* 迷 辶	迷 辶	*mí*	confound /kənˈfaʊnd/
1390	* 壅 土	壅 土	*yōng*	congestion /kənˈdʒɛstʃən/
1391	* 射 身	射 寸	*shè*	shoot /ʃut/

复合词 Compounds:

1803. 风寒犯肺 *fēng hán fàn fèi*, wind-cold invading the lung

1804. 风寒束肺 *fēng hán shù fèi*, wind-cold fettering the lung

1805. 风热袭肺 *fēng rè xí fèi*, wind-heat assailing the lung

1806. 风热犯肺 *fēng rè fàn fèi*, wind-heat invading the lung

1807. 风邪入侵经络 *fēng xié rù qīn jīng luò*, wind evil invading the channels and network vessels

1808. 寒痹 *hán bì*, cold impediment

1809. 寒疝 *hán shàn*, cold mounting

1810. 寒痛 *hán tòng*, cold pain

1811. 寒泻 *hán xiè*, cold diarrhea

1812. 寒邪犯胃 *hán xié fàn wèi*, cold evil invading the stomach

1813. 外寒犯胃 *wài hán fàn wèi*, external cold invading the stomach

1814. 寒痰阻肺 *hán tán zǔ fèi*, cold phlegm obstructing the lung

1815. 寒滞肝脉 *hán zhì gān mài*, cold stagnating in the liver vessel

1816. 寒湿困脾 *hán shī kùn pí*, cold-damp encumbering the spleen

1817. 寒湿中阻 *hán shī zhōng zǔ*, cold-damp obstructing the center

1818. 暑热 *shǔ rè*, summerheat-heat

1819. 暑湿 *shǔ shī*, summerheat-damp

1820. 湿阻 *shī zǔ*, damp obstruction

1821. 湿浊困心 *shī zhuó kùn xīn*, damp turbidity encumbering the heart

1822. 湿热 *shī rè*, damp-heat

1823. 湿热蕴脾 *shī rè yùn pí*, damp-heat brewing in the spleen

1824. 湿热蕴结肝胆 *shī rè yùn jié gān dǎn*, damp-heat brewing [and binding] in the liver and gallbladder

1825. 湿热阻滞脾胃 *shī rè zǔ zhì pí wèi*, damp-heat obstructing the spleen and stomach

1826. 湿热下注膀胱 *shī rè xià zhù páng guāng*, damp-heat pouring down into the bladder

1827. 湿热下注大肠 *shī rè xià zhù dà cháng*, damp-heat pouring down into the large intestine

1828. 风痰 *fēng tán*, wind phlegm

1829. 寒痰 *hán tán*, cold phlegm

1830. 热痰 *rè tán*, heat phlegm

1831. 燥痰 *zào tán*, dryness phlegm

1832. 湿痰 *shī tán*, damp phlegm

1833. 痰气互结 *tán qì hù jié*, phlegm and qì binding together

1834. 痰浊上扰 *tán zhuó shàng rǎo*, phlegm turbidity harassing the upper body

1835. 痰火扰心 *tán huǒ rǎo xīn*, phlegm-fire harassing the heart
1836. 痰迷心窍 *tán mí xīn qiào*, phlegm confounding the orifices of the heart
1837. 痰蒙蔽心包 *tán méng bì xīn bāo*, phlegm clouding the pericardium
1838. 燥邪犯肺 *zào xié fàn fèi*, dryness evil invading the lung
1839. 痰浊阻肺 *tán zhuó zǔ fèi*, phlegm turbidity obstructing the lung
1840. 痰热壅肺 *tán rè yōng fèi*, phlegm-heat congesting the lung
1841. 水寒射肺 *shuǐ hán shè fèi*, water-cold shooting into the lung
1842. 食伤脾胃 *shí shāng pí wèi*, damage to the spleen and stomach by food
1843. 伤食 *shāng shí*, food damage
1844. 食滞胃脘 *shí zhì wèi wǎn*, food stagnating in the stomach duct
1845. 瘀血结胃 *yū xuè jié wèi*, static blood binding in the stomach

---

第四节　第十一组   **SECTION 4: SET 11**

伤寒辩证   **Cold Damage Pattern Identification**

1392	* 迫辶　迫辵	*pò*	distress /dɪˈstrɛs/
1393	* 蓄艹　蓄艸	*xù*	amassment /əˈmæsmənt/
1394	* 扰扌　擾手	*rǎo*	harass /həˈræs, ˈhærəs/
1395	* 合人入　合口	*hé*	combination /kɑmbɪˈneʃ͵n/
1396	* 结纟　結糸	*jié*	bind /baɪnd/
1397	* 痞疒　痞疒	*pǐ*	glomus /ˈɡloməs/
1398	* 约纟　約糸	*yuē*	straitened /ˈstretṇd/

注 Note:

The terms presented in this set are from the *Shāng Hán Lùn* (伤寒论, "On Cold Damage"), China's first major monograph on the subject of febrile disease. Quite a number of terms in this set may be unfamiliar to students, such as 脾约 *pí yuē*, denoting constipation arising when splenic movement and transformation is impaired and the stool becomes dry. These terms are all discussed in *Shāng Hán Lùn, On Cold Damage: Translation and Commentaries* by Mitchell, Féng, and Wiseman, Paradigm Publications, 1999.

复合词 Compounds:

1846. 太阳病 *tài yáng bìng*, greater yáng (*tài yáng*) disease

1847. 太阳蓄水 *tài yáng xù shuǐ*, greater yáng (*tài yáng*) water amassment

1848. 太阳蓄血 *tài yáng xuè xuè*, greater yáng (*tài yáng*) blood amassment

1849. 太阳热邪迫肺 *tài yáng rè xié pò fèi*, greater yáng (*tài yáng*) heat evil distressing the lung

1850. 太阳热迫大肠 *tài yáng rè pò dà cháng*, greater yáng (*tài yáng*) heat distressing the large intestine

1851. 太阳热扰胸膈 *tài yáng rè rǎo xiōng gé*, greater yáng (*tài yáng*) heat harassing the chest and diaphragm

1852. 阳明病 *yáng míng bìng*, yáng brightness (*yáng míng*) disease

1853. 阳明经热 *yáng míng jīng rè*, yáng brightness (*yáng míng*) channel heat

1854. 阳明腑实 *yáng míng fǔ shí*, yáng brightness (*yáng míng*) bowel repletion

1855. 阳明湿热里实 *yáng míng shī rè lǐ shí*, yáng brightness (*yáng míng*) damp-heat interior repletion

1856. 阳明瘀血 *yáng míng yū xuè*, yáng brightness (*yáng míng*) static blood

1857. 阳明湿热 *yáng míng shī rè*, yáng brightness (*yáng míng*) damp-heat

1858. 阳明湿热兼表 *yáng míng shī rè jiān biǎo*, yáng brightness (*yáng míng*) damp-heat with an exterior pattern

1859. 少阳病 *shào yáng bìng*, lesser yáng (*shào yáng*) disease

1860. 少阳半表半里 *shào yáng bàn biǎo bàn lǐ*, lesser yáng (*shào yáng*) half-exterior half-interior pattern

1861. 热入血室 *rè rù xuè shì*, heat entering the blood chamber

1862. 太阴病 *tài yīn bìng*, greater yīn (*tài yīn*) disease

1863. 少阴病 *shào yīn bìng*, lesser yīn (*shào yīn*) disease

1864. 厥阴病 *jué yīn bìng*, reverting yīn (*jué yīn*) disease

1865. 厥阴蛔厥 *jué yīn huí jué*, reverting yīn (*jué yīn*) roundworm reversal

1866. 热厥 *rè jué*, heat reversal

1867. 三阳合病 *sān yáng hé bìng*, triple-yáng combination disease

1868. 上热下寒 *shàng rè xià hán*, upper body heat and lower body cold

1869. 脾约 *pí yuē*, straitened spleen

1870. 大结胸 *dà jié xiōng*, major chest bind

1871. 小结胸 *xiǎo jié xiōng*, minor chest bind

1872. 寒实结胸 *hán shí jié xiōng*, repletion cold chest bind

1873. 脏结 *zàng jié*, visceral bind

1874. 寒热互结痞 *hán rè hù jié pǐ*, glomus due to binding cold and heat

1875. 热痞 *rè pǐ*, heat glomus

1876. 下焦滑脱 *xià jiāo huá tuō*, lower burner efflux desertion

1877. 痰阻胸膈 *tán zǔ xiōng gé*, phlegm obstructing the chest and diaphragm

1878. 太阳与少阳合病 *tài yáng yǔ shào yáng hé bìng*, greater yáng and lesser yáng combination disease

1879. 太阳与阳明合病 *tài yáng yǔ yáng míng hé bìng*, greater yáng and yáng brightness combination disease

---

第四节　第十二组				**SECTION 4: SET 12**

温病辨证				**Warm-Disease Pattern Identification**
1399	* 伤亻 傷人	*shāng*	damage /ˈdæmɪdʒ/
1400	* 遏辶 遏辵	*è*	obstruction /əbˈstrʌkʃən/
1401	* 阻阝 阻阜	*zǔ*	obstruction /əbˈstrʌkʃən/
1402	* 壅土 壅土	*yōng*	congestion /kənˈdʒestʃən/
1403	* 扰扌 擾手	*rǎo*	harass /həˈræs, ˈhærəs/
1404	* 结纟 結糸	*jié*	bind /baɪnd/
1405	* 燔火 燔火	*fán*	blaze /blez/
1406	* 蒸艹 蒸艸	*zhēng*	steam /stim/
1407	* 蒙艹 蒙艸	*méng*	cloud /klaʊd/
1408	* 搏扌 搏手	*bó*	contend /kənˈtend/ *vi.*
1409	* 炽火 熾火	*chì*	intense /ɪnˈtens/
1410	* 动力 動力	*dòng*	stir /stɝ/

复合词 Compounds:

1880. 邪伤肺卫 *xié shāng fèi wèi*, evil damaging lung-defense

1881. 湿遏卫阳 *shī è wèi yáng*, dampness obstructing defense yáng

1882. 湿遏热伏 *shī è rè fú*, dampness trapping hidden (deep-lying) heat

1883. 湿阻气分 *shī zǔ qì fèn*, dampness obstructing the qì aspect

1884. 湿热弥漫三焦 *shī rè mí màn sān jiāo*, damp-heat spreading through the triple burner

1885. 湿热化燥 *shī rè huà zào*, damp-heat transforming into dryness

1886. 上焦燥热 *shàng jiāo zào rè*, upper burner dryness-heat

1887. 毒壅上焦 *dú yōng shàng jiāo*, toxin congesting the upper burner

1888. 热扰胸膈 *rè rǎo xiōng gé*, heat harassing the chest and diaphragm

1889. 热入气分 *rè rù qì fèn*, heat entering the qì aspect

1890. 热伤气阴 *rè shāng qì yīn*, heat damaging qì and yīn

1891. 热耗真阴 *rè hào zhēn yīn*, heat wearing true yīn

1892. 热结胃肠 *rè jié wèi cháng*, heat binding in the stomach and intestines

1893. 液乾便结 *yè gān biàn jié*, dry humor bound stool (bound stool due to dry humor); dry humor and bound stool

1894. 热入营分 *rè rù yíng fēn*, heat entering the construction aspect

1895. 气营两燔 *qì yíng liǎng fán*, qì and construction both ablaze; dual blaze of qì and construction

1896. 热炽毒盛 *rè chì dú shèng*, intense heat and exuberant toxin

1897. 热入血分 *rè rù xuè fēn*, heat entering the blood aspect

1898. 暑兼寒湿 *shǔ jiān hán shī*, summerheat with cold-damp

1899. 暑湿困阻中焦 *shǔ shī kùn zǔ zhōng jiāo*, summerheat-damp encumbering the middle burner

1900. 暑湿郁蒸 *shǔ shī yù zhēng*, depressed steaming summerheat-damp

1901. 暑热伤气 *shǔ rè shāng qì*, summerheat-heat damaging qì

1902. 暑伤心肾 *shǔ shāng xīn shèn*, summerheat damaging the heart and kidney

1903. 逆传心包 *nì chuán xīn bāo*, abnormal passage to the pericardium

1904. 痰浊内蒙心包 *tán zhuó nèi méng xīn bāo*, phlegm turbidity clouding the pericardium

1905. 瘀热相搏 *yū rè xiāng bó*, stasis and heat contending with each other

1906. 邪留阴分 *xié liú yīn fēn*, evil lodged in the yīn aspect

1907. 阴虚火炽 *yīn xū huǒ chì*, intense yīn vacuity fire

1908. 阴虚风动 *yīn xū fēng dòng*, yīn vacuity stirring wind

习题 Exercise:

535. when evil qì is exuberant, there is repletion ....

536. 阳盛则外热 ....

537. *hán shèng zé fú* ....

538. liver is often in superabundance ....

539. 浊阴不降 ....

540. *qì huà bú lì* ....

541. impaired depurative downbearing ....

542. 肝失疏泄 ....

543. *shí rè* ....

544. vacuity cold ....

545. 虚热 ....

546. *xū shí* ....

547. yīn and yáng, yīn-yáng ....

548. 真热假寒 ....

549. *zhēn shí jiǎ xū* ....

550. exterior and interior, exterior-interior ....

551. 寒热 ....

552. *shí hán* ....

553. vacuity heat ....

554. 虚实 ....

555. *biǎo xū* ....

556. truth and falsity ....

557. 夹杂 ....

558. *bàn biǎo bàn lǐ* ....

559. true vacuity and false repletion ....

560. 表里同病 ....

561. *yáng xū* ....

562. yīn collapse ....

563. 虚实夹杂 ....

564. *qì xū* ....

565. qì fall ....

566. 气脱 ....

567. *qì nì* ....

568. qì deserting with the blood desertion ....

569. 气滞血瘀 ....

570. *xīn qì xū* ....

571. heart blood vacuity ....

572. 心阳虚 ....

573. *xīn qì yīn liǎng xū* ....

574. exuberant heart fire ....

575. 水气凌心 ....

576. *gān xuè xū* ....

577. liver yīn vacuity ....

578. 肝火上炎 ....

579. *gān yáng shàng kàng* ....

580. liver wind stirring internally ....

581. 热极生风 ....

582. *pí qì xū* ....
583. spleen failing to control the blood ....
584. 脾虚湿困 ....
585. *fèi qì xū* ....
586. lung yīn vacuity ....
587. 肺气衰绝 ....
588. *fèi qì bù xuān* ....
589. impaired depurative downbearing ....
590. 肺津不布 ....
591. *shèn yīn xū* ....
592. insufficiency of kidney qì ....
593. 肾阴阳两虚 ....
594. *xīn gān xuè xū* ....
595. heart-lung qì vacuity ....
596. 心脾两虚 ....
597. *xīn shèn qì xū* ....
598. non-interaction of the heart and kidney ....
599. 心胆不宁 ....
600. *pí shī gān yù* ....
601. liver-stomach disharmony ....
602. 肝火犯肺 ....
603. *pí shèn yáng xū* ....
604. spleen-stomach yáng vacuity ....
605. *dǎn qì xū* ....
606. stomach qì vacuity ....
607. 胃寒 ....
608. *wèi xū hán* ....
609. stomach fire ....
610. 胃火炽盛 ....
611. *dà cháng jié rè* ....
612. large intestinal liquid depletion ....
613. 大肠虚寒 ....
614. *xiǎo cháng qì zhì* ....

615. bladder damp-heat ....

616. 风寒犯肺 ....

617. *fēng hán shù fèi* ....

618. wind-heat invading the lung ....

619. 寒痹 ....

620. *hán tòng* ....

621. cold evil invading the stomach ....

622. 寒滞肝脉 ....

623. *hán shī zhōng zǔ* ....

624. summerheat-heat ....

625. 暑湿 ....

626. *hán shī zhōng zǔ* ....

627. damp-heat brewing in the spleen ....

628. 湿热下注膀胱 ....

629. *shī rè xià zhù dà cháng* ....

630. cold phlegm ....

631. 燥痰 ....

632. *tán zhuó shàng rǎo* ....

633. phlegm clouding the pericardium ....

634. 痰浊阻肺 ....

635. *shuǐ hán shè fèi* ....

636. food stagnating in the stomach duct ....

637. 太阳蓄水 ....

638. *tài yáng rè xié pò fèi* ....

639. heat entering the blood chamber ....

640. 阳明经热 ....

641. *yáng míng fǔ shí* ....

642. greater yīn disease ....

643. 厥阴蛔厥 ....

644. *pí yuē* ....

645. minor chest bind ....

646. 少阳半表半里 ....

647. *tài yáng xù shuǐ* ....

648. evil damaging lung-defense ....

649. 湿遏卫阳 ....

650. *shī zǔ qì fèn* ....

651. heat entering the qì aspect ....

652. 热耗真阴 ....

653. *qì yíng liǎng fán* ....

654. intense heat and exuberant toxin ....

655. 逆传心包 ....

656. *yīn xū fēng dòng* ....

第五节：治疗法则

Section 5: Principles and Method of Treatment

The general approach to treatment in Chinese medicine is allopathic, as manifest in the principles 'supplement insufficiency' and 'drain superabundance'. The first set in the present section introduces terms relating to the principles of treatment. The following four sets, 'supplementing', 'draining', 'freeing and effusing', and 'securing and settling', present terms relating to methods of treatment. These groups correspond to the sets 'vacuity', 'repletion', 'stagnation', and 'insecurity' of the previous previous section. After this basic introduction to the characters used in therapeutic terms there follows a systematic presentation of therapeutic terms.

第五节　第一组				SECTION 5: SET 1

治则 — **Principles of Treatment**

1411-n881	* 治 氵	治 水	zhì	treat /trit/ vt. treatment /ˈtritmənt/ n. therapy /ˈθɛrəpɪ/ n. therapeutic /ˌθɛrəˈpjutɪk/ adj.
1412-n882	* 疗 疒	療 疒	liáo	treat /trit/ vt. treatment /ˈtritmənt/ n. therapy /ˈθɛrəpɪ/ n. therapeutic /ˌθɛrəˈpjutɪk/ adj.
1413-n883	* 法 氵	法 水	fǎ	method /ˈmɛθəd/
1414	* 则 貝	則 刀	zé	principle /ˈprɪnsɪpl/
1415	* 辨 辛	辨 辛	biàn	identify /aɪˈdɛntɪˌfaɪ/ vi. identification /aɪˌdɛntɪfɪˈkeʃən/ n.
1416	* 证 讠	證 言	zhèng	pattern /ˈpætən/
1417-n884	论 讠	論 言	lùn	discuss
1418-n885	施 方	施 方	shī	carry out
1419-n886	必 丶	必 心	bì	must; necessary
1420-n887	求 丶	求 水	qiú	seek; plead
1421	* 本 木	本 木	běn	root /rut/
1422-n888	* 标 木	標 木	biāo	tip /tɪp/
1423-n889	异 巳	異 田	yì	different; unlike
1424	* 反 厂	反 又	fǎn	paradoxical /ˌpærəˈdɑksɪkl/ adj.
1425-n890	同 冂	同 口	tóng	same; like

1426	* 正 止	正 止	*zhèng*	straight /stret/ *adj.*
1427	* 逆 辶	逆 辵	*nì*	counteract /ˌkaʊntəˈrækt/ *vi.*
				counteraction /ˌkaʊntəˈrækʃən/ *n.*
1428-n891	* 从 人	從 彳	*cóng*	coact /koˈækt/ *vi.*
				coaction /koˈækʃən/ *n.*
1429-n892	取 耳	取 又	*qǔ*	*take*
1430	因 口	因 口	*yīn*	*because; responding to*
1431	* 用 冂	用 用	*yòng*	use /juz/
1432-n893	未 木	未 木	*wèi*	*not yet*
1433-n894	* 扶 扌	扶 手	*fú*	support /səˈpɔrt/
1434-n895	* 祛 礻	祛 衣	*qū*	dispel /dɪsˈpɛl/

注 Notes:

1. The terms 疗法 *liáo fǎ* and 治法 *zhì fǎ* can both be translated as 'method of treatment'. However, the former generally means an independent system of treatment (e.g., moxibustion, cupping), while the latter usually refers to any of the various techniques used within a therapeutic system. This section presents the methods of treatment (治法 *zhì fǎ*) used in Chinese medicinal therapy.

2. 逆治 *nì zhì*, counteracting treatment, also called 正治 *zhèng zhì*. is the principle whereby the nature and pathomechanism are addressed directly, as when a cold pattern is treated with hot medicinals and a heat pattern is treated with cold medicinals, or when vacuity patterns are treated by supplementing or repletion patterns are treated by attack. It stands in opposition to 从治 *cóng zhì*, which is the nonroutine principle of treating false signs with medicinals of the same nature, e.g., treating heat with heat, cold with cold, the stopped by stopping, and flow by promoting flow.

复合词 Compounds:

1909. 治法 *zhì fǎ*, method of treatment
1910. 疗法 *liáo fǎ*, treatment; therapy
1911. 辨证施治 *biàn zhèng shī zhì*, identify patterns and administer treatment; administer treatment according to pattern
1912. 辨证论治 *biàn zhèng lùn zhì*, identify patterns and determine treatment; determine treatment by patterns identified
1913. 辨病论治 *biàn bìng lùn zhì*, identify diseases and determine treatment; determine treatment by diseases identified
1914. 同病异治 *tóng bìng yì zhì*, unlike treatment of like disease

1915. 治病必求於本 *zhì bìng bì qiú yú běn*, to treat disease, it is necessary to seek the root

1916. 异病同治 *yì bìng tóng zhì*, like treatment of unlike disease

1917. 治未病 *zhì wèi bìng*, treat disease before it arises

1918. 因时因地因人制宜 *yīn shí yīn dì yīn rén zhì yí*, act according to time, place, and person

1919. 标本 *biāo běn*, root and tip

1920. 扶正祛邪 *fú zhèng qū xié*, support right and dispel evil

1921. 标本同治 *biāo běn tóng zhì*, treating the root and tip simultaneously; simultaneous treatment of root and tip

1922. 逆治 *nì zhì*, counteracting treatment

1923. 逆从 *nì cóng*, counteraction and coaction

1924. 从治 *cóng zhì*, coacting treatment

1925. 正治 *zhèng zhì*, straight treatment

1926. 反治 *fǎn zhì*, paradoxical treatment

1927. 反佐 *fǎn zuǒ*, paradoxical assistant

1928. 热因热用 *rè yīn rè yòng*, treating heat with heat

1929. 上病下取 *shàng bìng xià qǔ*, treating upper body disease through the lower body

1930. 下病上取 *xià bìng shàng qǔ*, treating lower body disease through the upper body

1931. 通因通用 *tōng yīn tōng yòng*, treating the free by freeing

1932. 寒因寒用 *hán yīn hán yòng*, treating cold with cold

1933. 塞因塞用 *sāi yīn sāi yòng*, treating the stopped by stopping

1934. 阴病治阳 *yīn bìng zhì yáng*, yīn disease is treated through yáng

1935. 阳病治阴 *yáng bìng zhì yīn*, yáng disease is treated through yīn

1936. 虚者补其母 *xū zhě bǔ qí mǔ*, in vacuity, supplement the mother; vacuity is treated by supplementing the mother

1937. 实者泻其子 *shí zhě xiè qí zǐ*, in repletion, drain the child; repletion is treated by draining the child

1938. 酸可收之 *suān kě shōu zhī*, sourness can cause contraction

1939. 涩可固脱 *sè kě gù tuō*, astringency can stem desertion

1940. 通可去滞 *tōng kě qù zhì*, freeing can eliminate stagnation

第五节　第二组　　　　　　SECTION 5: SET 2

「补」类字词　　　　　　　'Supplement' Terms

1435-n896	*	补 衤	補 衣	*bǔ*	supplement /ˈsʌplimənt/
1436-n897	*	益 皿	益 皿	*yì*	boost /bust/
1437	*	化 亻	化 匕	*huà*	form /ˈfɔrm/
1438	*	养 丷	養 食	*yǎng*	nourish /ˈnɝɪʃ/
1439-n898	*	育 月	育 肉	*yù*	foster /ˈfɔstər/
1440-n899	*	滋 氵	滋 水	*zī*	enrich /ɪnˈrɪtʃ/
1441	*	涵 氵	涵 水	*hán*	moisten /ˈmɔɪsn̩/
1442	*	填 土	塡 土	*tián*	replenish /rɪˈplɛnɪʃ/
1443	*	润 氵	潤 水	*rùn*	moisten /ˈmɔɪsn̩/
1444	*	滑 氵	滑 水	*huá*	lubricate /ˈlubrɪket/
1445	*	生 丿	生 生	*shēng*	engender /ɪnˈgɛndər/
1446-n900	*	存 𠂇	存 子	*cún*	preserve /prɪˈzɝv/ safeguard /ˈsefgɑrd/
1447-n901	*	增 土	增 土	*zēng*	increase /ɪnˈkris/
1448	*	柔 矛	柔 木	*róu*	emolliate /ɪˈmɑlɪˌet/
1449	*	扶 扌	扶 手	*fú*	support /səˈpɔrt/
1450-n902	*	复 𠂇	復 彳	*fù*	restore /rɪˈstɔr, rɪˈstor/
1451-n903	*	培 土	培 土	*péi*	bank up /bænk ʌp/
1452	*	温 氵	溫 水	*wēn*	warm /wɔrm/
1453-n904	*	暖 火	煖 火	*nuǎn*	warm /wɔrm/
1454-n905	*	助 力	助 力	*zhù*	assist /əˈsɪst/
1455	*	强 弓	強 弓	*qiáng*	strengthen /ˈstrɛŋθən/
1456	*	壮 丬	壯 士	*zhuàng*	invigorate /ɪnˈvɪgəˌret/
1457-n906	*	回 口	回 口	*huí*	return /rɪˈtɝn/
1458-n907	*	救 攵	救 攴	*jiù*	rescue /ˈrɛskju/
1459	*	健 亻	健 人	*jiàn*	fortify /ˈfɔrtəˌfaɪ/
1460-n908	*	建 廴	建 廴	*jiàn*	fortify /ˈfɔrtəˌfaɪ/
1461-n909	*	醒 酉	醒 酉	*xǐng*	arouse /əˈraʊz/
1462	*	振 扌	振 手	*zhèn*	vitalize /ˈvaɪtəˌlaɪz/
1463	*	升 丿	升 十	*shēng*	upbear /ˈʌpbɛr/
1464-n910	*	提 扌	提 手	*tí*	raise /rez/
1465	*	举 丶	擧 臼	*jǔ*	lift /lɪft/

注 Notes:

1. The most generic of terms used to describe actions aimed at treating vacuity is 补 *bǔ*, to supplement. This character has the signific meaning cloth,

clearly indicating that its primary meaning is 'to patch' (clothing). It subsequently came to be used in the general sense of 'to supplement', 'to make up', 'to complete', etc., the sense in which it is used in Chinese medicine. In this text, 补 *bǔ* is systematically translated as 'supplement'. We rejected the commonly used term 'tonify', a verb created from 'tonic', a medicine that restores vigor. This word comes from the Greek *teinein*, to stretch, a meaning reflected in the term 'muscle tone'. 'Tonify' implies invigoration, and hence is more appropriate when applied to yáng than to yīn. 'Supplement', by contrast, is neutral just as the Chinese 补 *bǔ*.

2. The language of Chinese medicine has a series of words that are close synonyms of 补 *bǔ*. Some are applied to yīn or yáng entities, e.g., 益阴 *yì yīn* (boost yīn) and 益气 *yì qì* (boost qì). Some are usually applied to one or the other, e.g., 养阴 *yǎng yīn* (nourish yīn) and 养血 *yǎng xuè* (nourish the blood). The yīn-yáng connotations are carried over onto a viscus that is the subject of treatment. Thus 养肝 *yǎng gān*, 'nourish the liver', means to supplement the yīn-blood of the liver. The word 滋 *zī*, 'to enrich', is normally applied to yīn, 滋阴 *zī yīn*, 'enrich yīn'; hence 滋肾 *zī shèn*, 'enrich the kidney', means to enrich kidney yīn.

3. The word 滋 *zī* has no exact equivalent in English; it means 'to enrich', 'to moisten', or 'to nourish'. We chose the term 'enrich' because there are other words with stronger connotations of moistening and nourishing, and because a feature of yīn-enriching medicinals is that they are 'rich' in flavor 厚味 *hòu wèi*.

4. The word 柔 *róu* means 'soft' or to 'soften'. 柔肝 *róu gān*, 'emolliating the liver', is a method of treatment that addresses liver yīn vacuity (or insufficiency of liver blood), characterized by loss of visual acuity, dry eyes, night blindness, periodic dizzy head and tinnitus, and pale nails, or poor sleep, profuse dreaming, dry mouth with lack of fluid, and a fine, weak pulse. We rejected 'soften' in preference for the low-frequency word 'emolliate', which essentially means nothing more than to soften, only to highlight the fact that the method of treatment does not address any physical induration (such as cirrhosis).

5. The word 明 *míng*, 'brighten' (elsewhere rendered as 'brightness'), appears in the compound 明目 *míng mù*, to 'brighten the eyes', i.e., to improve visual acuity. The literal translation 'brighten the eyes' may not be as clear to the English reader as 'enhance vision'.

6. We consistently render 益 *yì* as 'boost'. The lexical meanings are to 'increase', 'enhance', 'benefit'. Bensky et al., have rendered this term as 'augment' with justification. Note that *yì* most commonly appears in the compound 益气 *yì qì*, to 'boost qì' (as in Center-Supplementing Qì-Boosting De-

coction (*bǔ zhōng yì qì tāng*)), and less frequently in the compound 益阴 *yì yīn*, to 'boost yīn'.

7. The term 健脾 *jiàn pí* is here rendered as 'fortifying the spleen'. The word 健 *jiàn* literally means 'to strengthen', '(make) healthy', 'constant'.

8. Some supplementation terms are used very specifically. The character 增 *zēng*, 'increase', is normally only used in the combination 增液 *zēng yè*, 'increase humor'. It could be rendered with the generic term 'supplement', yet in 增液行舟 *zēng yè xíng zhōu*, 'increase humor to move the [grounded] ship', 'increase' makes more sense (although the metaphor would be clearer even in Chinese if the bodily fluid 'humor' had been replaced with the natural 'water').

9. A few other supplementation terms should be commented upon briefly: 育 *yù*, 'foster', is used exclusively with yīn (foster yīn); 填 *tián*, 'replenish', is used almost exclusively with essence; 复 *fù*, 'restore', is used most in the compound 复脉 *fù mài*, 'restore the pulse' (after it has all but expired).

10. Chinese compounds describing therapeutic action naturally translate into verb + object constructions in English (e.g., 'supplement the spleen'). Gerund constructions (e.g., 'supplementing the spleen') can be used where necessary. Noun forms have been included for some actions (e.g., 'exterior resolution'). Adjectives are formed by inverting the verb and object (e.g., 'spleen-supplementing formula'). Multiple adjectives derived from multiple verb + object couplets can be unseparated by commas or the word 'and' to preserve the original unity of the compound (e.g., 'center-supplementing qì-boosting formula').

复合词 Compounds:

1941. 补阴 *bǔ yīn*, supplement yīn
1942. 补脾 *bǔ pí*, supplement the spleen
1943. 益气 *yì qì*, boost qì
1944. 益阴 *yì yīn*, boost yīn
1945. 酸甘化阴 *suān gān huà yīn*, form yīn with sweetness and sourness; sweet and sour yīn formation
1946. 养血 *yáng xuè*, nourish the blood
1947. 养肝 *yǎng gān*, nourish the liver
1948. 育阴 *yù yīn*, foster yīn
1949. 滋阴 *zī yīn*, enrich yīn
1950. 滋养 *zī yǎng*, enrich (and nourish)
1951. 涵木 *hán mù*, moisten wood
1952. 填精补髓 *tián jīng bǔ suǐ*, replenish essence and supplement marrow

1953. 生津 *shēng jīn*, engender liquid

1954. 润肺 *rùn fèi*, moisten the lung

1955. 润燥 *rùn zào*, moisten dryness

1956. 增液 *zēng yè*, increase humor

1957. 柔肝 *róu gān*, emolliate the liver

1958. 扶正 *fú zhèng*, support right

1959. 存正 *cún zhèng*, preserve right

1960. 助阳 *zhù yáng*, assist yáng

1961. 强阴 *qiáng yīn*, strengthen yīn

1962. 强筋壮骨 *qiáng jīn zhuàng gǔ*, strengthen sinew and bone

1963. 壮阳 *zhuàng yáng*, invigorate yáng

1964. 回阳 *huí yáng*, return yáng

1965. 健脾 *jiàn pí*, fortify the spleen

1966. 健中 *jiàn zhōng*, fortify the center

1967. 醒脾 *xǐng pí*, arouse the spleen

1968. 温振心阳 *wēn zhèn xīn yáng*, warm and vitalize heart yáng

1969. 升阳 *shēng yáng*, upbear yáng

第五节　第三组				**SECTION 5: SET 3**

「泻」类字词				**'Drain' Terms**
1466	* 泻 氵	瀉 水	*xiè*	drain /dren/
1467	* 泄 氵	泄 水	*xiè*	discharge /dɪˈtʃɑrdʒ/
1468	* 祛 礻	祛 衣	*qū*	dispel /dɪsˈpɛl/
1469-n911	* 除 阝	除 阜	*chú*	eliminate /ɪˈlɪmɪˌnet/
1470-n912	* 去 去	去 厶	*qù*	eliminate /ɪˈlɪmɪˌnet/
1471	* 解 角	解 角	*jiě*	resolve /rɪˈzɑlv/
1472-n913	* 却 去	卻 卩	*què*	eliminate /ɪˈlɪmɪˌnet/
1473-n914	* 退 辶	退 辵	*tuì*	abate /əˈbet/
1474	* 化 亻	化 匕	*huà*	transform /trænsˈfɔrm/
1475	* 燥 火	燥 火	*zào*	dry /draɪ/
1476-n915	* 驱 馬	驅 馬	*qū*	expel /ɪksˈpɛl/
1477-n916	* 逐 辶	逐 辵	*zhú*	expel /ɪksˈpɛl/
1478-n917	* 搜 扌	搜 手	*sōu*	track down /træk daʊn/
1479-n918	* 辟 辛	辟 辛	*bì*	repel /rɪˈpɛl/
1480	* 清 氵	清 水	*qīng*	clear /klɪr/
1481	* 凉 氵	涼 水	*liáng*	cool /kul/
1482	* 消 氵	消 水	*xiāo*	disperse /dɪˈspɝs/

1483-n919	*	导 已	導 寸	*dǎo*	abduct /əbˈdʌkt/
1484	*	软 車	軟 車	*ruǎn*	soften /ˈsɔfən/
1485-n920	*	渗 氵	滲 水	*shèn*	percolate /ˈpɝkəˌlet/
1486	*	利 禾	利 刀	*lì*	disinhibit /ˌdɪsɪnˈhɪbɪt/
1487	*	破 石	破 石	*pò*	break /brek/
1488-n921	*	排 扌	排 手	*pái*	expel /ɪksˈɛl/
1489	*	散 攵	散 攴	*sàn*	dissipate /ˈdɪsɪˌpet/
1490-n922	*	涤 氵	滌 水	*dí*	flush /flʌʃ/
1491-n923	*	豁 谷	豁 谷	*huò*	sweep /swip/
1492	*	下 卜	下 一	*xià*	precipitate /prɪˈsɪpɪˌtet/
1493-n924	*	攻 工	攻 攴	*gōng*	attack /əˈtæk/ offensive /əˈfɛnsɪv/
1494	*	洁 氵	潔 水	*jié*	cleanse /klɛnz/
1495	*	净 氵	淨 水	*jìng*	clean /klin/
1496-n925	*	伐 亻	伐 人	*fá*	quell /kwɛl/
1497-n926	*	抑 扌	抑 手	*yì*	repress /rɪˈprɛs/
1498-n927	*	熄 火	熄 火	*xī*	extinguish /ɪksˈtɪŋgwɪʃ/
1499-n928	*	杀 乂	殺 殳	*shā*	kill /kɪl/
1500-n929	*	治 氵	治 水	*zhì*	control /kənˈtrol/
1501-n930	*	截 弋	截 戈	*jié*	interrupt /ˌɪntəˈrʌpt/ *vt.*, interruption /ˌɪntəˈrʌpʃən/ *n.*
1502-n931	*	透 辶	透 辵	*tòu*	outthrust /ˈautθrʌst/

注 Notes:

　　1. The Chinese 泻 *xiè*, which has water as its signific, literally means 'to flow', 'cause to flow', 'to drain'. In the acupuncture context, *xiè* is a needle stimulus used to free accumulations of evils (邪 *xié*) or stagnant qì. By extension, is also a generic term for the elimination of evil qì by any means. The *Nèi Jīng* states that repletion is treated by draining. The channels and network vessels (经络 *jīng luò*) in their original conception were rivers and waterways traversing the body and providing the necessary transportation links between the various internal organs and body parts. In accordance with this conception, when qì, for one reason or another, stagnates in part of the channel system, *xiè*, a 'draining' stimulus, is used to restore normal free flow.

　　2. Instead of a literal translation such as 'drain', which preserves the original Chinese metaphor, much English literature uses the term 'sedate', and this is the term that many English-speaking teachers, students, and practitioners of acupuncture and Chinese medicine use. The term 'sedate', whose literal meaning is far removed from that of the Chinese term, can be traced to a mod-

ern interpretation that the channel system corresponds to the nervous system, and that the condition of stagnation corresponds to an excitation of the nervous system that is to be treated by a relaxing or sedating stimulus. The shift in framework of reference introduces a contradiction. 'Sedate' comes from the Latin 'sedare', 'to settle', 'to soothe'. (Both the Latin and the English 'settle' come from a common root meaning 'to sit' and 'to seat'; the English word 'sediment' shares the same root.) 'Sedate' implies a calming or settling action. When applied to the streams of fluid-like qì in the body, it suggests slowing down of activity and movement. To apply a 'sedating' stimulus to qì stagnation would therefore be, not to relieve it, but to aggravate it. Of course, the underlying problem here is that the channel system has not been identified as described by the Chinese, and correspondences to the nervous system are only partial. However, the purpose of translating Chinese medical texts is to convey the traditional Chinese understanding of the mechanisms of health and disease, not any modern reinterpretation of it.

The contradiction between the literal meaning of 'sedate' and the meaning of the Chinese term can be seen in instances of its usage. We might adduce the 开阖补泻法 *kāi hé bǔ xiè fǎ*, 'open and closed supplementation and drainage method', which involves pressing (closing) the hole in the skin left after the extraction of the needle to prevent the qì from escaping from the body in order to produce a supplementing stimulus, or which involves waggling the needle on extraction so as to widen the hole and facilitate the discharge of qì in order to produce a draining stimulus. The concept underlying this method, which is clearly reflected in it name, is that a *xiè* stimulus is achieved by allowing qì to drain out of the body. It is difficult to see how the word 'sedate', with its connotations of calming, tranquilizing, and settling, could meaningfully describe what the traditional Chinese healer understood himself to be performing.

3. The term 泻 *xiè*, 'drain', is a generic term. Another relatively generic term is 祛 *qū*, 'dispel'. The removal of specific evils, especially in drug therapy, uses a variety of other terms besides 'drain', e.g., 'transform phlegm', 'kill worms', 'extinguish wind'. However, 'drain' also has a specific application in 泻火 *xiè huǒ*, 'drain fire', that is, to eliminate internal fire.

4. Some of the draining verbs have specific objects. 散 *sàn*, 'dissipate', is used in the context of cold (散寒 *sàn hán*), but never in that of phlegm; 消 *xiāo*, 'disperse' is used almost exclusively for food accumulation, hardness, and phlegm. The choice of verb is not arbitrary, and often connotes a specificity. For example, 祛风 *qū fēng*, 'dispel wind', means to eliminate externally contracted wind and 熄风 *xī fēng*, 'extinguish wind', means to eliminate liver wind.

5. Sometimes, the verb hints at the strength of the action. For example, 祛痰 *qū tán*, 'dispel phlegm', generally denotes any action to eliminate phlegm; 化痰 *huà tán*, 'transform phlegm', is a mild action, while 豁痰 *huò tán*, 'sweep phlegm', or 攻痰 *gōng tán*, 'attack phlegm', represent more powerful actions. A similar difference of degree is observed between 化瘀 *huà yū*, 'transform stasis', and 破血 *pò xuè*, 'break blood'.

6. Special attention should be drawn to 化 *huà*, to 'transform'. In all its usages, *huà* means to change gently or gradually (hence the contrast above between 'transform phlegm' and 'attack phlegm'). It often contrasts with 变 *biàn*, 'mutate', which means a sudden or untoward change. 化 *huà* can mean both creative or destructive change. In the therapeutic context, it is most commonly used in the destructive sense: 化痰 *huà tán*, 'transform phlegm', 化湿 *huà shī*, 'transform dampness', and 化痞 *huà pǐ*, 'transform glomus'; it is used less frequently in the creative sense: 化阴 *huà yīn*, 'form yīn'.

7. The terminology for eliminating dampness varies according to the location of the dampness: 化湿 *huà shī*, 'transform dampness', means eliminating dampness from the upper burner (lung); 燥湿 *zào shī*, 'dry dampness', means eliminating dampness from the middle burner (spleen and stomach); and 利湿 *lì shī*, 'disinhibit dampness', means eliminating dampness from the lower burner (bladder). Of course, in each case the implication for treatment is different. Transforming dampness involves the use of medicinals such as atractylodes (*cāng zhú*), magnolia bark (*hòu pò*), agastache/patchouli (*huò xiāng*), eupatorium (*pèi lán*); drying dampness involves the use of warm medicinals such as magnolia bark (*hòu pò*), atractylodes (*cāng zhú*), pinellia (*bàn xià*), and cardamom (*bái dòu kòu*), or hot medicinals such as coptis (*huáng lián*), scutellaria (*huáng qín*), and phellodendron (*huáng bǎi*); disinhibiting dampness involves the use of poria (*fú líng*), polyporus (*zhū líng*), alisma (*zé xiè*), and coix (*yì yǐ rén*).

The literal meaning of the terms 化湿 *huà shī*, 'transform dampness', 燥湿 *zào shī*, 'dry dampness', and 利湿 *lì shī*, 'disinhibit dampness', provide no indication of the location of the dampness. Some translators have suggested that the burner in each case should be made explicit in translation. This is problematic because the terms are not systematically used in the specific senses. In particular, 化湿 *huà shī*, 'transform dampness', is often used in a generic sense in the same way as 祛湿 *qū shī*, 'dispel dampness'. Here, accurate translation, that is, translation that is as precise or as imprecise as the original, can only be ensured by systematic literal renderings.

8. The character 清, to clear, describes action to eliminate heat. When it is applied to an organ name, the notion of heat is implicit. Thus 清肺 *qīng fèi*, 'clear the lung', means to eliminate lung heat (or fire).

9. The Chinese 下 *xià* literally means 'down', 'go down', 'cast down'. In the context of treatment, it is mostly used in the sense of 'cast down', i.e., force the contents of the intestines down and out of the body. This notion is normally expressed in English as 'purgation', whose literal meaning is 'cleansing'. The term 'precipitation' (to cast down) is used instead to reflect the Chinese notion. It is therefore applicable to other uses of 下 outside the context of the bowels, namely 下气 *xià qì*, to send qi downward.

复合词 Compounds:

1970. 泻火 *xiè huǒ*, drain fire
1971. 泻肝 *xiè gān*, drain the liver
1972. 泄卫 *xiè wèi*, discharge defense
1973. 泄热 *xiè rè*, discharge heat
1974. 祛风 *qū fēng*, dispel wind
1975. 祛痰 *qù tán*, dispel phlegm
1976. 除湿 *chú shī*, eliminate dampness
1977. 除热 *chú rè*, eliminate heat
1978. 去热 *qù rè*, eliminate heat
1979. 驱虫 *qū chóng*, expel worms
1980. 驱蛔 *qū huí*, expel roundworm
1981. 逐水 *zhú shuǐ*, expel water
1982. 逐瘀 *zhú yū*, expel stasis
1983. 搜风逐寒 *sōu fēng zhú hán*, track wind and expel cold
1984. 辟秽 *bì huì*, repel fouless
1985. 辟瘟 *bì wēn*, repel scourge
1986. 清热 *qīng rè*, clear heat
1987. 清心 *qīng xīn*, clear the heart
1988. 凉血 *liáng xuè*, cool the blood
1989. 凉营 *liáng yíng*, cool construction
1990. 消食 *xiāo shí*, disperse food
1991. 消痰 *xiāo tán*, disperse phlegm
1992. 软坚除满 *ruǎn jiān chú mǎn*, soften hardness and eliminate fullness
1993. 渗湿 *shèn shī*, percolate dampness
1994. 利湿 *lì shī*, disinhibit dampness
1995. 破血 *pò xuè*, break blood
1996. 破瘀消癥 *pò yū xiāo zhēng*, break stasis and disperse concretions
1997. 排脓 *pái nóng*, expel pus
1998. 散寒 *sàn hán*, dissipate cold
1999. 散瘀 *sàn yū*, dissipate stasis

2000. 下气 *xià qì*, precipitate qì

2001. 泻下 *xiè xià*, draining precipitation

2002. 下燥屎 *xià zào shǐ*, precipitate dry stool

2003. 涤痰 *dí tán*, flush phlegm

2004. 清心涤热 *qing xīn dí rè*, clear the heart and flush heat

2005. 豁痰 *huò tán*, sweep phlegm

2006. 以毒攻毒 *yǐ dú gōng dú*, attacking toxin with toxin

2007. 攻下 *gōng xià*, offensive precipitation

2008. 伐肝 *fā gān*, quell the liver

2009. 抑肝 *yì gān*, repress the liver

2010. 熄风 *xī fēng*, extinguish wind

2011. 杀虫 *shā chóng*, kill worms

2012. 透热 *tòu rè*, outthrust heat

2013. 截疟 *jié nüè*, interrupt malaria

第五节　第四组				SECTION 5: SET 4

「通利」、「发散」字词　　'Free' & 'Effuse' Terms

1503	* 通 辶	通 辵	*tōng*	free /fri/
1504	* 利 禾	利 刀	*lì*	disinhibit /ˌdɪsɪnˈhɪbɪt/
1505	* 行 彳	行 彳	*xíng*	move /muv/
1506	* 运 辶	運 辵	*yùn*	move /muv/
1507-n932	* 活 氵	活 水	*huó*	quicken /ˈkwɪkən/
1508	* 宣 宀	宣 宀	*xuān*	diffuse /dɪˈfjuz/
1509	* 发 又	發 癶	*fā*	effuse /ɪˈfjuz/
1510	* 透 辶	透 辵	*tòu*	outthrust /ˈautθrʌst/
1511-n933	* 达 辶	達 辵	*dá*	outthrust /ˈautθrʌst/
1512	* 散 攵	散 攴	*sàn*	dissipate /ˈdɪsɪˌpet/
1513	* 解 角	解 角	*jiě*	resolve /rɪˈzɑlv/
1514	* 疏 乛	疏 疋	*shū*	course /kɔrs, kors/
1515	* 理 王	理 玉	*lǐ*	rectify /ˈrɛktɪˌfaɪ/
1516-n934	* 舒 人	舒 舌	*shū*	soothe /suð/
1517-n935	* 顺 页	順 頁	*shùn*	normalize /ˈnɔrmlˌaɪz/
1518	* 降 阝	降 阜	*jiàng*	downbear /ˈdaunbɛr/
1519	* 开 廾	開 門	*kāi*	open /ˈopən/
1520	* 下 卜	下 一	*xià*	precipitate /prɪˈsɪpɪˌtet/
1521-n936	* 宽 宀	寬 宀	*kuān*	loosen /ˈlusn̩/
1522	* 豁 谷	豁 谷	*huò*	sweep /swip/

1523	* 润 氵	潤 水	*rùn*	moisten /ˈmɔɪsn̩/
1524	* 滑 氵	滑 水	*huá*	lubricate /ˈlubrɪket/
1525-n937	* 托 扌	托 手	*tuō*	draw /drɔ/

注 Notes:

1. Freeing and effusing terms are terms that describe any action to free blockages and promote flow. Mostly, they are a subset of the draining terms discussed above.

2. The most generic term is 通 *tōng*, a word that has multiple senses in the everyday language (e.g., not blocked; open; communicate). In the context of Chinese medical therapy, the mostly commonly intended sense is 'to free'. It is the counterpart of 不通 *bù tōng*, 'stoppage'.

3. The word 利 *lì* has already been encountered in its negated form, 不利 *bú lì*, 'inhibited'. Here, as an active verb, it is rendered as 'disinhibit'. One of the most common combinations is 利水 *lì shuǐ*, 'disinhibit water', which treats inhibited, or disfluent urination. Other examples include 利湿 *lì shī*, 'disinhibit dampness' and 利咽 *lì yān*, 'disinhibit the throat'. In the everyday language, *lì* can mean 'going smoothly' (顺利 *shùn lì*) and to 'benefit' (to make something go smoothly). Rarely, it is used in Chinese medicine in this sense. 'Disinhibit' is something of a coinage (although the word 'disinhibition' and 'disinhibitory' are to be found in *Webster's*). However, no single word in English expresses what is meant by the Chinese so clearly. More natural English expressions would be lengthy (e.g., 'make urine flow smoothly') and would not serve our need for neat technical compounds (e.g., 'urine-disinhibiting medicinals').

A near synonym of 利水 *lì shuǐ*, 'disinhibit water', is 利尿 *lì niào*, 'disinhibit urine'. This Chinese term is used in Western medicine as the equivalent of 'diuresis' (利尿药 *lì niào yào* is a 'diuretic'). Note that we have not chosen 'diuresis' as the translation for the term as used in Chinese medicine because Western medicine deals in nouns and adjectives (diuresis, diuretic), while in Chinese medicine *lì niào* is used first and foremost as a verb phrase. Efforts have been made to translate Chinese therapeutic terminology into the noun/adjective terminology of Western medicine. Unfortunately there are very few genuine counterparts, and the translator is forced to deal with the problems created by different parts of speech in English.

4. The word 渗 *shèn* means ' to seep', 'to leech', or, as we render it, 'to percolate'. The Chinese term 淡渗利水 *dàn shèn lì shuǐ*, to 'disinhibit water by bland percolation', means to promote the flow of water (urine), with bland-

flavored medicinals that encourage water to seep downwards. It has been suggested, with reason, that 'seep' might be a clearer rendering for *shèn*.

5. The word 解 *jiě* literally means 'to separate', 'undo', 'untie', 'release', or 'liberate'. We render this in most Chinese medical contexts as 'resolve'. Thus, 解表 *jiě biǎo*, to 'resolve the exterior', means to free the exterior of external evils by making the patient sweat. There are other uses too: 解毒 *jiě dú*, to 'resolve toxin', and 解郁 *jiě yù*, to 'resolve depression'.

6. 发 *fā* is another word that has many meanings in the ordinary language, at the core of which is the notion of outward movement: 'to put out (or forth)', 'to distribute', 'to broadcast', 'to emanate'. 发 *fā* occurs in a number of terms describing outward movement: 发汗 *fā hàn*, '[effuse] sweat', 发疹 *fā zhěn*, '[effuse] papules', and 发表 *fā biǎo*, 'effuse the exterior' (more or less synonymous with 解表 *jiě biǎo*, resolve the exterior). 发 *fā* also appears in the term 发黄 *fā huáng*, 'yellowing' or 'turning yellow'.

7. Other words are used to describe the therapeutic interventions in the interior-exterior dynamics of the body. The word 透 *tòu*, lit. to 'get through', 'penetrate', 'appear', 'thoroughly', describes the process of forcing things to the exterior or bringing them out. We render this idea as to 'thrust outward' or 'outthrust': 透邪 *tòu xié*, 'outthrust evils', 透泄 *tòu xiè*, 'outthrust and discharge', 透斑 *tòu bān*, 'outthrust macules'. We bend English a little when we say 'outthrust the exterior' to match the Chinese 透表 *tòu biǎo*, which means to bring (evils) to and out of the surface.

8. The character 疏 *shū* originally meant to enhance or restore free flow along water courses, and is used in this sense in the therapeutic context. Many translators render it as 'to dredge', but we have chosen a less specific word, 'to course'. 疏表 *shū biǎo*, 'course the exterior', is similar to 解表 *jiě biǎo*, 'resolve the exterior', but different in that it implies that the action is performed without causing the patient to sweat. 疏风 *shū fēng*, 'course wind', is to eliminate wind by coursing the exterior. Note that the liver is said to 'govern free coursing' (肝主疏泄 *gān zhǔ shū xiè*), which means that it keeps qì flowing like a well-dredged watercourse.

9. The character 导 *dǎo* means 'to lead' or 'to guide'. It occurs in the compound term 消食导滞 *xiāo shí dǎo zhì*, which means to break up food accumulations in the digestive tract and conduct stagnating waste down the digestive tract. We have rendered this as 'disperse food and abduct stagnation'. The word 'abduct', which here renders 导 *dǎo*, is from the Latin *ab*, 'down', 'away', + *ducere*, to 'lead' or 'guide'. Readers who know the word abduct only in the sense of 'to kidnap' should note that it is used in Western medicine in the sense of to draw away from the median plane or axial line of the limb.

10. The term 活血 *huó xuè* is rendered in this text as 'quicken the blood'. The Chinese 活 *huó* means 'alive', 'active', to 'live', 'work', or to 'instill life into'. The English 'quick' also means alive and moving, as well as rapid (as in 'the quick and the dead' and 'quicksilver'). It is akin to Latin *vivus*, the Greek *bios*, and the Sanskrit *jivas*. Our verb 'quicken' does not only mean accelerate but also to bring to life (the spring rain quickens the earth; the breath of life quickens the fetus). In Chinese medicine, the term 活血 *huó xuè* has both the notions of bringing to life and speeding movement. The English word 'activate', which is often used to translate the Chinese, is from 'act', which means to perform a role or function. 'Activate' is normally used in the mechanical context (activate a machine) and chemical context (activated sludge). It is completely devoid of the connotations of life inherent in the Chinese 活 *huó* and the English 'quicken'. Our close translation faithfully preserves the original image in translation. This is important in Chinese medicine because many concepts lack clear definitions beyond the words used to describe them.

11. The difficulty of finding one-word equivalents is nowhere more pronounced than in the realm of freeing and effusing terms. The words 通 *tòng*, 利 *lì*, and 发 *fā*, are very commonly used words in the everyday Chinese language, but in their various contexts they correspond to a whole host of different expressions in English. Yet in Chinese medicine, these words are not simply descriptive, they also carry a technical content. A technical term that in the source language is always used in a specific sense has to be translated with a single equivalent in the foreign language, so that the equivalent appears in the translated text as the original term does in the original text. We have to remember that the source of all new information for Westerners comes through the medium of translation. At the present incomplete stage of transmission, the possibilities for Westerners to bring about new developments in China's art of healing are slight. We therefore need a systematic English terminology that the translator finds easy to handle. If we allow the *lì* in 利湿 *lì shī* to be translated in one way, while the 利水 *lì* in *lì shuǐ* is translated in another, the translator trying to keep to a strict terminology will never master all the equivalents. S/he will forever be consulting term lists. The only way we can avoid this problem is if, as far as possible, we have an English terminology that relates to the Chinese at the level of single characters. Furthermore, not only do we need a single English equivalent for a single Chinese character, but, if we are to handle all the compound terms, the English equivalents need to be single words. If we render '*lì* X' as 'to make X flow smoothly', we have a lengthy English phrase that becomes awkward in compounds. A single-word equivalent for a single character overcomes this problem: 利水剂 *lì shuǐ jì* translated as 'water-disinhibiting formula' is neater than 'a formula that makes the urine flow smoothly', which is eight words as opposed to

the three Chinese characters, and which looks like an occasional description rather than a fixed term.

复合词 Compounds:

2014. 通下 *tōng xià*, precipitation

2015. 利关节 *lì guān jié*, disinhibit the joints

2016. 利咽 *lì yān*, disinhibit the throat

2017. 利湿 *lì shī*, disinhibit dampness

2018. 行气 *xíng qì*, move qi

2019. 行血 *xíng xuè*, move the blood

2020. 宣肺 *xuān fèi*, diffuse the lung

2021. 宣通水道 *xuān tōng shuǐ dào*, free the waterways

2022. 发表 *fā biǎo*, effuse the exterior

2023. 发汗法 *fā hàn fǎ*, sweating

2024. 透疹 *tòu zhěn*, outthrust papules

2025. 透表 *tòu biǎo*, outthrust the exterior

2026. 达邪 *dá xié*, outthrust evils

2027. 解表 *jiě biǎo*, resolve the exterior

2028. 疏表 *shū biǎo*, course the exterior

2029. 理气 *lǐ qì*, rectify qi

2030. 理血 *lǐ xuè*, rectify the blood

2031. 舒筋 *shū jīn*, soothe the sinews

2032. 舒肝 *shū gān*, soothe the liver

2033. 顺气 *shùn qì*, normalize qi

2034. 降逆 *jiàng qì*, downbear counterflow

2035. 降浊 *jiàng zhuó*, downbear the turbid

2036. 下气 *xià qì*, precipitate qi

2037. 宽胸 *kuān xiōng*, loosen the chest

2038. 宽中 *kuān zhōng*, loosen the center

2039. 开鬼门 *kāi guǐ mén*, open the ghost gates

2040. 开窍 *kāi qiào*, open the orifices

2041. 辛开苦泄 *xīn kāi kǔ xiè*, open with acridity and discharge with bitterness; acrid opening and bitter discharge

2042. 豁痰 *huò tán*, sweep phlegm

2043. 润肠 *rùn fèi*, moisten the intestines

2044. 滑肠 *rùn cháng*, lubricate the intestine

2045. 滑利关节 *huá lì guān jié*, disinhibit the joints

2046. 托法 *tuō fǎ*, drawing

2047. 排脓托毒 *pái nóng tuō dú*, expel pus and draw toxin

第五节　第五组   **SECTION 5: SET 5**

「固涩」、「镇纳」类字词　'Secure' & 'Settle' Terms

1526	* 固 □　固 □	*gù*	secure /sɪˈkjʊr/
			stem /stɛm/ (desertion only)
1527-n938	* 止 止　止 止	*zhǐ*	stanch /stɔntʃ/ (bleeding)
			allay /əˈle/ (thirst)
			check /tʃɛk/ (sweating, emission)
			suppress /səˈprɛs/ (cough)
1528	* 救 攵　救 攴	*jiù*	stem /stɛm/
1529	* 缩 纟　縮 糸	*suō*	reduce /rɪˈdjus/
1530-n939	* 敛 攵　斂 攴	*liǎn*	constrain /kənˈstren/
1531-n940	* 摄 扌　攝 手	*shè*	contain /kənˈten/
1532	* 涩 氵　澀 水	*sè*	astringe /əˈstrɪndʒ/
1533	* 平 一　平 干	*píng*	calm /kɑm/
1534-n941	* 安 宀　安 宀	*ān*	quiet /ˈkwaɪət/
1535-n942	* 宁 宀　寧 宀	*níng*	quiet /ˈkwaɪət/
1536	* 定 宀　定 宀	*dìng*	stabilize /ˈstebəˌlaɪz/
1537-n943	* 镇 钅　鎮 金	*zhèn*	settle /ˈsɛtl̩/
1538-n944	* 潜 氵　潛 水	*qián*	subdue /səbˈdju/
1539	* 纳 纟　納 糸	*nà*	absorb /əbˈsɔrb/

复合词 Compounds:

2048. 固表 *gù biǎo*, secure the exterior
2049. 固精 *gù jīng*, secure essence
2050. 止血 *zhǐ xuè*, stanch bleeding
2051. 止汗 *zhǐ hàn*, check sweating
2052. 敛肺 *liǎn fèi*, constrain the lung
2053. 敛阴 *liǎn yīn*, constrain yīn
2054. 涩肠 *sè cháng*, astringe the intestines
2055. 涩精 *sè jīng*, astringe essence
2056. 缩尿 *suō niào*, reduce urine
2057. 平肝 *píng gān*, calm the liver
2058. 安中 *ān zhōng*, quiet the center
2059. 安神 *ān shén*, quiet the spirit
2060. 镇惊 *zhèn jīng*, settle fright
2061. 潜阳 *qián yáng*, subdue yáng
2062. 潜镇 *qián zhèn*, subdue and settle

2063. 纳气 *nà qì*, promote qì absorption

| 第五节　第六组 | | | | SECTION 5: SET 6 |

汗法　　　　　　　　　　　　　　　　　　Sweating

1540	* 汗 氵	汗 水	*hàn*	sweat /swɛt/
1541	* 发 又	發 癶	*fā*	effuse /ɪˈfjuz/
1542	* 解 角	解 角	*jiě*	resolve /rɪˈzɑlv/ *vt, vi.*
				resolution /rɛzəljʃən/ *n.*
1543	* 疏 マ	疏 疋	*shū*	course /kɔrs, kors/
1544	* 透 辶	透 辵	*tòu*	outthrust /ˈaʊtθrʌst/
1545	* 达 辶	達 辵	*dá*	outthrust /ˈaʊtθrʌst/
1546	* 开 廾	開 門	*kāi*	open /ˈopən/ *vt.*
				opening /ˈopənɪŋ/ *n.*
1547	* 泄 氵	泄 水	*xiè*	discharge /dɪˈtʃɑrdʒ/
1548	* 祛 衤	祛 衣	*qū*	dispel /dɪsˈpɛl/
1549	* 搜 扌	搜 手	*sōu*	track down /træk daʊn/

注 Note:

The term 解表 *jiě biǎo*, resolve the exterior, means to free the exterior of evils. It usually involves causing the patient to sweat. The term 解肌 *jiě jī*, resolve the flesh, specifically means to resolve the exterior in initial-stage external contraction patterns marked by sweating. The term 疏表 *shū biǎo*, course the exterior, means to resolve the exterior with minimum sweating in the case of mild exterior patterns. The term 透表 *tòu biǎo*, outthrust the exterior, means to resolve the exterior heat. Notice that 疏 and 透 may have objects other than 'exterior': 疏风 *shū fēng*, course wind; 透邪 *tòu xié*, outthrust evil; 透疹 *tòu zhěn*, outthrust macules.

复合词 Compounds:

2064. 汗法 *hàn fǎ*, sweating
2065. 发汗法 *fā hàn fǎ*, sweating
2066. 解表 *jiě biǎo*, resolve the exterior; exterior resolution
2067. 解肌 *jiě jī*, resolve the flesh
2068. 祛风解表 *qū fēng jiě biǎo*, dispel wind and resolve the exterior
2069. 辛凉解表 *xīn liáng jiě biǎo*, resolve the exterior with coolness and acridity; cool acrid exterior resolution

2070. 辛温解表 *xīn wēn jiě biǎo*, resolve the exterior with warmth and acridity; warm acrid exterior resolution

2071. 益气解表 *yì qì jiě biǎo*, boost qì and resolve the exterior

2072. 助阳解表 *zhù yáng jiě biǎo*, assist yáng and resolve the exterior

2073. 养阴解表 *yǎng yīn jiě biǎo*, nourish yīn and resolve the exterior

2074. 滋阴解表 *zī yīn jiě biǎo*, enrich yīn and resolve the exterior

2075. 养血解表 *yǎng xuè jiě biǎo*, nourish the blood and resolve the exterior

2076. 化饮解表 *huà yǐn jiě biǎo*, transform rheum and resolve the exterior

2077. 透疹解表 *tòu zhěn jiě biǎo*, outthrust papules and resolve the exterior

2078. 疏表化湿 *shū biǎo huà shī*, course the exterior and transform dampness

2079. 疏表 *shū biǎo*, course the exterior

2080. 疏风 *shū fēng*, course wind

2081. 疏风泄热 *shū fēng xiè rè*, course wind and discharge heat

2082. 祛风 *qū fēng*, dispel wind

2083. 祛风除湿 *qū fēng chú shī*, dispel wind and eliminate dampness

2084. 祛风散寒 *qū fēng sàn hán*, dispel wind and dissipate cold

2085. 搜风逐寒 *sōu fēng zhú hán*, track wind and expel cold

2086. 解肌 *jiě jī*, resolve the flesh

2087. 透表 *tòu biǎo*, outthrust the exterior

2088. 透疹 *tòu zhěn*, outthrust papules

2089. 透斑 *tòu bān*, outthrust macules

2090. 透邪 *tòu xié*, outthrust evils

2091. 达邪 *dá xié*, outthrust evils

2092. 透泄 *tòu xiè*, outthrust and discharge

2093. 开鬼门 *kāi guǐ mén*, open the ghost gates

2094. 轻清疏解 *qīng qīng shū jiě*, clear and course with light [medicinals]

2095. 调和营卫 *tiáo hé yíng wèi*, harmonize construction and defense; construction-defense harmonization

2096. 泄卫透热 *xiè wèi tòu rè*, discharge defense and outthrust heat

---

第五节 第七组				**SECTION 5: SET 7**

吐法   **Ejection**

1550	* 吐 口	吐 口	*tù*	ejection /ɪˈdʒɛkʃən/
1551-n945	涌 氵	湧 水	*yǒng*	*welling up*
1552-n946	催 亻	催 人	*cuī*	*hasten, promote, induce*
1553-n947	探 扌	探 手	*tàn*	*probe, poke*

注 Note:

To induce vomiting in order to expel food stagnating in the stomach or phlegm obstructing the throat. 'Ejection' has been chosen instead of 'emesis' since the goal of the therapy is not necessarily to expel the gastric contents.

复合词 Compounds:

2097. 吐法 *tù fǎ*, ejection
2098. 涌吐 *yǒng tù*, eject; ejection
2099. 催吐法 *cuī tù fǎ*, ejection
2100. 探吐 *tàn tù*, mechanical ejection

第五节　第八组				**SECTION 5: SET 8**

下法				**Precipitation**
1554	* 下 卜	下 一	*xià*	precipitate /prɪˈsɪpɪˌtet/
1555	* 泻 氵	瀉 水	*xiè*	drain /dren/
1556	* 泄 氵	泄 水	*xiè*	discharge /dɪsˈtʃɑrdʒ/
1557	* 逐 辶	逐 辵	*zhú*	expel /ɪksˈpɛl/
1558	* 通 辶	通 辵	*tōng*	free /fri/
1559	* 攻 工	攻 攴	*gōng*	attack /əˈtæk/
				offensive /əˈfɛnsɪv/
1560-n948	釜 父	釜 金	*fǔ*	*pot, cauldron*
1561-n949	底 广	底 广	*dī*	*bottom*
1562	抽 扌	抽 手	*chōu*	*pull*
1563-n950	薪 艹	薪 艸	*xīn*	*firewood*
1564-n951	宛 宀	宛 宀	*yù*	*depression*
1565-n952	陈 阝	陳 阜	*chén*	*old*
1566-n953	莝 艹	莝 艸	*cuò*	*grass cuttings*
1567-n954	* 舟 舟	舟 舟	*zhōu*	ship /ʃɪp/
1568-n955	* 峻 山	峻 山	*jùn*	drastic /ˈdræstɪk/ *adj.*
				drastically /ˈdræstɪklɪ/ *adv.*

注 Notes:

1. 下法 *xià fǎ*, 'precipitation', is a method of treatment involving the stimulation of fecal flow to expel repletion evils and remove accumulation and

stagnation. It is also called 泻下 *xiè xià*, 'draining precipitation', or 攻下 *gōng xià*, 'offensive precipitation'. The principal forms are 寒下 *hán xià*, cold precipitation, 温下 *wēn xià*, warm precipitation, and 润下 *rùn xià*, moist precipitation.

2. The terminology of precipitation includes several metaphorical terms. 增水行舟 *zēng shuǐ xíng zhōu*, 'increase water to refloat the [grounded] ship', that is, to free the stool by increasing fluid, is a method of moist precipitation applied in warm disease to treat constipation due to heat bind and desiccation of humor and presenting as half vacuity, half repletion patterns. 去宛陈莝 *qù yù chén cuò*, 'eliminate depression stale water', is a method of treatment used to address stagnation and old fluid accumulations using medicinals such as kansui (*gān suì*) and morning glory (*qiān niú zǐ*). The character 宛 normally means 'meandering', in which sense it is pronounced *wǎn*, but here it is said to be synonymous with 郁 *yù*, depression, and pronounced *yù*; 莝 *cuò* means grass cuttings or hay, and is used to refer to stale accumulations of water. 釜底抽薪 *fǔ dǐ chōu xīn*, 'rake the firewood from beneath the cauldron', means using precipitation to eliminate repletion heat.

复合词 Compounds:

2101. 下法 *xià fǎ*, precipitation
2102. 泻下 *xiè xià*, draining precipitation
2103. 攻下 *gōng xià*, offensive precipitation
2104. 寒下 *hán xià*, cold precipitation
2105. 温下 *wēn xià*, warm precipitation
2106. 润下 *rùn xià*, moist precipitation
2107. 峻下 *jùn xià*, drastic precipitation
2108. 缓下 *huǎn xià*, mild precipitation
2109. 通下 *tōng xià*, precipitation
2110. 通里 *tōng lǐ*, free the interior
2111. 通泄 *tōng xiè*, free [the bowels] and discharge [heat]
2112. 通腑泄热 *tōng fǔ xiè rè*, free the bowels and discharge heat
2113. 通泄阳明腑实 *tōng xiè yáng míng fǔ shí*, free and discharge yáng brightness bowel repletion
2114. 导滞通腑 *dǎo zhì tōng fǔ*, abduct stagnation and free the bowels
2115. 润肠通便 *rùn cháng tōng biàn*, moisten the intestines and free the stool
2116. 增液泻下 *zēng yè xiè xià*, increase humor and precipitate with moistness; humor-increasing draining precipitation
2117. 增水行舟 *zēng shuǐ xíng zhōu*, refloat the grounded ship (i.e., to free the stool by increasing fluid)

2118. 咸寒增液 *xián hán zēng yè*, increase humor with cold and saltiness
2119. 急下存津 *jí xià cún jīn*, urgent precipitation to preserve liquid
2120. 急下存阴 *jí xià cún yīn*, urgent precipitation to preserve yīn
2121. 引火下行 *yǐn huǒ xià xíng*, conduct fire downwards
2122. 攻寒积 *gōng hán jī*, attack cold accumulations
2123. 逐水 *zhú shuǐ*, expel water
2124. 逐水饮 *zhú shuǐ yǐn*, expel water-rheum
2125. 泻水逐饮 *xiè shuǐ zhú yǐn*, drain water and expel rheum
2126. 去宛陈莝 *qù yù chén cuò*, eliminate stale water
2127. 釜底抽薪 *fǔ dǐ chōu xīn*, rake the firewood from beneath the cauldron
2128. 软坚除满 *ruǎn jiān chú mǎn*, soften hardness and eliminate fullness

---

第五节　第九组				**SECTION 5: SET 9**

和法				**Harmonization**
1569	* 和 禾	和 口	*hé*	harmonize /ˈhɑrməˌnaɪz/ *vt.*, harmonization /ˌhɑrməˌnaɪˈzeʃən/ *n.*
1570	* 调 讠	調 言	*tiáo*	regulate /ˈrɛgjəˌlet/ *vt.*, regulation /ˌrɛgjəˈleʃən/ *n.*
1571	* 解 角	解 角	*jiě*	resolve /rɪˈzɑlv/ *vt, vi.*, resolution /rɛzəljˈʃən/ *n.*

注 Notes:

1. 和法 *hé fǎ*, 'harmonization', is the method of adjusting functions within the human body that is used when an evil is at midstage penetration (half exterior and half interior) or when there is disharmony between qì and blood or between the organs, and such methods as sweating (diaphoresis), ejection, precipitation, warming, clearing, dispersion, and supplementation cannot be applied.

2. The Chinese 半表半里 *bàn biǎo bàn lǐ* is literally translated as 'half exterior half interior'. In actual fact, it is not half exterior half interior, but in the lesser yáng (*shào yáng*) between the exterior and interior. The translation 'midstage penetration' is less literal, but expresses the concept more precisely.

复合词 Compounds:

2129. 和解法 *hé fǎ*, harmonization
2130. 和解少阳 *hé jiě shào yáng*, harmonize the lesser yáng

2131. 和解表里 *hé jiě biǎo lǐ*, harmonize the exterior and interior
2132. 调和肝脾 *tiáo hé gān pí*, harmonize the liver and spleen
2133. 调和肝胃 *tiáo hé gān wèi*, harmonize the liver and stomach
2134. 调和肠胃 *tiáo hé cháng wèi*, harmonize the stomach and intestines
2135. 和肝 *hé gān*, harmonize the liver
2136. 和胃 *hé wèi*, harmonize the stomach
2137. 和胃止痛 *hé wèi zhǐ tòng*, harmonize the stomach and relieve pain
2138. 和中 *hé zhōng*, harmonize the center

第五节　第十组　　　　SECTION 5: SET 10

清法　　　　　　　Clearing

1572	* 清 氵	清 水	*qīng*	clear /klɪr/
1573	* 泄 氵	泄 水	*xiè*	discharge /ˈdɪstʃɑrdʒ/
1574	* 解 角	解 角	*jiě*	resolve /rɪzɑlv/
1575	* 凉 氵	凉 水	*liáng*	cool /kul/
1576	* 除 阝	除 阜	*chú*	eliminate /ɪˈlɪmɪˌnet/

注 Notes:

1. 清法 *qīng fǎ*, clearing, also called 清热法 *qīng rè fǎ*, is the method of treatment used to address heat.

2. In 清宫 *qīng gōng*, 'clear the palace', 宫 *gōng* denotes the heart; in other contexts, it denotes the uterus.

3. The term 凉燥 *liáng zào* in the therapeutic context means 'cooling dryness', a method of treating warm dryness. In warm disease terminology, the same two characters mean 'cool dryness', i.e., dryness with cold signs.

4. In this section, 补阳 *bǔ yáng*, supplementing yáng, overlaps with the warming method.

复合词 Compounds:

2139. 清法 *qīng fǎ*, clearing
2140. 清热法 *qīng rè fǎ*, heat-clearing method
2141. 清实热 *qīng shí rè*, clear repletion heat
2142. 清虚热 *qīng xū rè*, clear vacuity heat
2143. 清热泻火 *qīng rè xiè huǒ*, clear heat and drain fire
2144. 清热解毒 *qīng rè jiě dú*, clear heat and resolve toxin

2145. 清热凉血 *qīng rè liáng xuè*, clear heat and cool the blood

2146. 清热化湿 *qīng rè huà shī*, clear heat and transform dampness

2147. 清热利湿 *qīng rè lì shī*, clear heat and disinhibit dampness

2148. 清热利湿通淋 *qīng rè lì shī tōng lín*, clear heat, disinhibit dampness, and free strangury

2149. 清热润燥 *qīng rè rùn zào*, clear heat and moisten dryness

2150. 清热解暑 *qīng rè jiě shǔ*, clear heat and resolve summerheat

2151. 滋阴清热 *zī yīn qīng rè*, enrich yīn and clear heat

2152. 清络保阴 *qīng luò bǎo yīn*, clear the network vessels and preserve yīn

2153. 清心 *qīng xīn*, clear the heart

2154. 清心涤热 *qing xīn dí rè*, clear the heart and flush heat

2155. 清心泻火 *qīng xīn xiè huǒ*, clear the heart and drain fire

2156. 泻心 *xiè xīn*, drain the heart

2157. 清肝火 *qīng gān huǒ*, clear liver fire

2158. 清肝泻火 *qīng gān xiè huǒ*, clear the liver and drain fire

2159. 清肝泻肺 *qīng gān xiè fèi*, clear the liver and drain the lung

2160. 清泻肝胆实热 *qīng xiè gān dǎn shí rè*, clear and drain liver-gallbladder repletion heat

2161. 清热利胆 *qīng rè lì dǎn*, clear heat and disinhibit the gallbladder

2162. 清泄少阳 *qīng xiè shào yáng*, clear and discharge the lesser yáng

2163. 泻肝 *xiè gān*, drain the liver

2164. 清肺热 *qīng fèi rè*, clear lung heat

2165. 清金 *qīng jīn*, clear metal

2166. 清金降火 *qīng jīn jiàng huǒ*, clear metal and depurate fire

2167. 泻肺 *xiè fèi*, drain the lung

2168. 泻白 *xiè bái*, drain the white

2169. 清胃热 *qīng wèi rè*, clear stomach heat

2170. 清肠润燥 *qīng cháng rùn zào*, clear the intestines and moisten dryness

2171. 清化大肠湿热 *qīng huà dà cháng shī rè*, clear and transform large intestine damp-heat

2172. 清燥 *qīng zào*, clear dryness

2173. 凉燥 *liáng zào*, cool dryness

2174. 清气 *qīng qì*, clear qì

2175. 清气分热 *qīng qì fèn rè*, clear qì-aspect heat

2176. 辛寒清气 *xīn hán qīng qì*, clear qì with cold and acridity

2177. 苦寒清气 *kǔ hán qīng qì*, clear qì with cold and bitterness

2178. 清营 *qīng yíng*, clear construction

2179. 清营分热 *qīng yíng fēn rè*, clear construction-aspect heat
2180. 清营泄热 *qīng yíng xiè rè*, clear construction and discharge heat
2181. 透营转气 *tòu yíng zhuǎn qì*, outthrust construction heat through qì
2182. 气营两清 *qì yíng liǎng qīng*, clear both qì and construction; dual clearing of qì and construction
2183. 清血分热 *qīng xuè fēn rè*, clear blood-aspect heat
2184. 凉血 *liáng xuè*, cool the blood
2185. 凉血散血 *liáng xuè sàn xuè*, cool the blood and dissipate the blood
2186. 凉血解毒 *liáng xuè jiě dú*, cool the blood and resolve toxin
2187. 化斑 *huà bān*, transform macules
2188. 清宫 *qīng gōng*, clear the palace
2189. 苦寒清热 *kǔ hán qīng rè*, clear heat with cold and bitterness
2190. 苦寒泄热 *kǔ hán xiè rè*, discharge heat with cold and bitterness
2191. 甘温除（大）热 *gān wēn chú (dà) rè*, eliminate (great) heat with warmth and sweetness (a method of treating vacuity heat)

第五节　第十一组				**SECTION 5: SET 11**

温法				**Warming**
1577	* 温 氵	溫 水	*wēn*	warm /wɔrm/
1578	* 暖 火	煖 火	*nuǎn*	warm /wɔrm/
1579	* 救 扌	救 手	*jiù*	rescue /ˈrɛskju/ stem /stɛm/
1580	* 固 囗	固 囗	*gù*	secure /sɪˈkjʊr/ stem /stɛm/ (desertion only)
1581	* 回 囗	回 囗	*huí*	return /rɪˈtɝn/

注 Notes:

1. 温法 *wēn fǎ*, warming, is the method of treatment used to address cold patterns. It involves the use of warm or hot medicinals to supplement yáng qì and expel cold evil.

2. The character 救 *jiù* can usually be rendered as 'rescue' (救阳 *jiù yáng*, rescue yáng; 救肺 *jiù fèi*, rescue the lung), but the compound 救逆 *jiù nì* is rendered as 'stem counterflow'. Similarly, 固 *gù* in this text is usually rendered as 'secure' (固表 *gù biǎo*, secure the exterior; 固本 *gù běn*, secure the root), but the compound 固脱 *gù tuō* is rendered as 'stem desertion'.

3. The terms 助阳 *zhù yáng*, 'assist yáng', 补阳 *bǔ yáng*, 'supplement yáng', and 温阳 *wēn yáng*, 'warm yáng', are all equivalent, meaning to enhance the warming power of yáng qì. The term 回阳 *huí yáng*, 'return yáng', differs in that it denotes the supplementing of yáng in conditions of 'yáng desertion' (阳脱 *yáng tuō*), as we see in the fuller compound 回阳就逆 *huí yáng jiù nì*, 'return yáng and stem counterflow'. The term 壮阳 *zhuàng yáng*, 'invigorate yáng', means to supplement kidney yáng in the treatment of impotence. Here, the sexual connotations of 'invigorate' parallel those of 壮 *zhuàng* perfectly. In the therapeutic context, 回 *huí*, 'return', 助 *zhù*, 'assist', and 壮 *zhuàng*, 'invigorate' are only applied to 阳 *yáng*. A synonym of 温 *wēn*, warm, is 暖 *nuǎn*, which occurs in the term 暖胃 *nuǎn wèi*, to warm the stomach.

复合词 Compounds:

2192. 温法 *wēn fǎ*, warming
2193. 祛寒法 *qū hán fǎ*, dispelling cold
2194. 温阳 *wēn yáng*, warm yáng
2195. 温阳救逆 *wēn yáng jiù nì*, warm yáng and stem counterflow
2196. 温里 *wěn lǐ*, warm the interior
2197. 温中 *wēn zhōng*, warm the center
2198. 温中祛寒 *wēn zhōng qū hán*, warm the center and dispel cold
2199. 温中回阳 *wēn zhōng huí yáng*, warm the center and return yáng
2200. 温运中阳 *wēn yùn zhōng yáng*, warm and move center yáng
2201. 温化寒湿 *wēn huà hán shī*, warm and transform cold-damp
2202. 理中 *lǐ zhōng*, rectify the center
2203. 温肝散寒 *wēn gān sàn hán*, warm the liver and dissipate cold
2204. 暖肝散寒 *nuǎn gān sàn hán*, warm the liver and dissipate cold
2205. 益气温胆 *yì qì wēn dǎn*, boost qì and warm the gallbladder
2206. 温振心阳 *wen zhèn xīn yáng*, warm and vitalize heart yáng
2207. 温补心肾 *wēn bǔ xīn shèn*, warm and supplement the heart and kidney
2208. 温脾 *wēn pí*, warm the spleen
2209. 温脾截疟 *wēn pí jié nüè*, warm the spleen and interrupt malaria
2210. 温阳 *wēn yáng*, warm yáng
2211. 温经 *wēn jīng*, warm the channels
2212. 暖胃 *nuǎn wèi*, warm the stomach
2213. 温胃止呕 *wēn wèi zhǐ ǒu*, warm the stomach and check vomiting
2214. 温胃建中 *wēn wèi jiàn zhōng*, warm the stomach and fortify the center
2215. 温肺 *wēn fèi*, warm the lung

2216. 温肺化痰 *wēn fèi huà tán*, warm the lung and transform phlegm
2217. 温肺化饮 *wēn fèi hào yǐn*, warm the lung and transform rheum
2218. 温肾 *wēn shèn*, warm the kidney
2219. 温肾补火 *wēn shèn bǔ huǒ*, warm the kidney and supplement fire
2220. 温补肾阳 *wēn bǔ shèn yáng*, warm and supplement kidney yáng
2221. 温补命门 *wēn bǔ mìng mén*, warm and supplement the life gate
2222. 温肾固脬 *wēn shèn gù pāo*, warm the kidney and secure the bladder
2223. 暖水脏 *nuǎn shuǐ zàng*, warm the water viscus
2224. 温水脏 *wēn shuǐ zàng*, warm the water viscus
2225. 温经祛寒 *wēn jīng qū hán*, warm the channels and dispel cold
2226. 温经散寒 *wēn jīng sàn hán*, warm the channels and dissipate cold
2227. 温经止血 *wēn jīng zhǐ xuè*, warm the channels and stanch bleeding
2228. 温血 *wēn xuè*, warm the blood
2229. 温补血分 *wēn bǔ xuè fēn*, warm and supplement the blood aspect
2230. 回阳 *huí yáng*, return yáng
2231. 回阳救逆 *huí yáng jiù nì*, return yáng and stem counterflow
2232. 通阳 *tōng yáng*, free yáng
2233. 救阳 *jiù yáng*, rescue yáng
2234. 救脱 *jiù tuō*, stem desertion

第五节　第十二组				**SECTION 5: SET 12**

消法				**Dispersion**
1582	* 消 氵	消 水	*xiāo*	disperse /dɪˈspɝs/
1583	* 导 已	導 寸	*dǎo*	abduct /əbˈdʌkt/
1584	* 化 亻	化 匕	*huà*	transform /trænsˈfɔrm/
1585	* 开 卅	開 門	*kāi*	open /ˈopən/
1586	* 通 辵	通 辶	*tōng*	free /fri/

注 Note:

消法 *xiāo fǎ*, dispersion, is a group of methods of treatment used to gently break up accumulations in the body, including concretions and conglomerations, lump glomus, food accumulations, water amassment, calculi (stones), scrofula, and phlegm nodes.

复合词 Compounds:

2235. 消法 *xiāo fǎ*, dispersion

2236. 消导 *xiāo dǎo*, abductive dispersion

2237. 消食导滞 *xiāo shí dǎo zhì*, disperse food and abduct stagnation; abductive dispersion of food stagnation

2238. 消食化滞 *xiāo shí huà zhì*, disperse food and transform stagnation

2239. 消食通腑 *xiāo shí tōng fǔ*, disperse food and free the bowels

2240. 消食健脾 *xiāo shí jiàn pí*, disperse food and fortify the spleen

2241. 消补兼施 *xiāo bǔ jiān shī*, disperse and supplement simultaneously; simultaneous dispersion and supplementation

2242. 温中化食 *wēn zhōng huà shí*, warm the center and transform food

2243. 清热化食 *qīng hè huà shí*, clear heat and transform food

2244. 消痞 *xiāo pǐ*, disperse glomus

2245. 消痞化积 *xiāo pǐ huà jī*, disperse glomus and transform accumulation

2246. 化痞 *huà pǐ*, transform glomus

2247. 开痞 *kāi pǐ*, relieve glomus

2248. 开胃 *kāi wèi*, open the stomach; increase the appetite

2249. 开胃进食 *kāi wèi jìn shí*, open the stomach and increase the appetite

---

第五节　第十三组				**SECTION 5: SET 13**

祛痰法　　　　　　　　　　　　　Dispelling Phlegm

1587	* 祛 礻	祛 衣	*qū*	dispel /dɪsˈpɛl/
1588	* 化 亻	化 匕	*huà*	transform /trænsˈfɔrm/
1589	* 涤 氵	滌 水	*dí*	flush /flʌʃ/
1590	* 豁 谷	豁 谷	*huò*	sweep /swip/

注 Note:

祛痰 *qū tán*, 'dispelling phlegm', refers to any method of eliminating phlegm. 化痰 *huà tán*, 'transforming phlegm', is a synonym. Phlegm occurs with heat or cold, and the treatment is varied accordingly: 清热化痰 *qīng rè huà tán*, 'clearing heat and transforming phlegm'; 祛寒化痰 *qū hán huà tán*, 'dispelling cold and transforming phlegm'. Action to dispel stubborn phlegm or phlegm-rheum is often called 涤痰 *dí tán*, 'flushing phlegm'.

复合词 Compounds:

2250. 祛痰 *qū tán*, dispel phlegm

2251. 化痰 *huà tán*, transform phlegm; phlegm transformation

2252. 宣肺化痰 *xuān fèi huà tán*, diffuse the lung and transform phlegm

2253. 清热化痰 *qīng rè huà tán*, clear heat and transform phlegm
2254. 润肺化痰 *rùn fèi huà tán*, moisten the lung and transform phlegm
2255. 燥湿化痰 *zào shī huà tán*, dry dampness and transform phlegm
2256. 祛寒化痰 *qū hán huà tán*, dispel cold and transform phlegm
2257. 治风化痰 *zhì fēng huà tán*, control wind and transform phlegm
2258. 消痰 *xiāo tán*, disperse phlegm
2259. 消痰平喘 *xiāo tán píng chuǎn*, disperse phlegm and calm panting
2260. 消痰软坚 *xiāo tán ruǎn jiān*, disperse phlegm and soften hardness
2261. 涤痰 *dí tán*, flush phlegm
2262. 豁痰 *huò tán*, sweep phlegm

第五节　第十四组				**SECTION 5: SET 14**

祛**湿**法				**Dispelling Dampness**
1591	* 化 亻	化 匕	*huà*	transform /trænsˈfɔrm/
1592	* 燥 火	燥 火	*zào*	dry /draɪ/
1593	* 利 禾	利 刀	*lì*	disinhibit /ˌdɪsɪnˈhɪbɪt/
1594	* 洁 氵	潔 水	*jié*	cleanse /klɛnz/

注 Note:

Different terms are used to denote the removal of dampness: 祛湿 *qū shī*, 'dispel dampness', is a general term; 化湿 *huà shī*, transform dampness, usually denotes the removal of dampness from the upper burner, but like 祛湿 *qū shī* it is also a general term; 燥湿 *zào shī*, dry dampness, usually denotes the removal of dampness from the middle burner; and 利湿 *lì shī*, disinhibit dampness, denotes removal of dampness from the lower burner.

复合词 Compounds:

2263. 祛湿 *qū shī*, dispel dampness
2264. 化湿 *huà shī*, transform dampness
2265. 化湿浊 *huà shī zhuó*, transform damp turbidity
2266. 行气化湿 *xíng qì huà shī*, move qì and transform dampness
2267. 清热化湿 *qīng rè huà shī*, clear heat and transform dampness
2268. 温中化湿 *wēn zhōng huà shī*, warm the center and transform dampness
2269. 疏表化湿 *shū biǎo huà shī*, course the exterior and transform dampness

2270. 芳香化湿 *fāng xiāng huà shī*, transform dampness with aroma

2271. 芳香化浊 *fāng xiāng huà zhuó*, transform turbidity with aroma

2272. 辛香化浊 *xīn xiāng huà zhuó*, transform turbidity with acridity and aroma

2273. 燥湿 *zào shī*, dry dampness

2274. 健脾燥湿 *jiàn pí zào shī*, fortify the spleen and transform dampness

2275. 温中燥湿 *wēn zhōng zào shī*, warm the center and dry dampness

2276. 燥湿除满 *zào shī chú mǎn*, dry dampness and eliminate fullness

2277. 燥湿化痰 *zào shī huà tán*, dry dampness and transform phlegm

2278. 苦温燥湿 *kǔ wēn zào shī*, dry dampness with warmth and bitterness

2279. 苦寒燥湿 *kǔ hán zào shī*, dry dampness with cold and bitterness

2280. 利湿 *lì shī*, disinhibit dampness

2281. 清热利湿 *qīng rè lì shī*, clear heat and disinhibit dampness

2282. 清暑利湿 *qīng shǔ lì shī*, clear summerheat and disinhibit dampness

2283. 温阳利湿 *wēn yáng lì shī*, warm yáng and disinhibit dampness

2284. 化气利湿 *huà qì lì shī*, transform qì and disinhibit dampness; promote qì transformation and disinhibit water

2285. 滋阴利湿 *zī yīn lì shī*, enrich yīn and disinhibit dampness

2286. 利湿退黄 *lì shī tuì huáng*, disinhibit dampness and abate jaundice

2287. 淡渗利湿 *dàn shèn lì shī*, disinhibit dampness by bland percolation

2288. 温肾利水 *wēn shèn lì shuǐ*, warm the kidney and disinhibit water

2289. 渗湿於热下 *shèn shī yú rè xià*, percolate dampness through the heat; heat-releasing dampness percolation

2290. 利小便，实大便 *lì xiǎo biàn, shí dà biàn*, disinhibit urine and harden the stool

2291. 宣通水道 *xuān tōng shuǐ dào*, free the waterways

2292. 洁净腑 *jié jìng fǔ*, cleansing the clean bowel

第五节　第十五组				**SECTION 5: SET 15**

理气开郁法				**Rectifying Qì & Opening Depression**
1595	* 理 王	理 玉	*lǐ*	rectify /ˈrɛktɪˌfaɪ/
1596	* 通 辶	通 辵	*tōng*	free /fri/
1597	* 开 廾	開 門	*kāi*	open /ˈopən/
1598	* 利 禾	利 刀	*lì*	disinhibit /ˌdɪsɪnˈhɪbɪt/
1599	* 行 彳	行 彳	*xíng*	move /muv/
1600	* 解 角	解 角	*jiě*	resolve /rɪˈzɑlv/
1601	* 疏 マ	疏 疋	*shū*	course /kɔrs, kors/

1602	* 舒 人	舒 舌	*shū*	soothe /suð/
1603	* 順 页	順 頁	*shùn*	normalize /ˈnɔrml͵aɪz/
1604	* 降 阝	降 阜	*jiàng*	downbear /ˈdaʊnbɛr/
1605	* 下 卜	下 一	*xià*	precipitate /prɪˈsɪpɪ͵tet/
1606	* 宽 宀	宽 宀	*kuān*	loosen /ˈlusn̩/
1607	* 宣 宀	宣 宀	*xuān*	diffuse /dɪˈfjuz/

注 Notes:

1. 理气开郁 *lǐ qì kāi yù*, 'rectify qì and open depression', is any method of treating qì stagnation or qì counterflow. It includes 行气 *xíng qì*, 'moving qì', and 降逆下气 *jiàng nì xià qì*, 'downbear counterflow and precipitate qì'.

行气 *xíng qì*, 'moving qì', 利气 *lì qì*, 'disinhibiting qì', 通气 *tōng qì*, 'freeing qì', and 调气 *tiáo qì*, 'regulating qì', all mean dissipating qì stagnation in the treatment of distention, oppression, and pain in the chest and abdomen. This includes a) 疏郁理气 *shū yù lǐ qì*, 'coursing depression and rectifying qì' (also called 宽胸 *kuān xiōng*, 'loosening the chest', 宽中 *kuān zhōng*, 'loosening the center', and 解郁 *jiě yù*, 'resolving depression'), which is used to treat glomus and oppression in the chest and diaphragm, and pain and distention in the both rib-side and lesser abdomen; and b) 和胃理气 *hé wèi lǐ qì*, 'harmonizing the stomach and rectifying qì', which is used to treat qì stagnation and phlegm-damp giving rise to distention and oppression in the stomach duct, acid regurgitation, vomiting of sour fluid, and belching.

降逆下气 *jiàng nì xià qì*, 'downbearing counterflow and precipitating qì', includes: a) 降逆止呕 *jiàng nì zhǐ ǒu*, 'downbearing counterflow and checking vomiting', a method of treatment used to downbear counterflow and precipitate qì to treat stomach vacuity cold causing persistent hiccup, and discomfort in the chest; b) 降逆平喘 *jiàng nì píng chuǎn*, 'downbearing qì and calming panting', a method used to downbear counterflow and precipitate qì in the treatment of wheezing and panting or rapid panting breathing, and copious phlegm.

2. 破气 *pò qì*, breaking qì, means rectifying qì with drastic medicinals such as unripe tangerine peel (*qīng pí*) and unripe bitter orange (*zhǐ shí*), which dissipate binds and abduct stagnation.

复合词 Compounds:

2293. 理气 *lǐ qì*, rectify qì
2294. 顺气 *shùn qì*, normalize qì
2295. 行气 *xíng qì*, move qì
2296. 行气止痛 *xíng qì zhǐ tòng*, move qì and relieve pain

2297. 利气 *lì qì*, disinhibit qì

2298. 通气 *tōng qì*, free qì

2299. 降气 *jiàng qì*, downbear qì

2300. 下气 *xià qì*, precipitate qì

2301. 调气 *tiáo qì*, regulate qì

2302. 破气 *pò qì*, break qì

2303. 疏郁理气 *shū yù lǐ qì*, course depression and rectify qì

2304. 宽胸 *kuān xiōng*, loosen the chest

2305. 宽中 *kuān zhōng*, loosen the center

2306. 解郁 *jiě yù*, resolve depression

2307. 开郁 *kāi yù*, open depression

2308. 疏肝 *shū gān*, course the liver

2309. 疏肝理气 *shū gān lǐ qì*, course the liver and rectify qì

2310. 疏肝解郁 *shū gān jiě yù*, course the liver and resolve depression

2311. 健脾疏肝 *jiàn pí shū gān*, fortify the spleen and course the liver

2312. 舒肝 *shū gān*, soothe the liver

2313. 降逆下气 *jiàng nì xià qì*, downbear counterflow and precipitate qì

2314. 和胃理气 *hé wèi lǐ qì*, harmonize the stomach and rectify qì

2315. 降逆止呕 *jiàng nì zhǐ ǒu*, downbear counterflow and check vomiting

2316. 降逆平喘 *jiàng nì píng chuǎn*, downbear counterflow and calm panting

2317. 宣肺 *xuān fèi*, diffuse the lung

2318. 宣肺止咳 *xuān fèi zhǐ ké*, diffuse the lung and suppress cough

2319. 宣白 *xuān bái*, diffuse the white

2320. 宣降肺气 *xuān jiàng fèi qì*, diffuse and downbear lung qì

2321. 轻宣肺气 *qīng xuān fèi qì*, diffuse lung qì with light [medicinals]

2322. 清肃肺气 *qīng sù fèi qì*, clear and depurate lung qì

2323. 辛开苦降 *xīn kāi kǔ jiàng*, open with acridity and downbear with bitterness; acrid opening and bitter downbearing

2324. 辛开苦泄 *xīn kāi kǔ xiè*, open with acridity and discharge with bitterness; acrid opening and bitter discharge

2325. 开泄 *kāi xiè*, opening and discharging

第五节　第十六组   **SECTION 5: SET 16**

活血化瘀法   **Quickening the Blood &**
                                       Transforming Stasis

1608	* 活 氵	活 水	*huó*	quicken /ˈkwɪkən/
1609	* 化 亻	化 匕	*huà*	transform /trænsˈfɔrm/
1610	* 行 彳	行 彳	*xíng*	move /muv/
1611	* 祛 礻	祛 衣	*qū*	dispel /dɪsˈpɛl/
1612	* 散 攵	散 攴	*sàn*	dissipate /ˈdɪsɪˌpet/
1613	* 破 石	破 石	*pò*	break /brek/
1614	* 逐 辶	逐 辵	*zhú*	expel /ɪksˈpɛl/
1615	* 通 辶	通 辵	*tōng*	free /fri/
1616	* 消 氵	消 水	*xiāo*	disperse /dɪˈspɝs/

注 **Note:**

Different expressions are used to denote action to remove static blood and enhance the movement of blood: 祛血 *qū xuè* is a general term for the removal of static blood; 活血 *huó xuè* denotes a mild action; 化血 *huà xuè* implies a stronger action; 破血 *pò xuè* (or 破瘀 *pò yū*) denotes a forceful action; 逐瘀 *zhú yū* is the removal of internal static blood giving rise to signs such as black stool or menstrual block.

复合词 **Compounds:**

2326. 活血化瘀 *huó xuè huà yū*, quicken the blood and transform phlegm
2327. 温化祛瘀 *wēn huà qū yū*, warming transformation of static blood
2328. 祛瘀活血 *qū yū huó xuè*, dispel stasis and quicken the blood
2329. 去瘀生新 *qù yū shēng xīn*, eliminate stasis and engender the new
2330. 活血生新 *huó xuè shēng xīn*, quicken the blood and engender the new
2331. 化瘀行血 *huà yū xíng xuè*, transform stasis and move the blood
2332. 破瘀消癥 *pò yū xiāo zhēng*, break stasis and disperse concretions
2333. 散瘀 *sàn yū*, dissipate stasis
2334. 通瘀破结 *tōng yū pò jié*, free stasis and break binds
2335. 逐瘀 *zhú yū*, expel stasis
2336. 祛瘀消肿 *qū yū xiāo zhǒng*, dispel stasis and disperse swelling
2337. 行血 *xíng xuè*, move the blood
2338. 破血 *pò xuè*, break blood
2339. 通脉 *tōng mài*, free the vessels

第五节　第十七组 **SECTION 5: SET 17**

止血法 **Stanching Bleeding**

1617	*	止 止	止 止	*zhǐ*	stanch /stɔntʃ/
1618	*	摄 扌	攝 手	*shè*	contain /kənˈten/
1619-n956	*	归 彐	歸 止	*guī*	return /rɪˈtɜ˞n/

复合词 Compounds:

2340. 止血 *zhǐ xuè*, stanch bleeding
2341. 清热止血 *qīng rè zhǐ xuè*, clear heat and stanch bleeding
2342. 补气止血 *bǔ qì zhǐ xuè*, supplement qì and stanch bleeding
2343. 补气摄血 *bǔ qì shè xuè*, supplement qì and contain the blood
2344. 祛瘀止血 *qū yū zhǐ xuè*, dispel stasis and stanch bleeding
2345. 引血归经 *yǐn xuè guī jīng*, return blood to the channels

第五节　第十八组 **SECTION 5: SET 18**

开窍法 **Opening the Orifices**

1620	*	开 卝	開 門	*kāi*	open /ˈopən/
1621	*	化 亻	化 匕	*huà*	transform /trænsˈfɔrm/
1622	*	宣 宀	宣 宀	*xuān*	diffuse /dɪˈfjuz/
					perfuse /pɚˈfjuz/
1623	*	醒 酉	醒 酉	*xǐng*	arouse /əˈrauz/

注 Note:

开窍 *kāi qiào*, opening the orifices, also called 开闭 *kāi bì*, is a method of treatment used to address clouded spirit and coma due to evil obstructing the orifices of the heart. It employs acrid aromatic penetrating medicinals that penetrate the heart and free the orifices, repel foulness, and open blocks. Opening the orifices is also called 开闭 *kāi bì*, opening blocks, 醒神 *xǐng shén*, arousing the spirit, and 醒脑 *xǐng nǎo*, arousing the brain.

复合词 Compounds:

2346. 开窍 *kāi qiào*, open the orifices; orifice opening
2347. 开闭 *kāi bì*, open block

2348. 宣窍 *xuān qiào*, perfuse the orifices
2349. 凉开 *liáng kāi*, cool opening
2350. 温开 *wēn kāi*, warm opening
2351. 清热开窍 *qīng rè kāi qiào*, clear heat and open the orifices
2352. 清心开窍 *qīng xīn kāi qiào*, clear the heart and open the orifices
2353. 清热化痰开窍 *qīng rè huà tán kāi qiào*, clear heat, transform phlegm, and open the orifices
2354. 逐寒开窍 *zhú hán kāi qiào*, expel cold and open the orifices
2355. 化痰开窍 *huà tán kāi qiào*, transform phlegm and open the orifices
2356. 开窍通神 *kāi qiào tōng shén*, open the orifices and free the spirit
2357. 醒脑 *xǐng nǎo*, arouse the brain
2358. 豁痰醒脑 *huò tán xǐng nǎo*, sweep phlegm and arouse the brain
2359. 涌痰醒脑 *yǒng tán xǐng nǎo*, eject phlegm and arouse the brain
2360. 醒神 *xǐng shén*, arouse the spirit
2361. 开噤通关 *kāi jìn tōng guān*, open the jaws

第五节　第十九组	**SECTION 5: SET 19**

安神法				**Quieting the Spirit**
1624	* 安 ⌒	安 ⌒	*ān*	quiet /ˈkwaɪət/
1625	* 宁 ⌒	寧 ⌒	*níng*	quiet /ˈkwaɪət/
1626	* 定 ⌒	定 ⌒	*dìng*	stabilize /ˈstebəˌlaɪz/
1627	* 镇 钅	鎮 金	*zhèn*	settle /ˈsɛtl̩/

注 Note:

安神 *ān shén*, quiet the spirit, denotes any method of treatment used to address disquieted spirit, that is, palpitation, insomnia, agitation, mania. The main forms are 养心安神 *yǎng xīn ān shén*, nourish the heart and quiet the spirit, which treats heart blood depletion, and 重镇安神 *zhòng zhèn ān shén*, quiet the spirit with heavy settlers, which treats palpitation, fearful throbbing, insomnia, or fright mania with heavy mineral and shell medicinals.

复合词 Compounds:

2362. 安神 *ān shén*, quiet the spirit
2363. 养心安神 *yǎng xīn ān shén*, nourish the heart and quiet the spirit
2364. 重镇安神 *zhòng zhèn ān shén*, quiet the spirit with heavy settlers
2365. 镇心 *zhèn xīn*, settle the heart

2366. 镇惊 *zhèn jīng*, settle fright

2367. 定志 *dìng zhì*, stabilize the mind

2368. 宁志 *níng zhì*, quiet the mind

2369. 宁神安魂 *níng shén ān hún*, quiet the spirit and ethereal soul

2370. 交通心肾 *jiāo tōng xīn shèn*, promote heart-kidney interaction

---

第五节　第二十组 — SECTION 5: SET 20

固涩法 — Securing & Astriction

1628	* 固 口	固 口	*gù*	secure /sɪˈkjʊr/	
1629	* 止 止	止 止	*zhǐ*	suppress /səˈprɛs/ (cough) check /tʃɛk/ (sweating, emission)	
1630	* 缩 纟	縮 糸	*suō*	reduce /rɪˈdjus/	
1631	* 敛 攵	斂 攴	*liǎn*	constrain /kənˈstren/	
1632	* 摄 扌	攝 手	*shè*	contain /kənˈten/	
1633	* 涩 氵	澀 水	*sè*	astringe /əˈstrɪndʒ/	

复合词 Compounds:

2371. 固涩 *gù sè*, securing and astriction

2372. 固摄 *gù shè*, securing and containing

2373. 收涩 *shōu sè*, astriction

2374. 敛汗固表 *liàn hàn gù biǎo*, constrain sweat and secure the exterior

2375. 敛肺止咳 *liàn fèi zhǐ ké*, constrain the lung and suppress cough

2376. 涩肠止泻 *sè cháng zhǐ xiè*, astringe the intestines and check diarrhea

2377. 涩肠固脱 *sè cháng gù tuō*, astringe the intestines and stem desertion

2378. 固肾涩精 *gù shèn sè jīng*, secure the kidney and astringe essence

2379. 涩精止遗 *sè jīng zhǐ yí*, astringe essence and check emission

2380. 摄精 *shè jīng*, contain essence

2381. 固精 *gù jīng*, secure essence

2382. 固崩止带 *gù bēng zhǐ dài*, stem flooding and check discharge

2383. 缩尿 *suō niào*, reduce urine

第五节　第二十一组	**SECTION 5: SET 21**

潜镇熄风法	**Subduing, Settling &** **Extinguishing Wind**

1634	* 潜 氵	潛 水	*qián*	subdue /səbˈdju/
1635	* 镇 钅	鎮 金	*zhèn*	settle /ˈsɛtl̩/
1636	* 熄 火	熄 火	*xī*	extinguish /ɪksˈtɪŋgwɪʃ/
1637	* 平 一	平 干	*píng*	calm /kɑm/

注 Notes:

1. 熄风 *xī fēng*, 'extinguishing wind', is a method of treatment addressing liver wind stirring internally.

2. 伐肝 *fá gān*, 'quelling the liver', is a method of treatment used to control excessively exuberant liver qì invading the spleen using medicinals such as bupleurum (*chái hú*), unripe tangerine peel (*qīng pí*), costusroot (*guǎng mù xiāng*), and Buddha's hand (*fó shǒu gān*). It is also called 抑肝 *yì gān*, 'repressing the liver'.

复合词 Compounds:

2384. 潜阳 *qián yáng*, subdue yáng

2385. 滋阴平肝潜阳 *zī yīn píng gān qián yáng*, enrich yīn, calm the liver, and subdue yáng

2386. 潜镇 *qián zhèn*, subdue and settle

2387. 镇潜 *zhèn qián*, subdue and settle

2388. 熄风 *xī fēng*, extinguish wind

2389. 滋阴熄风 *zī yīn xī fēng*, enrich yīn and extinguish wind

2390. 平肝熄风 *píng gān xī fēng*, calm the liver and extinguish wind

2391. 镇肝熄风 *zhèn gān xī fēng*, settle the liver and extinguish wind

2392. 泻火熄风 *xiè huǒ xī fēng*, drain fire and extinguish wind

2393. 清热凉肝熄风 *qīng rè liáng gān xī fēng*, clear heat, cool the liver, and extinguish wind

2394. 养血熄风 *yǎng xuè xī fēng*, nourish the blood and extinguish wind

2395. 和血熄风 *hé xuè xī fēng*, harmonize the blood and extinguish wind

2396. 泄肝 *xiè gān*, discharge the liver

2397. 伐肝 *fá gān*, quell the liver

2398. 抑肝 *yì gān*, repress the liver

2399. 解痉 *jiě jìng*, resolve tetany

2400. 镇痉 *zhèn jìng*, settle tetany

| 第五节　第二十二组 | | | | SECTION 5: SET 22 |

妇产科治法　　　　　　　　Women's Treatment Methods

1638	* 调 讠	調 言	*tiáo*	regulate /ˈrɛgjə،let/ *vt.*
				regulation /،rɛgjəˈʃən/ *n.*
1639	* 通 辶	通 辶	*tōng*	free /fri/
1640	催 亻	催 人	*cuī*	*hasten, promote, induce*
1641-n957	* 暖 火	煖 火	*nuǎn*	warm /wɔrm/

注 Note:

In 暖宫 *nuǎn gōng*, 'warm the palace', 宫 *gōng* denotes the uterus. Earlier in this book, it appeared in the term 清宫 *qīng gōng* in the meaning of heart.

复合词 Compounds:

2401. 调经 *tiáo jīng*, regulate menstruation
2402. 通经 *tōng jīng*, free menstruation; promote menstruation
2403. 催乳 *cuī rǔ*, promote lactation
2404. 通乳 *tōng rǔ*, promote lactation; free milk
2405. 下乳 *xià rǔ*, promote lactation
2406. 止带 *zhǐ dài*, check vaginal discharge
2407. 补益冲任 *bǔ yì chōng rèn*, supplement (and boost) the thoroughfare and controlling vessels
2408. 补肾固冲 *bǔ shèn gù chōng*, supplement the kidney and secure the thoroughfare vessel
2409. 扶阳暖宫 *fú yáng nuǎn gōng*, support yáng and warm the palace
2410. 暖宫行滞 *nuǎn gōng xíng zhì*, warm the palace and move stagnation
2411. 清热安胎 *qīng rè ān tāi*, clear heat and quiet the fetus
2412. 暖宫安胎 *nuǎn gōng ān tāi*, warm the palace and quiet the fetus

| 第五节　第二十三组 | | | | SECTION 5: SET 23 |

外科治法　　　　　　　　External Medical Treatment Methods

1642	* 托 扌	托 手	*tuō*	draw /drɔ/
1643	* 排 扌	排 手	*pái*	expel /ɪksˈɛl/
1644	* 攻 工	攻 攴	*gōng*	attack /əˈtæk/

				offensive /ə'fɛnsɪv/
1645-n958	* 拔 扌	拔 手	*bá*	draw /drɔ/
1646	* 枯 木	枯 木	*kū*	desiccate /'dɛsɪˌket/ *vt.* desiccation* /ˌdɛsɪ'keʃən/ *n.*

注 Note:

内托 *nèi tuō*, internal expression, means pushing the toxin outward from within in the treatment of sores. It involves the use of qì and blood-supplementing medicinals to support right qì, express the toxin, and prevent it from falling inward.

复合词 Compounds:

2413. 内消 *nèi xiāo*, internal dispersion-thirst
2414. 内托 *nèi tuō*, internal expression
2415. 托法 *tuō fǎ*, drawing
2416. 排脓托毒 *pái nóng tuō dú*, expel pus and draw toxin
2417. 排托 *pái tuō*, expulsion
2418. 攻溃 *gōng kuì*, offensive bursting
2419. 外科补法 *wài kē bǔ fǎ*, external medical supplementation
2420. 以毒攻毒 *yǐ dú gōng dú*, attacking toxin with toxin
2421. 拔脓 *bá nóng*, draw pus
2422. 枯痔法 *kū zhì fǎ*, desiccate hemorrhoids; hemorrhoid desiccation

---

第五节　第二十四组　　　　SECTION 5: SET 24

驱虫法　　　　Expelling Worms

1647	* 驱 马	驅 馬	*qū*	expel /ɪks'pɛl/
1648	* 杀 乂	殺 殳	*shā*	kill /kɪl/
1649	* 安 宀	安 宀	*ān*	quiet /'kwaɪət/

复合词 Compounds:

2423. 驱虫 *qū chóng*, expel worms; worm expulsion
2424. 杀虫 *shā chóng*, kill worms
2425. 安虫 *ān chóng*, quiet worms
2426. 安虫止痛 *ān chóng zhǐ tòng*, quiet worms and relieve pain

习题 Exercise:

657. administer treatment according to pattern ....

658. 辨证论治 ....

659. *tóng bìng yì zhì* ....

660. like treatment of unlike disease ....

661. 因时因地因人制宜 ....

662. *biāo běn tóng zhì* ....

663. paradoxical assistant ....

664. 正治 ....

665. *cóng zhì* ....

666. treating the stopped by stopping ....

667. 阳病治阴 ....

668. *hàn fǎ* ....

669. sweating ....

670. 解表 ....

671. *xīn liáng jiě biǎo* ....

672. assist yáng and resolve the exterior ....

673. 滋阴解表 ....

674. *tòu zhěn jiě biǎo* ....

675. course the exterior ....

676. 疏风 ....

677. *qū fēng* ....

678. dispel wind and dissipate cold ....

679. 透表 ....

680. *tòu xié* ....

681. open the ghost gates ....

682. 调和营卫 ....

683. *yǒng tù* ....

684. mechanical ejection ....

685. 下法 ....

686. *xiè xià* ....

687. offensive precipitation ....

688. 润下 ....

689. *jùn xià* ....
690. free and discharge yáng brightness bowel repletion ....
691. 增液泻下 ....
692. *zēng shuǐ xíng zhōu* ....
693. urgent precipitation to preserve liquid ....
694. 逐水 ....
695. *qù yù chén cuò* ....
696. soften hardness and eliminate fullness ....
697. 和解法 ....
698. *hé jiě biǎo lǐ* ....
699. harmonize the liver and stomach ....
700. 和肝 ....
701. *hé wèi zhǐ tòng* ....
702. clearing ....
703. 清实热 ....
704. *qīng rè xiè huǒ* ....
705. clear heat and transform dampness ....
706. 清心 ....
707. *qīng gān huǒ* ....
708. clear the liver and drain the lung ....
709. 清泄少阳 ....
710. *qīng jīn* ....
711. clear the intestines and moisten dryness ....
712. 清气分热 ....
713. *qīng yíng fèn rè* ....
714. clear both qì and construction; dual clearing of qì and construction
715. 凉血解毒 ....
716. *kǔ hán xiè rè* ....
717. eliminate (great) heat with warmth and sweetness ....
718. 温法 ....
719. *qū hán fǎ* ....
720. warm yáng and stem counterflow ....
721. 温中祛寒 ....

722. *lǐ zhōng* ....
723. warm the liver and dissipate cold ....
724. 温振心阳 ....
725. *wēn fèi* ....
726. warm the lung and transform rheum ....
727. 温肾补火 ....
728. *nuǎn shuǐ zàng* ....
729. warm the channels and dissipate cold ....
730. 温补血分 ....
731. *huí yáng jiù nì* ....
732. rescue yáng ....
733. 补法 ....
734. *bǔ yǎng* ....
735. nourish yīn ....
736. 滋心阴 ....
737. *zī bǔ gān shèn* ....
738. rescue yīn ....
739. 助阳 ....
740. *zhuàng yáng* ....
741. warm and nourish ....
742. 补脾气 ....
743. *shēng tí zhōng qì* ....
744. boost qì and engender liquid ....
745. 双补气血 ....
746. *yǎng xuè róu gān* ....
747. engender liquid with cold and sweetness ....
748. 益气生津 ....
749. *zī shuǐ hán mù* ....
750. fortify the spleen; splenic fortification ....
751. 培土 ....
752. *bǔ huǒ shēng tǔ* ....
753. supplement the kidney ....
754. 肺肾同治 ....

755. *yǐn huǒ guī yuán* ....
756. warm and supplement the life gate ....
757. 消法 ....
758. *xiāo dǎo* ....
759. disperse food and abduct stagnation; abductive dispersion of food stagnation ....
760. 消食化滞 ....
761. *wēn zhōng huà shí* ....
762. disperse glomus and transform accumulation ....
763. 开痞 ....
764. *kāi wèi* ....
765. open the stomach and increase the appetite ....
766. 祛痰 ....
767. *xuān fèi huà tán* ....
768. clear head and transform phlegm ....
769. 燥湿化痰 ....
770. *zhì fēng huà tán* ....
771. disperse phlegm and calm panting ....
772. 涤痰 ....
773. *huò tán* ....
774. rectify qì ....
775. 行气 ....
776. *lì qì* ....
777. downbear qì ....
778. 破气 ....
779. *kāi yù* ....
780. course depression and rectify qì ....
781. course the liver ....
782. 疏肝解郁 ....
783. *shū gān* ....
784. diffuse the lung ....
785. 宣降肺气 ....
786. *xīn kāi kǔ jiàng* ....

787. open with acridity and discharge with bitterness; acrid opening and bitter discharge ....

788. 开泄 ....

789. *huó xuè huà yū* ....

790. warming transformation of static blood ....

791. 去瘀生新 ....

792. *pò yū xiāo zhēng* ....

793. expel stasis ....

794. 破血 ....

795. *zhǐ xuè* ....

796. supplement qì and contain the blood ....

797. 引血归经 ....

798. *kāi qiào* ....

799. perfuse the orifices ....

800. 温开 ....

801. *qīng xīn kāi qiào* ....

802. expel cold and open the orifices ....

803. 开窍通神 ....

804. *xǐng shén* ....

805. open the jaws ....

806. 安神 ....

807. settle the heart ....

808. 定志 ....

809. *níng shén ān hún* ....

810. dispel dampness ....

811. 化湿 ....

812. *fāng xiāng huà shī* ....

813. transform turbidity with acridity and aroma ....

814. 燥湿除满 ....

815. *lì shī* ....

816. clear summerheat and disinhibit dampness ....

817. 利湿退黄 ....

818. *xuān tōng shuǐ dào* ....

819. cleansing the clean bowel ....

820. 固涩 ....

821. *gù shè* ....

822. constrain sweat and secure the exterior ....

823. 涩肠止泻 ....

824. *shè jīng* ....

825. reduce urine ....

826. 固崩止带 ....

827. *sè kě gù tuō* ....

828. subdue yáng ....

829. 潜镇 ....

830. *xī fēng* ....

831. calm the liver and extinguish wind ....

832. 泻火熄风 ....

833. *yǎng xuè qū fēng* ....

834. quell the liver ....

835. 解痉 ....

836. *tiáo jīng* ....

837. free milk ....

838. 补益冲任 ....

839. *fú yǎng nuǎn gōng* ....

840. clear heat and quiet the fetus ....

841. 暖宫安胎 ....

842. *pái nóng tuō dú* ....

843. draw pus ....

844. 驱虫 ....

845. *shā chóng* ....

846. quiet worms ....

第六节：中药学
Section 6: Chinese Pharmaceutics

第六节　第一组				SECTION 6: SET 1

药性 　　　　　　　　　　　　　　　　Drug Nature

1650-n959	* 药 艹	藥 艸	yào	drug /drʌg/
				medicinal /mə'dɪsɪnəl/
1651-n960	* 性 忄	性 心	xìng	nature /'netʃɚ/
1652	* 味 口	味 口	wèi	flavor /'flevɚ/
1653	* 寒 宀	寒 宀	hán	cold /kold/
1654	* 热 灬	熱 火	rè	hot /hɑt/
1655	* 温 氵	溫 水	wēn	warm /wɔrm/
1656	* 凉 氵	涼 水	liáng	cool /kul/
1657	* 平 一	平 干	píng	balanced /'bælənst/
1658	* 微 彳	微 彳	wēi	slightly /'slaɪtlɪ/
1659	* 酸 酉	酸 酉	suān	sour /saʊr/
1660	* 苦 艹	苦 艸	kǔ	bitter /'bɪtɚ/
1661	* 甘 甘	甘 甘	gān	sweet /swit/
1662	* 辛 辛	辛 辛	xīn	acrid /'ækrɪd/
1663	* 咸 戊	鹹 鹵	xián	salty /'sɔltɪ/
1664	* 香 香	香 香	xiāng	aromatic /ˌærə'mætɪk/
1665-n961	* 芳 艹	芳 艸	fāng	aromatic /ˌærə'mætɪk/
1666	* 淡 氵	淡 水	dàn	bland /blænd/
1667	* 厚 厂	厚 厂	hòu	rich /rɪtʃ/
1668	* 薄 艹	薄 艸	bó	mild /maɪld/
1669	* 升 丿	升 十	shēng	upbear /'ʌpbɛr/
1670	* 降 阝	降 阜	jiàng	downbear /'daʊnbɛr/
1671	* 浮 氵	浮 水	fú	float /flot/
1672	* 沉 氵	沉 水	chén	sinking /'sɪŋkɪŋ/ adj.
1673	* 毒 龶	毒 毋	dú	toxic /'tɑksɪk/ adj.
				toxicity /tɑks'ɪsətɪ/ n.
1674	* 入 入	入 入	rù	enter /'ɛntɚ/ vi.
				entry /'ɛntrɪ/ n.
1675	归 彐	歸 止	guī	home to, return to

注 Notes:

1. The Chinese 药 *yào* has the natural equivalent in the English 'drug'. Some translate the term as 'herb', although by no means are all Chinese drugs derived from herbs or even plants in general. In view of modern objections to applying the word drug outside the Western pharmacopoeia, the term 'medicinal' is used in this text instead.

2. The 'four natures', also called the 'four qì', are cold, hot, warm, and cool. Cold and cool are yīn, and hot and warm are yáng. The 'five flavors' are sour, bitter, sweet, acrid, and salty, associated with wood, fire, earth, metal, and water, respectively among the five phases.

复合词 Compounds:

2427. 四性 *sì xìng*, four natures
2428. 性味 *xìng wèi*, nature and flavor
2429. 四气 *sì qì*, four qì
2430. 气味 *qì wèi*, qì and flavor
2431. 五味 *wǔ wèi*, the five flavors
2432. 苦寒 *kǔ hán*, cold and bitter
2433. 寒凉 *hán liáng*, cold and cool
2434. 温热 *wēn rè*, warm and hot
2435. 性寒味苦 *xìng hán wèi kǔ*, cold in nature and bitter in flavor
2436. 性热味苦 *xìng rè wèi kǔ*, hot in nature and bitter in flavor
2437. 辛温无毒 *xīn wēn wú dú*, warm, acrid, and non-toxic
2438. 味甘性温 *wèi gān xìng wēn*, sweet in flavor and warm in nature
2439. 味厚 *wèi hòu*, rich flavor
2440. 味薄 *wèi bó*, mild flavor
2441. 气厚 *qì hòu*, rich qì
2442. 气薄 *qì bó*, mild qì
2443. 味苦辛 *wèi kǔ xīn*, bitter and acrid in flavor
2444. 升降浮沉 *shēng jiàng fú chén*, upbearing, downbearing, floating, and sinking
2445. 沉降药 *chén jiàng yào*, downbearing and sinking medicinal; downsinking medicinal
2446. 升浮药 *shēng fú yào*, upbearing and floating medicinal; upfloating medicinal
2447. 入经 *rù jīng*, channel entry
2448. 归经 *guī jīng*, channel entry

第六节　第二组 | **SECTION 6: SET 2**

炮制

Processing of Medicinals

1676-n962	* 炮 火	炮 火	*páo*	blast-fry /ˈblæstfraɪ/
1677-n963	* 制 刂	製 衣	*zhì*	process /ˈprɑsɛs/
1678-n964	* 炙 火	炙 火	*zhì*	mix-fry /ˈmɪksfraɪ/
1679	* 切 刀	切 刀	*qiē*	cut /kʌt/
1680	* 去 去	去 厶	*qù*	remove /rɪˈmuv/
1681-n965	* 镑 钅	鎊 金	*bàng*	flake /flek/
1682	为 丶	爲 火	*wèi*	*make as, make into*
1683-n966	* 末 木	末 木	*mò*	powder /ˈpaʊdɚ/
1684	* 粗 米	粗 米	*cū*	rough /rʌf/
1685-n967	* 磨 麻	磨 石	*mó*	grind /graɪnd/
1686-n968	成 戊	成 戈	*chéng*	*become, into*
1687-n969	* 粉 米	粉 米	*fěn*	powder /ˈpaʊdɚ/
1688	* 细 纟	細 糸	*xì*	fine /faɪn/
1689-n970	* 捣 扌	搗 手	*dǎo*	pound /paʊnd/
1690-n971	* 浸 氵	浸 水	*jìn*	steep /stip/
1691	* 泡 氵	泡 水	*pào*	soak /sok/
1692-n972	* 洗 氵	洗 水	*xǐ*	wash /wɑʃ, wɔʃ/
1693-n973	* 漂 氵	漂 水	*piāo*	long-rinse /ˈlɔŋrɪns/
1694-n974	* 炒 火	炒 火	*chǎo*	stir-fry /ˈstɝ—fraɪ/
1695	* 清 氵	清 水	*qīng*	plain /plen/
1696	* 微 彳	微 彳	*wēi*	light /laɪt/
1697-n975	* 炭 山	炭 山	*tàn*	char /tʃɑr/ *vt, vi.* charred /tʃɑrd/ *adj.*
1698-n976	* 煨 火	煨 火	*wēi*	roast /rost/
1699-n977	* 焙 火	焙 火	*bèi*	stone-bake /ˈstonbek/
1700	* 烧 火	燒 火	*shāo*	burn /bɝn/
1701	* 存 ナ	存 子	*cún*	preserve /prɪˈzɝv/
1702-n978	* 煅 火	煅 火	*duàn*	calcine /kælˈsaɪn/
1703-n979	* 淬 氵	淬 水	*cuì*	dip /dɪp/
1704-n980	* 熬 灬	熬 火	*áo*	boil /bɔɪl/
1705-n981	* 煮 灬	煮 火	*zhǔ*	boil /bɔɪl/
1706	* 蒸 艹	蒸 艸	*zhēng*	steam /stim/
1707-n982	* 炖 火	燉 火	*dùn*	double-boil /ˈdʌbl̩-bɔɪl/
1708-n983	* 霜 雨	霜 雨	*shuāng*	frost /frɔst/
1709	* 水 水	水 水	*shuǐ*	water /ˈwɔtɚ/
1710-n984	飞 乙	飛 飛	*fēi*	*fly*
1711	饮 饣	飲 食	*yǐn*	*drink*

1712-n985	片 片 片 片	*piàn*	strip, piece
1713	* 生 丿 生 生	*shēng*	raw /rɔ/ (plants)
			crude /crud/ (minerals)
1714	* 熟 灬 熟 火	*shú*	cooked /kʊkt/
			processed /ˈprɑsɛst/

注 Note:

The character 切 *qiē*, to cut, has already been encountered in the four examinations where it is used in the meaning of palpation and is read in the fourth tone as *qiè*.

复合词 Compounds:

2449. 炮制 *páo zhì*, processing of medicinals
2450. 炮炙 *páo zhì*, processing of medicinals
2451. 制法 *zhì fǎ*, processing method
2452. 切片 *qiē piàn*, cut into slices
2453. 去皮 *qì pí*, remove the skin
2454. 为末 *wéi mò*, grind to a powder (lit. 'make into a powder')
2455. 为粗末 *wéi cū mò*, grind to a rough powder
2456. 为细末 *wéi xì mò*, grind to a fine powder
2457. 磨成粉 *mó chéng fěn*, grind to a powder (the Chinese term is a colloquial expression not often used in medical texts)
2458. 煅淬 *duàn cuì*, dip-calcine
2459. 漂洗 *piǎo xǐ*, long-rinse
2460. 泡水 *pào shuǐ*, soak in water
2461. 烧存性 *shāo cún xìng*, nature-preservative burning
2462. 制霜 *zhì shuāng*, to frost; make a frost
2463. 微炒 *wēi chǎo*, stir-fry lightly; light stir-frying
2464. 清炒 *qīng chǎo*, plain stir-frying
2465. 炒黄 *chǎo huáng*, stir-fry until yellow
2466. 炒炭 *chǎo tàn*, char-fry
2467. 饮片 *yǐn piàn*, decocting pieces
2468. 水飞 *shuǐ fēi*, water-grind

第六节　第三组　　　　　　　　　　**SECTION 6: SET 3**

剂型　　　　　　　　　　　　　Preparations

1715-n986	*	汤 氵	湯 水	*tāng*	decoction /dɪˈkɑkʃən/
1716	*	饮 饣	飲 食	*yǐn*	beverage /ˈbɛvərɪdʒ/
1717-n987	*	煎 灬	煎 火	*jiān*	decoction /dɪˈkɑkʃən/
					brew /bru/ (in formula names)
1718	*	膏 高	膏 肉	*gāo*	paste /pest/ (soft)
					plaster /ˈplæstəˌ/ (hard)
1719	*	露 雨	露 雨	*lù*	distillate /ˈdɪstɪlət/
					dew /dju/
1720	*	散 夂	散 夊	*sǎn*	powder /ˈpaʊdəˌ/
1721	*	丸 丸	丸 丶	*wán*	pill /pɪl/
1722	*	丹 丿	丹 丶	*dān*	elixir /ɪˈlɪksɪr/
1723	*	酒 氵	酒 水	*jiǔ*	liquor /ˈlɪkəˌ/ (general)
					wine /waɪn/ (low alcohol)
1724-n988	*	锭 钅	錠 金	*dìng*	lozenge /ˈlɑzɪndʒ/
1725	*	胶 月	膠 肉	*jiāo*	glue /glu/
1726-n989	*	茶 艹	茶 艸	*chá*	tea /ti/
1727	*	油 氵	油 水	*yóu*	oil /ɔɪl/
1728	*	片 片	片 片	*piàn*	tablet /ˈtæblɪt/

注 Notes:

1. Most of the characters in this set such as 汤 *tāng*, 膏 *gāo*, and 散 *sǎn* are often used singly. They also very often appear in formula names such as 桂枝汤 *guì zhī tāng*, Cinnamon Twig Decoction, and 平胃散 *píng wèi sǎn*, Stomach-Calming Powder.

2. The character 散 is read as *sǎn* in the meaning of powder, but as 散 *sàn* in the meaning of dissipate.

3. The term 煎 *jiān*, used as a verb, means to brew or decoct; used as a noun, it is identical in meaning to 汤 *tāng*, a decoction. In formula names, 煎 is rendered as 'brew' to avoid possible confusion with a 汤 of the same name. Note that in the common language, 煎 is most commonly used in the sense of to fry (with a small amount of oil, without stirring). The term 饮 *yǐn*, beverage, denotes a decoction taken after it has cooled, and one originally prescribed to be taken at any time is called 饮子 *yǐn zǐ*, a drink.

复合词 Compounds:

2469. 膏药 *gāo yào*, plaster; medicinal paste

2470. 药膏 *yào gāo*, medicinal paste

2471. 膏滋 *gāo zī*, rich paste

2472. 汤剂 *tāng jì*, decoction

2473. 水丸 *shuǐ wán*, water pill

2474. 药酒 *yào jiǔ*, medicinal wine

2475. 酒剂 *jiǔ jì*, wine

2476. 钉剂 *dìng jì*, lozenge

2477. 玉女煎 *yù nǚ jiān*, Jade Lady Brew

2478. 大青龙汤 *dà qīng lóng tāng*, Major Green-Blue Dragon Decoction

2479. 补中益气汤 *bǔ zhōng yì qì tāng*, Center-Supplementing Qì-Boosting Decoction

2480. 清肺饮 *qīng fèi yǐn*, Lung-Clearing Beverage

2481. 三生饮 *sān shēng yǐn*, Three Raw Agents Beverage

2482. 清脾饮 *qīng pí yǐn*, Spleen-Clearing Beverage

2483. 清凉饮 *qīng liáng yǐn*, Cool Clearing Beverage

2484. 清肺饮子 *qīng fèi yǐn zǐ*, Lung-Clearing Drink

2485. 驱风散热饮子 *qū fēng sàn rè yǐn zǐ*, Wind-Expelling Heat-Dissipating Drink

2486. 五积散 *wǔ jī sǎn*, Five Accumulations Powder

2487. 导赤散 *dǎo chì sǎn*, Red-Abducting Powder

2488. 清胃散 *qīng wèi sǎn*, Stomach-Clearing Powder

2489. 润肠丸 *rùn cháng wán*, Intestine-Moistening Pill

2490. 理中丸 *lǐ zhōng wán*, Center-Rectifying Pill

2491. 甘露消毒丹 *gān lù xiāo dú dān*, Sweet Dew Toxin-Dispersing Elixir

2492. 小活络丹 *xiǎo huó luò dān*, Minor Network-Quickening Elixir

2493. 紫雪丹 *zǐ xuě dān*, Purple Snow Elixir

2494. 甘露饮 *gān lù yǐn*, Sweet Dew Beverage

2495. 截疟七宝饮 *jié nüè qī bǎo yǐn*, Malaria-Interrupting Seven-Jewel Beverage

2496. 清空膏 *qīng kōng gāo*, Clear Sky Paste

2497. 清凉膏 *qīng liáng gāo*, Cool Clearing Paste

2498. 止带片 *zhǐ dài piàn*, Discharge-Checking Tablet

2499. 滋补片 *zī bǔ piàn*, Enriching Supplementation Tablet

第六节　第四组				**SECTION 6: SET 4**

药物用法   **Directions for Use of Medicinals**

1729-n990	*	服 月	服 月	*fú*	take /tek/
1730	*	冲 冫	沖 冫	*chōng*	drench /drɛntʃ/
1731	*	调 讠	調 言	*tiáo*	mix /mɪks/
1732	*	频 页	頻 頁	*pín*	frequent /ˈfrikwənt/
1733	*	顿 页	頓 頁	*dùn*	quaff /kwɔf/
1734-n991		送 辶	送 辵	*sòng*	*send, deliver, take*
1735-n992		饭 饣	飯 食	*fàn*	*rice, food, meal*
1736	*	前 丷	前 八	*qián*	before /bɪˈfɔr, bɪˈfor/
1737		后 厂	後 彳	*hòu*	*after*
1738		远 辶	遠 辵	*yuǎn*	*far, distant*
1739-n993		临 丨	臨 臣	*lín*	*face (a situation); come up to (a time)*
1740	*	空 穴	空 穴	*kōng*	empty /ˈɛmptɪ/
1741-n994	*	敷 攵	敷 攴	*fū*	apply /əˈplaɪ/
1742	*	撒 扌	撒 手	*sǎ*	sprinkle /ˈsprɪŋkl̩/ (powder)
1743	*	洒 冫	灑 水	*sǎ*	sprinkle /ˈsprɪŋkl̩/ (liquids)
1744-n995	*	嗅 口	嗅 口	*xiù*	insufflation /ˌɪnsʌfˈleʃən/

注 Notes:

1. The character 撒 is read here as *sǎ* in the third tone to mean sprinkle. It is given earlier with the pronunciation *sā* in the first tone to mean limp (introduced in the Four Examinations).

2. The term 调 *tiáo* has already been encountered in the meaning of regulate. Another meaning is to mix, and in Chinese medicine it specifically means to mix (a powder) with a small amount of fluid. The character 冲 *chōng* in its common usage means flush, drench, wash with running water, or to wash away. In pharmaceutics, it means to mix (a powder or soluble substance) so that it dissolves or can be swallowed. This usage is translated as 'drench'. For other comments on the character 冲, see Section 1, Channels and Network Vessels.

复合词 Compounds:

2500. 服药 *fú yào*, take medicine
2501. 冲服 *chōng fú*, take drenched
2502. 调服 *tiáo fú*, take mixed (with fluid)
2503. 频服 *pín fú*, take in small frequent doses

2504. 顿服 *dùn fú*, quaff; take in a single dose

2505. 饭前服 *fàn qián fú*, take before meals

2506. 饭后服 *fàn hòu fú*, take after meals

2507. 食远服 *shí yuǎn fú*, take between meals

2508. 临睡前服 *lín shuì qián fú*, take before sleeping

2509. 空腹服 *kōng fù fú*, take on an empty stomach

2510. 送服 *sòng fú*, take with fluid

2511. 调敷 *tiáo fū*, apply mixed (with fluid)

第六节　第五组　　　　　　　　　SECTION 6: SET 5

方剂组成　　　　　　　　Formula Construction

1745-n996	* 方 方	方 方	*fāng*	formula /ˈfɔrmjələ/
1746	* 君 口	君 口	*jūn*	sovereign /ˈsavərin/
1747-n997	* 臣 臣	臣 臣	*chén*	minister /ˈmɪnɪstər/
1748-n998	* 佐 亻	佐 人	*zuǒ*	assistant /əˈsɪstənt/
1749-n999	* 使 亻	使 人	*shǐ*	courier /ˈkʊrɪər/

习题 Exercise:

847. 甘寒 ....

848. *wēi hán* ....

849. bitter in flavor and balanced in nature ....

850. 酸平 ....

851. *xìng hán wèi kǔ yǒu dú* ....

852. sweet and slightly acrid ....

853. 苦甘 ....

854. *suān wēn* ....

855. warm and salty ....

856. 性凉味苦 ....

857. *xīn wēn wú dú* ....

858. rich flavor ....

859. 味薄 ....

860. *shēng jiàng fú chén* ....

861. upbearing and floating medicinal; upfloating medicinal ....

862. 入经 ....

863. *páo zhì* ....

864. cut into slices ....

865. 为末 ....

866. *wéi cū mò* ....

867. grind to a powder ....

868. 漂洗 ....

869. *shāo cún xìng* ....

870. to frost; make a frost ....

871. 微炒 ....

872. *chǎo huáng* ....

873. water-grind ....

874. 饮片 ....

875. *gāo yào* ....

876. medicinal paste ....

877. 丹 ....

878. *wán* ....

879. powder ....

880. 汤 ....

881. *yǐn* ....

882. drink ....

883. 冲服 ....

884. *tiáo fú* ....

885. quaff; take in a single dose ....

886. 食远服 ....

887. *kōng fù fú* ....

888. apply mixed (with fluid) ....

第七节：针灸
Section 7: Acumoxatherapy

第七节　第一组				SECTION 7: SET 1

针灸器材 — Acumoxatherapy Equipment

1750	* 针 钅	針 金	*zhēn*	needle /nidl̩/
1751-n1000	* 灸 火	灸 火	*jiǔ*	moxibustion /ˈmɑksɪˌbʌstʃən/
1752-n1001	毫 毛	毫 毛	*háo*	*filiform*
1753-n1002	* 棱 木	稜 禾	*léng*	edge /ɛdʒ/
1754	* 梅 木	梅 木	*méi*	plum /plʌm/
1755	* 花 艹	花 艸	*huā*	blossom /ˈblɑsəm/
1756	* 星 日	星 日	*xīng*	star /stɑr/
1757-n1003	* 电 雨	電 雨	*diàn*	electricity /ˌɪlɛkˈtrɪsɪtɪ/ *n.* electrical /ɪˈlɛktrɪkl̩/ *adj.* electro- /ɪˈlɛktro/
1758-n1004	* 艾 艹	艾 艸	*ài*	moxa /ˈmɑksə/
1759-n1005	* 绒 纟	絨 糸	*róng*	floss /flɔs/
1760	* 条 夂	條 木	*tiáo*	stick /stɪk/ pole /pol/
1761-n1006	炷 火	炷 火	*zhù*	*wick, candle*
1762	* 壮 丬	壯 士	*zhuàng*	cone /kon/ (with a number)
1763-n1007	拔 扌	拔 手	*bá*	*pull up, pull out*
1764	* 火 火	火 火	*huǒ*	fire /faɪr/
1765-n1008	* 罐 缶	罐 缶	*guàn*	cup /kʌp/

复合词 Compounds:

2512. 毫针 *háo zhēn*, filiform needle
2513. 三棱针 *sān léng zhēn*, three-edged needle
2514. 电针 *diàn zhēn*, electroacupuncture
2515. 艾条 *ài tiáo*, moxa pole
2516. 艾炷 *ài zhù*, moxa cone
2517. 状数 *zhuàng shù*, number of cones
2518. 五壮 *wǔ zhuàng*, five cones
2519. 拔火罐 *bá huǒ guàn*, cupping

2520. 梅花针 *méi huā zhēn*, plum-blossom needle
2521. 七星针 *qī xīng zhēn*, seven-star needle

第七节　第二组　　　　　　　　　SECTION 7: SET 2

针刺法　　　　　　　　　　　　Needle Manipulation

1766	* 刺 刂	刺 刀	*cì*	needle /nidl̩/
1767	* 刺 刂	刺 刀	*cì*	insert /in'sɜ˞t/
1768-n1009	进 辶	進 辵	*jìn*	*advance, enter, insert*
1769-n1010	* 捻 扌	捻 手	*niǎn*	twirl /twɜ˞l/
1770	* 捣 扌	搗 手	*dǎo*	pound /paʊnd/
1771	* 留 田	留 田	*liú*	retain /rɪ'ten/
1772	* 摇 扌	搖 手	*yáo*	waggle /'wægl̩/
1773-n1011	* 搓 扌	搓 手	*cuō*	twist /twɪst/
1774	* 退 辶	退 辵	*tuì*	retract /rɪ'trækt/
1775-n1012	出 屮	出 凵	*chū*	*remove*
1776	* 直 十	直 目	*zhí*	perpendicular /ˌpɜ˞pən'dɪkjələ˞/
1777	* 斜 斗	斜 斗	*xié*	oblique /ə'blik/
1778-n1013	* 横 木	横 木	*héng*	transverse /'trænzvɜ˞s/
1779	透 辶	透 辵	*tòu*	*go all the way through, transpierce penetrate*
1780	* 烧 火	燒 火	*shāo*	burn /bɜ˞n/
1781	* 泻 氵	瀉 水	*xiè*	drain /dren/
1782	* 补 衤	補 衣	*bǔ*	supplement /'sʌplɪmənt/
1783	* 开 卅	開 門	*kāi*	open /'opən/
1784	* 阖 門	闔 門	*hé*	closed /'klozd/
1785	迎 辶	迎 辵	*yíng*	*go toward, against*
1786-n1014	随 阝	隨 阜	*suí*	*follow, go with*
1787	* 疾 疒	疾 疒	*jí*	quick /kwɪk/
1788-n1015	* 徐 彳	徐 彳	*xú*	slow /slo/
1789	呼 口	呼 口	*hū*	*exhale*
1790	吸 口	吸 口	*xī*	*inhale*
1791	* 提 口	提 手	*tí*	lift /lɪft/
1792-n1016	* 插 扌	插 手	*chā*	thrust /θrʌst/
1793	* 转 车	轉 車	*zhuǎn*	twirl /twɜ˞l/
1794	* 搓 扌	搓 手	*cuō*	twist /twɪst/ (between the fingers)
1795	得 彳	得 彳	*dé*	*get, obtain*
1796-n1017	* 至 至	至 至	*zhì*	arrival /ə'raɪvəl/
1797-n1018	灵 彐	靈 雨	*líng*	*magical*

1798-n1019 * 龟 龟　龜 龜　*guī*　tortoise /ˈtɔrtəs/

复合词 Compounds:

2522. 进针 *jìn zhēn*, insert the needle, needle insertion
2523. 捻针 *niǎn zhēn*, needle
2524. 捣针 *dǎo zhēn*, pound the needle; needle pounding
2525. 留针 *liú zhēn*, retain the needle; needle retention
2526. 退针 *tuì zhēn*, retract the needle; needle retraction
2527. 出针 *chū zhēn*, remove the needle; needle removal
2528. 起针 *qǐ zhēn*, remove the needle; needle removal
2529. 搓针 *cuō zhēn*, twist the needle; needle twisting
2530. 开阖补泻 *kāi hé bǔ xiè*, open and closed supplementation and drainage
2531. 迎随补泻 *yíng suí bǔ xiè*, directional supplementation and drainage
2532. 呼吸补泻 *hū xī bǔ xiè*, respiratory supplementation and drainage
2533. 疾徐补泻 *jí xú bǔ xiè*, quick and slow supplementation and drainage
2534. 提插补泻 *tí chā bǔ xiè*, lift-and-thrust supplementation and drainage
2535. 捻转补泻 *niǎn zhuǎn bǔ xiè*, twirling supplementation and drainage
2536. 透天凉 *tòu tiān liáng*, heaven-penetrating cooling method
2537. 烧山火 *shāo shān huǒ*, burning mountain fire method
2538. 灵龟八法 *líng guī bā fǎ*, eightfold method of the magical tortoise
2539. 气至 *qì zhì*, arrival of qì
2540. 得气 *dé qì*, obtain qì

第七节　第三组				**SECTION 7: SET 3**

灸法				**Moxibustion**
1799	* 灸 火	灸 火	*jiǔ*	moxibustion /ˈmɑksɪˌbʌstʃən/
1800	* 条 夊	條 木	*tiáo*	stick /stɪk/
				pole /pol/
1801	炷 火	炷 火	*zhù*	*wick, candle*
1802	直 十	直 目	*zhí*	*straight*
1803-n1020	间 门	間 門	*jiān*	*interval*
1804	接 扌	接 手	*jiē*	*receive*
1805-n1021 *	瘢 疒	瘢 疒	*bān*	scar /skɑr/
1806	痕 疒	痕 疒	*hén*	*mark*
1807-n1022	隔 阝	隔 阜	*gé*	*separate, insulate*

1808-n1023 *	姜 羊	薑 艸	*jiāng*	ginger	/ˈdʒɪndʒəʳ/
1809-n1024 *	蒜 艸	蒜 艸	*suàn*	garlic	/ˈɡɑrlɪk/
1810-n1025 *	盐 皿	鹽 鹵	*yán*	salt	/sɔlt/
1811-n1026	附 阝	附 阜	*fù*	append, appendage	
1812-n1027 *	饼 饣	餅 食	*bǐng*	cake	/kek/

复合词 Compounds:

2541. 艾炷灸 *ài zhù jiǔ*, cone moxibustion
2542. 艾条灸 *ài tiáo jiǔ*, poll moxibustion, moxa poling
2543. 直接灸 *zhí jiē jiǔ*, direct moxibustion
2544. 间接灸 *jiān jiē jiǔ*, indirect moxibustion
2545. 瘢痕灸 *bān hén jiǔ*, scarring moxibustion
2546. 隔姜灸 *gé jiāng jiǔ*, moxibustion on ginger
2547. 隔蒜灸 *gé suàn jiǔ*, moxibustion on garlic
2548. 隔盐灸 *gé yán jiǔ*, moxibustion on salt
2549. 隔附子饼灸 *gé fù zǐ bǐng jiǔ*, moxibustion on aconite cake
2550. 附子 *fù zǐ*, aconite (the Chinese literally means an appendage, describing the part of the root of the aconite plant used as the drug)
2551. 雀啄灸 *què zhuó jiǔ*, pecking sparrow moxibustion
2552. 温针灸 *wēn zhēn jiǔ*, warm needle moxibustion
2553. 天灸 *tiān jiǔ*, natural moxibustion
2554. 药物灸 *yào wù jiǔ*, medicinal moxibustion
2555. 发泡灸 *fā pào jiǔ*, blister moxibustion

习题 Exercise:

889. 毫针 ....
890. *sān léng zhēn* ....
891. moxa pole ....
892. 状数 ....
893. *méi huā zhēn* ....
894. seven-star needle ....
895. 进针 ....
896. *niǎn zhēn* ....
897. retain the needle; needle retention ....
898. 起针 ....
899. *yíng suí bǔ xiè* ....

900. respiratory supplementation and drainage ....

901. 疾徐补泻 ....

902. *tòu tiān liáng* ....

903. burning mountain fire method ....

904. 得气 ....

905. *ài zhù jiǔ* ....

906. poll moxibustion, moxa poling ....

907. 间接灸 ....

908. *gé jiāng jiǔ* ....

909. moxibustion on salt ....

910. 天灸 ....

附录1：习题答案
Appendix 1: Answers to Questions

1. wood engenders fire [*mù shēng huǒ*]
2. 木克土 wood restrains earth
3. 土克水 [*tǔ kè shuǐ*]
4. water restrains fire [*shuǐ kè huǒ*]
5. 金克木 metal restrains wood
6. 土生金 [*tǔ shēng jīn*]
7. metal restrains wood [*jīn kè mù*]
8. 土乘水 earth restrains water
9. 火乘金 [*huǒ kè jīn*]
10. metal restrains wood [*jīn kè mù*]
11. 火反侮水 fire rebels against water
12. 水侮土 [*shuǐ wǔ tǔ*]
13. earth rebels again wood [*tǔ fǎn wǔ mù*]
14. 东北 northeast
15. 东南 [*dōng nán*]
16. south belongs to fire [*nán shǔ huǒ*]
17. 西属金 west belongs to metal
18. 四时 [*sì shí*]
19. winter [*dōng tiān*]
20. 春属木 spring belongs wood
21. 秋属金 [*qiū shǔ jīn*]
22. winter belongs to water [*dōng shǔ shuǐ*]
23. 六腑 six bowels
24. 心阳 [*xīn yáng*]
25. heart yīn [*xīn yīn*]
26. 肺金 lung-metal

27. 胃肠 [*wèi cháng*]
28. heart and spleen, heart-spleen [*xīn pí*]
29. 心肝 heart and liver, heart-liver
30. 心包 [*xīn bāo*]
31. lung and kidney, lung-kidney [*fèi shèn*]
32. 心肾 heart and kidney, heart-kidney
33. 肝胃 [*gān wèi*]
34. liver and kidney, liver-kidney [*gān shèn*]
35. 肝脾 liver and spleen, liver-spleen
36. 肝阴 [*gān yīn*]
37. kidney yīn [*shèn yīn*]
38. 肾阳 kidney yáng
39. 心属火 [*shī shǔ huǒ*]
40. the spleen belongs to earth [*pí shǔ tǔ*]
41. 肺属金 the lung belongs to metal
42. 肾属水 [*shèn shǔ shuǐ*]
43. middle burner [*zhōng jiāo*]
44. 下焦 lower burner
45. 上焦 [*shàng jiāo*]
46. the lung is in the upper burner [*fèi zài shàng jiāo*]
47. 胃在中焦 the stomach is in the middle burner
48. 肾在下焦 [*shèn zài xià jiāo*]
49. spleen qì [*pí qì*]
50. 肺气 lung qì
51. 肾气 [*shèn qì*]

52. liver blood [*gān xuè*]
53. 心血 heart blood
54. 皮毛 [*pí máo*]
55. sinew and bone [*jīn gǔ*]
56. 筋肉 sinew and flesh
57. 肝属木，主筋 [*gān shǔ mù, zhǔ jīn*]
58. the spleen belongs to earth, and governs the flesh [*pí shǔ tǔ, zhǔ jī ròu*]
59. 肺属金，主皮毛 the lung belongs to metal, and governs the skin and [body] hair
60. 肾属水，主骨 [*shèn shǔ shuǐ, zhǔ gǔ*]
61. right qì [*zhèng qì*]
62. 君火 sovereign fire
63. 宗气 [*zōng qì*]
64. ancestral sinew [*zōng jīn*]
65. 真元 true origin
66. 原气 [*yuán qì*]
67. life gate [*mìng mén*]
68. 肺为水之上源 the lung is the upper source of water
69. 肾为先天之本 [*shèn wéi xiān tiān zhī běn*]
70. qì is the commander of the blood [*qì wéi xuè zhī shuāi*]
71. 血为气之母 blood is the mother of qì
72. the kidney, its bloom is in the hair [*shèn, qí huá zài fà*]
73. 心藏神 the heart stores the spirit
74. 心主血脉 [*xīn zhǔ xuè mài*]
75. the heart opens into the tongue [*xīn kāi qiào yú shé*]
76. 大肠主津 the large intestine governs liquid
77. 小肠主液 [*xiǎo cháng zhǔ yè*]
78. the kidney stores essence [*shèn cáng jīng*]
79. 肾主水 kidney governs water
80. 肾开窍于耳 [*shèn kāi qiào yú ěr*]
81. the liver opens into the eyes [*gān kāi qiào yú mù*]
82. 胃主受纳 the stomach governs intake
83. 肾主骨生髓 [*shèn zhǔ gǔ shēng suǐ*]
84. the spleen governs the flesh [*pí zhǔ ròu*]
85. uterus
86. 少腹 [*shào fù*]
87. smaller abdomen [*xiǎo fù*]
88. 咽喉 throat
89. 表里 [*biǎo lǐ*]
90. teeth [*yá chǐ*]
91. 齿牙 teeth
92. 腰膝 [*yāo xī*]
93. chest and rib-side [*xiōng xié*]
94. 腠理 interstices
95. 鬼门 [*guǐ mén*]
96. the lumbus is the house of the kidney [*yāo zhě, shèn zhī fǔ*]
97. 腰为肾之府 the lumbus is the house of the kidney
98. 膝者，筋之府 [*xī zhě, jīn zhī fǔ*]
99. 手少阳经 [*shǒu shào yáng jīng*]
100. yáng brightness (*yáng míng*) channel [*shǒu yáng míng jīng*]
101. 手太阴经 hand greater yīn (*tài yīn*) channel
102. 手少阴经 [*shǒu shào yīn jīng*]

103. hand reverting (*jué yīn*) yīn channel [*shǒu jué yīn jīng*]

104. 足太阳经 foot greater yáng (*tài yáng*) channel

105. 足少阳经 [*zú shào yáng jīng*]

106. yáng brightness (*yáng míng*) channel [*zú yáng míng jīng*]

107. 足太阴经 foot greater yīn (*tài yīn*) channel

108. 足少阴经 [*zú shào yīn jīng*]

109. foot reverting yīn (*jué yīn*) channel [*zú jué yīn jīng*]

110. 肝经 liver channel

111. 心经 [*xīn jīng*]

112. spleen channel [*pí jīng*]

113. 肺经 lung channel

114. 肾经 [*shèn jīng*]

115. 胃经 [*wèi jīng*]

116. the lesser yīn (*shào yīn*) has copious qì and scant blood [*shào yīn duō qì shǎo xuè*]

117. 厥阴多血少气 the reverting yīn (*jué yīn*) has copious blood and scant qì

118. 太阴多气多血 [*tài yīn duō qì duō xuè*]

119. eight meeting points [*bā huì xuè*]

120. 交会穴 intersection point

121. 下合穴 [*xià hé xuè*]

122. back transport points [*bèi shū xuè*]

123. 募穴 alarm point

124. 会穴 [*huì xuè*]

125. five transport points [*wǔ shū xuè*]

126. 荥穴 brook point

127. 气会 [*qì huì*]

128. meeting point of the bone [*gǔ huì*]

129. 四总穴 four command points

130. 郄穴 [*xī xué*]

131. a) drink; b) rheum

132. 外因 external cause

133. 风热 [*fēng rè*]

134. liver fire [*gān huǒ*]

135. 伤阴 damage to yīn

136. 伤食 [*shāng shí*]

137. liquor damage [*shāng jiǔ*]

138. 伤风 wind damage

139. 饮酒过多 [*yǐn jiǔ guò duō*]

140. snake bite [*shé yǎo*]

141. 虫咬 insect bite

142. 病因 [*bìng yīn*]

143. miasma, miasmic qì [*shān lán zhàng qì*]

144. 痰火 phlegm-fire

145. 痰饮 [*tán yǐn*]

146. voracious eating and drinking [*bào yǐn bào shí*]

147. 过食肥甘 excessive consumption of sweet and fatty foods

148. 得神 [*dé shén*]

149. spiritlessness [*wú shén*]

150. 假神 false spiritedness

151. 肥胖 [*féi pàng*]

152. deviated eyes and mouth [*kǒu yǎn wāi xié*]

153. 口噤 clenched jaw

154. 半身不遂 [*bàn shēn bú suì*]

155. arched-back rigidity [*jiǎo gōng fǎn zhāng*]

156. 拘急 hypertonicity

157. 挛急 [*luán jí*]

158. sinew hypertonicity [*jīn jí*]

159. 四肢拘急 hypertonicity of the limbs
160. 手舞足蹈 [shǒu wǔ zú dào]
161. convulsion of the limbs [sì zhī chōu chù]
162. 手足蠕动 wriggling of the extremities
163. 肩不举 [jiān bù jǔ]
164. groping in the air and pulling at [invisible] threads [cuō kōng lǐ xiàn]
165. 循衣摸床 picking at bedclothes; carphology
166. 头面红肿 [tóu miàn hóng zhǒng]
167. puffy face [miàn fú]
168. 口噤 clenched jaw
169. 面赤 [miàn chì]
170. yellow face [miàn huáng]
171. 面色㿠白 bright white facial complexion
172. 面色淡白 [miàn sè dàn bái]
173. somber white facial complexion [miàn sè cāng bái]
174. 面色萎黄 withered-yellow complexion
175. 面色无华 [miàn sè wú huá]
176. maculopapular eruption [bān zhěn]
177. 白痦 miliaria alba
178. 舌裂 [shé liè]
179. enlarged tongue [shé pàng]
180. 舌歪 deviated tongue
181. 舌疮 [shé chuāng]
182. prickles [máng cì]
183. 舌生芒刺 prickly tongue
184. 舌边齿痕 [shé biān chǐ hén]
185. smooth bare tongue [shé guāng]
186. 舌干 dry tongue
187. 舌淡白 [shé dàn bái]
188. pale tongue [shé dàn bái]
189. 舌红 red tongue
190. 舌绛 [shé jiàng]
191. purple tongue [shé zǐ]
192. 白苔 white fur
193. 黄苔 [huáng tāi]
194. slimy yellow tongue fur [shé tāi huáng nì]
195. 舌苔焦黄 burnt-yellow tongue fur
196. 舌苔老黄 [shé tāi lǎo huáng]
197. mealy white tongue fur [shé tāi bái rú jī fěn]
198. 舌苔焦黑 burnt-black tongue fur
199. 舌苔薄白 [shé tāi bó bái]
200. no phlegm; absence of phlegm [wú tán]
201. 痰清白稀薄 clear thin white phlegm
202. 痰黄黏稠 [tán huáng nián chóu]
203. thick sticky turbid yellow phlegm [tán huáng zhuó nián chóu]
204. 痰如败絮 phlegm like rotten wadding
205. 咳痰清稀 [ké tán qīng xī]
206. coughing of thick sticky phlegm [ké tán nián chóu]
207. 痰中带血丝 phlegm streaked with blood
208. 流涎清稀 [liú xián qīng xī]
209. runny nose with turbid snivel [bí liú zhuó tì]
210. 呕吐痰涎 vomiting of phlegm-drool

211. 呕吐黄绿苦水 [*ǒu tù huáng lǜ kǔ shuǐ*]
212. vomiting of dark purple blood [*ǒu xuè zǐ àn*]
213. 大便色黑 black stool
214. 粪便干燥 [*fèn biàn gān zào*]
215. thick sticky stool [*dà biàn nián chóu*]
216. 大便稀溏 thin sloppy stool
217. 完谷不化 [*wán gǔ bú huà*]
218. stool containing blood [*dà biàn dài xuè*]
219. 便血黑 black blood in the stool
220. 小便 [*xiǎo biàn*]
221. reddish urine [*xiǎo biàn sè chì*]
222. 小便浑浊 turbid urine
223. 小便如米泔状 [*xiǎo biàn rú mǐ gān zhuàng*]
224. semen in the urine [*niào jīng*]
225. 声音嘶哑 hoarse voice
226. 声音轻微细弱 [*shēng yīn qīng wēi xì ruò*]
227. hoarse voice [*shēng yīn cū yǎ*]
228. 声音低怯 hoarse voice
229. 呻吟 [*shēn yín*]
230. loss of voice [*shī yīn*]
231. 谵语 delirious speech
232. 郑声 [*zhèng shēng*]
233. confused speech [*cuò yǔ*]
234. 语无伦次 incoherent speech
235. 错言妄语 [*cuò yán wàng yǔ*]
236. difficult sluggish speech [*yǔ yán jiǎn sè*]
237. 呼吸 breathing
238. 气粗 [*qì cū*]
239. shortness of breath [*duǎn qì*]
240. 气急 rapid breathing
241. 喘不得卧 [*chuǎn bù dé wò*]
242. cough and panting [*ké chuǎn*]

243. 咳嗽无力 forceless cough
244. 鼻鼾 [*bí hān*]
245. yawning [*hē qiàn*]
246. 善太息 frequent sighing
247. 喷嚏 [*pēn tì*]
248. 怕冷 fear of cold
249. 憎寒 [*zēng hán*]
250. abhorrence of cold and vigorous heat [effusion] [*zēng hán zhuàng rè*]
251. 畏恶风寒 aversion to wind and cold
252. 形寒肢冷 [*xíng hán zhī lěng*]
253. alternating heat [effusion] and [aversion to] cold [*hán rè wǎng lái*]
254. 潮热 tidal heat [effusion]
255. 日晡潮热 [*rì bū cháo rè*]
256. absence of sweating [*wú hàn*]
257. 汗多 copious sweat
258. 战汗 [*zhàn hàn*]
259. spontaneous sweating [*zì hàn*]
260. 盗汗 night sweating
261. 头晕 [*tóu yūn*]
262. dizzy vision [*mù xuàn*]
263. 头重 heavy-headedness
264. 头重如裹 [*tóu zhòng rú guǒ*]
265. shaking of the head [*tóu yáo*]
266. 目痛 eye pain
267. 目眩 [*mù xuàn*]
268. dry eyes [*mù sè*]
269. 视一为二 seeing one as two
270. 流泪 [*liú lèi*]
271. ear pain [*ěr tòng*]
272. 鼻痛 pain in the nose
273. 喉咙肿痛 [*hóu lóng tòng*]
274. fatigue [*juàn dài*]
275. 疲劳 fatigue
276. 体倦乏力 [*tǐ juàn fá lì*]

277. drowsiness after eating [*shí hòu kùn dùn*]
278. 周身酸楚 generalized pain
279. 肢倦乏力 [*zhī juàn fá lì*]
280. back pain [*bèi tòng*]
281. 腰膝无力 lack of strength in the lumbus and knees
282. 腰膝酸软 [*yāo xī suān ruǎn*]
283. chest pain [*xiōng tòng*]
284. 胸闷 oppression in the chest
285. 胸胁满 [*xiōng xié mǎn*]
286. painful distention in the chest and rib-side [*xiōng xié zhàng mǎn*]
287. 胁肋隐痛 dull rib-side pain
288. 两胁拘急 [*liǎng xié jū jí*]
289. palpitation below the heart [*xīn xià jì*]
290. 呃逆 hiccup
291. 恶心 [*ě xīn*]
292. blood ejection and spontaneous external bleeding [*tǔ nǜ*]
293. 痛有定处 pain of fixed location
294. 窜痛 [*cuàn tòng*]
295. pain around the umbilicus [*rào qí tòng*]
296. 少腹痛 lesser-abdominal pain
297. 肠鸣 [*cháng míng*]
298. thirst [*kǒu kě*]
299. 口渴引饮 thirst with taking of fluids
300. 口渴喜饮 [*kǒu kě xǐ yǐn*]
301. thirst without great intake of fluids [*kǒu kě bú yù yǐn*]
302. 食欲不振 poor appetite
303. 不思饮食 [*bù sī yǐn shí*]
304. predilection for strange foods [*xǐ shí yì wù*]

305. 异嗜 predilection for strange foods
306. 口酸 [*kǒu suān*]
307. slimy sensation in the mouth [*kǒu nì*]
308. a) pale; b) bland
309. 大便 stool
310. 粪便 [*fèn biàn*]
311. fecal stoppage; constipation [*dà biàn bù tōng*]
312. 便难 difficult defecation
313. 上吐下泻 [*shàng tù xià xiè*]
314. fecal incontinence [*dà biàn shī jìn*]
315. 泄泻 diarrhea
316. 水泻 [*shuǐ xiè*]
317. bloody stool [*biàn xuè*]
318. 矢气频频 frequent passing of flatus
319. 小便 [*xiǎo biàn*]
320. short voidings of reddish urine [*xiǎo biàn duǎn chì*]
321. 小便淋赤刺痛 dribbling urination with reddish urine and stinging pain
322. 小便频数 [*xiǎo biàn pín shuò*]
323. dribble after voiding [*niào hòu yú lì*]
324. 小便不通 urinary stoppage
325. 小便淋漓不禁 [*xiǎo biàn lín lí bú jìn*]
326. tendency to wake up easily [*yì xǐng*]
327. 失眠 insomnia
328. 健忘 [*jiàn wàng*]
329. vexation [*xīn fán*]
330. 善忧思 anxiety and preoccupation
331. 郁闷 [*yù mèn*]

332. clotted menstrual flow [*jīng xuè jiá kuài*]
333. 月经过多 profuse menstruation
334. 月经过少 [*yuè jīng guò shǎo*]
335. advanced menstruation [*jīng xíng xiān qī*]
336. 经行先后无定期 menstruation at irregular intervals
337. 恶风 [*wù fēng*]
338. yellow vaginal discharge [*dài xià sè huáng*]
339. 带下色青 green-blue vaginal discharge
340. 带下黏稠 [*dà xià nián chóu*]
341. fishy-smelling vaginal discharge [*dài xià wèi xīng*]
342. 阳萎 'yáng wilt'; impotence
343. 早泄 [*zǎo xiè*]
344. seminal emission [*yí jīng*]
345. 阴缩 retracted genitals
346. 梦失精 [*mèng jiāo shī jīng*]
347. inch, bar, and cubit [*cùn、guàn、chǐ*]
348. 右尺 right cubit
349. 左寸 [*zuǒ cùn*]
350. take the pulse, pulse-taking [*bǎ mài*]
351. 反关脉 pulse on the back of the wrist
352. 气口 [*qì kǒu*]
353. stirred pulse [*dòng mài*]
354. 伏脉 hidden pulse
355. 常脉 [*cháng mài*]
356. large pulse [*dà mài*]
357. 散脉 dissipated pulse
358. 浮脉 [*fú mài*]
359. slow pulse [*chí mài*]
360. 数脉 rapid pulse
361. 微脉 [*wēi mài*]
362. soggy pulse [*rú mài*]
363. 肝脉弦 liver pulse is stringlike
364. 心脉洪 [*xīn mài hóng*]
365. spleen pulse is moderate [*pí mài huǎn*]
366. 促脉 skipping pulse, rapid irregularly interrupted pulse
367. 虚脉 [*xū mài*]
368. replete pulse [*shí mài*]
369. 滑脉 slippery pulse
370. 涩脉 [*sè mài*]
371. stringlike pulse [*xián mài*]
372. 洪脉 surging pulse
373. 沉脉 [*chén mài*]
374. fine pulse [*xì mài*]
375. 脉小 small pulse
376. 弱脉 [*ruò mài*]
377. tight pulse [*jǐn mài*]
378. 芤脉 scallion-stalk pulse
379. 平脉 [*píng mài*]
380. long pulse [*cháng mài*]
381. 病脉 morbid pulse
382. 革脉 [*gé mài*]
383. confined pulse [*láo mài*]
384. 疾脉 racing pulse
385. 缓脉 [*huǎn mài*]
386. bound pulse [*jié mài*]
387. 代脉 regularly interrupted pulse
388. 短脉 [*duǎn mài*]
389. a rapid large surging pulse [*mài hóng dà ér shuō*]
390. 脉沉滑 a sunken slippery pulse
391. 脉沉弦 [*mài chén xián*]
392. a rapid pulse [*mài shuò*]
393. 脉沉滑 a sunken slippery pulse
394. 脉沉实有力 [*mài chén shí yǒu lì*]

395. a rapid soggy pulse [*mài rú shuò*]
396. 脉浮 floating pulse
397. 脉细数无力 [*mài xì shuò yǒu lì*]
398. faint at the inch, slippery at the bar, and slightly rapid at the cubit [*cùn wēi, guān huá, chǐ dài shuò*]
399. 左关脉弦 a stringlike left bar pulse; a pulse that is stringlike at the left bar
400. 右寸脉浮滑 [*yòu cùn mài fú huá*]
401. a) yawn; b) lack
402. palpation of the skin [*àn jī fū*]
403. 肌肤甲错 encrusted skin
404. 按手足 [*àn shǒu zú*]
405. vexing heat in the heart of the palms and soles [*shǒu zú xīn fán rè*]
406. 四肢欠温 lack of warmth in the limbs
407. 四肢清冷 [*sì zhī qīng lěng*]
408. counterflow cold of the limbs [*sì zhī nì lěng*]
409. 腹痛拒按 abdominal pain that rejects pressure
410. 按之柔软 [*àn zhī róu ruǎn*]
411. lump glomus that can be felt under pressure [*àn zhī yǒu pǐ kuài*]
412. 按之没指 engulfs the fingers when pressure is applied
413. cold damage [*shāng hán*]
414. 伤暑 summerheat damage
415. 时疫 [*shí yì*]
416. heaven-current red eye [*tiān xíng chì yǎn*]
417. 大头瘟 toad-head scourge
418. 疟疾 [*nüè jí*]
419. dysentery [*lì jí*]
420. 霍乱 cholera, sudden turmoil
421. 痉病 [*jìng bìng*]
422. hard tetany [*gāng jìng*]
423. 破伤风 lockjaw
424. 痿 [*wěi*]
425. consumption [*láo zhài*]
426. 夏痉 summer infixation
427. 胸痹 [*xiōng bì*]
428. dysphagia-occlusion [*yē gé*]
429. 黄疸 jaundice
430. 癥瘕积聚 [*zhēng jiǎ jī jù*]
431. wheezing [*xiāo*]
432. 喘 panting
433. 痰饮 [*tán yǐn*]
434. suspended rheum [*xuán yǐn*]
435. 溢饮 spillage rheum
436. 支饮 [*zhī yǐn*]
437. bloody stool [*biàn xuè*]
438. 心悸 palpitation
439. 惊悸 [*jīng jì*]
440. fearful throbbing [*zhēng chōng*]
441. 行痹 moving impediment
442. 寒痹 [*hán bì*]
443. fixed impediment [*zháo (zhuó) bì*]
444. 酒疸 liquor jaundice
445. 鼓胀 [*gǔ zhàng*]
446. damp diarrhea [*shī xiè*]
447. 脾泄 spleen diarrhea
448. 五更泄 [*wǔ gēng (jīng) xiè*]
449. early morning diarrhea [*chén xiè*]
450. 阳水 yáng water
451. 风水 [*fēng shuǐ*]
452. regular water [*zhèng shuǐ*]

453. 肉瘿 flesh goiter
454. 石瘿 [*shí yǐng*]
455. vacuity taxation [*xū láo*]
456. 洞泄 throughflux diarrhea
457. 濡泄 [*rú xiè*]
458. dribbling urinary block [*lóng bì*]
459. 五淋 five stranguries
460. 沙淋 [*shā lín*]
461. unctuous strangury [*gāo lín*]
462. 疝气 mounting qì
463. 痴呆 [*chī dāi*]
464. epilepsy [*xián*]
465. 疔疮 clove sore
466. 疔疮走黄 [*dīng chuāng zǒu huáng*]
467. swollen boil [*jié zhǒng*]
468. 发背 effusion
469. 圆癣 [*yuán xiǎn*]
470. pine bark lichen [*sōng pí xiǎn*]
471. 白秃疮 bald white scalp sore
472. 癞大风 [*lài dà fēng*]
473. loss-of-glory [*shī róng*]
474. 缠腰蛇丹 snake-girdle cinnabar
475. 脱肛 [*tuō gāng*]
476. scrofula [*luǒ li*]
477. 粉刺 acne
478. 耳聋 [*ěr lóng*]
479. spontaneous bleeding of the ear [*ěr nǜ*]
480. 鼻渊 deep-source nasal congestion
481. 鼻鼽 [*bí qiú*]
482. drinker's nose [*jiǔ zhā bí*]
483. 梅核气 plum-pit qì
484. 悬旗风 [*xuán qí fēng*]
485. fish bones stuck in the throat [*yú gǔ gěng hóu*]
486. 星翳 starry screen
487. 眼睑丹毒 [*yǎn jiǎn dān dú*]
488. phlegm node of the eye [*yǎn shēng tán hé*]
489. 拳毛倒睫 ingrown eyelash
490. ulceration of the eyelid rim [*yǎn xián chì làn*]
491. 胬肉攀睛 excrescence creeping over the eye
492. 蟹睛 [*xiè jīng*]
493. sparrow's vision [*què mù*]
494. 内障 internal obstruction
495. 青盲 [*qīng máng*]
496. 'yáng wilt,' impotence [*yáng wěi*]
497. 早泄 premature ejaculation
498. 阳强 [*yáng jiàng*]
499. testicular welling-abscess [*zǐ yōng*]
500. 子痰 testicular phlegm
501. 白淫 [*bái yín*]
502. red turbidity [*chì zhuó*]
503. 胎毒 fetal toxin
504. 解颅 [*jiě lú*]
505. pigeon chest [*jī xiōng*]
506. 齿迟 slowness to teethe
507. 百日咳 [*bǎi rì ké*]
508. mumps [*zhà sāi*]
509. 麻疹 measles
510. 水痘 [*shuǐ dòu*]
511. menstrual irregularities [*yuè jīng bù tiáo*]
512. 经乱 chaotic menstruation
513. 经行头痛 [*jīng xíng tóu tòng*]
514. menstrual lumbar pain [*jīng xíng yāo tòng*]
515. 崩漏 flooding and spotting
516. 赤带 [*chì dài*]

517. vomiting in pregnancy [*rèn shēn ǒu tù*]

518. 妊娠腹痛 abdominal pain in pregnancy

519. 妊娠喑哑 [*rèn shēn yīn yǎ*]

520. distention and fullness in the heart [region] and abdomen in pregnancy [*rèn shēn xīn fù zhàng mǎn*]

521. 胎动不安 stirring fetus

522. 胎水 [*tāi shuǐ*]

523. malposition of the fetus [*tāi wèi bú zhèng*]

524. 流产后闭经 post-miscarriage menstrual block

525. 乳汁不行 [*rǔ zhī bù xíng*]

526. postpartum leakage of breast milk [*rǔ zhī zì lòu*]

527. 胞衣不下 retention of the placenta

528. 恶露 [*è lù*]

529. infant's-pillow pain [*ér zhěn tòng*]

530. 产后腹痛 postpartum abdominal pain

531. 产后小便频数 [*chǎn hòu xiǎo biàn pín shuò*]

532. postpartum lumbar pain [*chǎn hòu yāo tòng*]

533. 阴户肿痛 painful swelling of the yīn door

534. puffy swelling in children [*xiǎo ér fú zhǒng*]

535. 邪气盛则实 [*xié qì shèng zé shí*]

536. when yáng is exuberant, there is external heat [*yáng shèng zé wài rè*]

537. 寒胜则浮 when cold prevails, there is swelling

538. 肝常有馀 [*gān cháng yǒu yú*]

539. turbid yīn failing to bear downward [*zhuó yīn bú jiàng*]

540. 气化不利 inhibited qì transformation

541. 肺失肃降 [*fèi shī sù jiàng*]

542. liver failing to course freely; impairment of the liver's free couring [*gān shī shū xiè*]

543. 实热 repletion heat

544. 虚寒 [*xū hán*]

545. vacuity heat [*xū rè*]

546. 虚实 vacuity and repletion, vacuity-repletion

547. 阴阳 [*yīn yáng*]

548. true heat and false cold [*zhēn rè jiǎ hán*]

549. 真实假虚 true repletion and false vacuity

550. 表里 [*biǎo lǐ*]

551. cold and heat, cold-heat [*hán rè*]

552. 实寒 repletion cold

553. 虚热 [*xū rè*]

554. vacuity and repletion, vacuity-repletion [*xū shí*]

555. 表虚 exterior vacuity

556. 真假 [*zhēn jiǎ*]

557. complex [*jiā zá*]

558. 半表半里 half interior half exterior; midstage penetration

559. 真虚假实 [*zhēn xū jiǎ shí*]

560. disease of both the exterior and interior [*biǎo lǐ tóng bìng*]

561. 阳虚 yáng vacuity

562. 亡阴 [*wáng yīn*]

563. vacuity-repletion complex [*xū shí jiā zá*]
564. 气虚 qì vacuity
565. 气陷 [*qì xiàn*]
566. qì desertion [*qì tuō*]
567. 气逆 qì counterflow
568. 气随血脱 [*qì suí xuè tuō*]
569. qì stagnation and blood stasis [*qì zhì xuè yū*]
570. 心气虚 heart qì vacuity
571. 心血虚 [*xīn xuè xū*]
572. heart yáng vacuity [*xīn yáng xū*]
573. 心气阴两虚 dual vacuity of heart qì and yīn; heart qì and yīn vacuity
574. 心火亢盛 [*xīn huǒ kàng shèng*]
575. water qì intimidating the heart [*shuǐ qì líng xīn*]
576. 肝血虚 liver blood vacuity
577. 肝阴虚 [*gān yīn xū*]
578. liver fire flaming upward [*gān huǒ shàng yán*]
579. 肝阳上亢 ascendant hyperactivity of liver yáng
580. 肝风内动 [*gān fēng nèi dòng*]
581. extreme heat engendering wind [*rè jí shēng fēng*]
582. 脾气虚 spleen qì vacuity
583. 脾不统血 [*pí bù tǒng xuè*]
584. spleen vacuity with damp encumbrance [*pí xū shī kùn*]
585. 肺气虚 lung qì vacuity
586. 肺阴虚 [*fèi yīn xū*]
587. expiration of lung qì [*fèi qì shuāi jué*]
588. 肺气不宣 lung qì failing to diffuse; non-diffusion of lung qì

589. 肺失肃降 [*fèi shī sù jiàng*]
590. lung liquid failing to distribute; non-distribution of lung liquid [*fèi jīn bú bù*]
591. 肾阴虚 kidney yīn vacuity
592. 肾气不足 [*shèn qì bù zú*]
593. dual vacuity of kidney yīn and yáng [*shèn yīn yáng liǎng xū*]
594. 心肝血虚 heart-liver blood vacuity
595. 心肺气虚 [*xīn fèi qì xū*]
596. dual vacuity of the heart and spleen; heart-spleen vacuity [*xīn pí liǎng xū*]
597. 心肾气虚 heart-kidney qì vacuity
598. 心肾不交 [*xīn shèn bù jiāo*]
599. disquieting of the heart and gallbladder [*xīn dǎn bù níng*]
600. 脾湿肝郁 spleen dampness and liver depression
601. 肝胃不和 [*gān wèi bù hé*]
602. liver fire invading the lung [*gān huǒ fàn fèi*]
603. 脾肾阳虚 spleen-kidney yáng vacuity
604. 脾胃阳虚 [*pí wèi yáng xū*]
605. 胆气虚 gallbladder qì vacuity
606. 胃气虚 [*wèi qì xū*]
607. stomach cold [*wèi hán*]
608. 胃虚寒 stomach vacuity cold
609. 胃火 [*wèi huǒ*]
610. intense stomach fire [*wèi huǒ chì shèng*]
611. 大肠结热 large intestinal heat bind
612. 大肠津亏 [*dà cháng jīn kuī*]
613. large intestinal vacuity cold [*dà cháng xū hán*]

614. 小肠气滞 small intestinal qì stagnation

615. 膀胱湿热 [páng guāng shī rè]

616. wind-cold invading the lung [fēng hán fàn fèi]

617. 风寒束肺 wind-cold fettering the lung

618. 风热犯肺 [fēng rè fàn fèi]

619. cold impediment [hán bì]

620. 寒痛 cold pain

621. 寒邪犯胃 [hán xié fàn wèi]

622. cold stagnating in the liver vessel [hán zhì gān mài]

623. 寒湿中阻 cold-damp obstructing the center

624. 暑热 [shǔ rè]

625. summerheat-damp [shǔ shī]

626. 寒湿中阻 cold-damp obstructing the center

627. 湿热蕴脾 [shī rè yùn pí]

628. damp-heat pouring down into the bladder [shī rè xià zhù páng guāng]

629. 湿热下注大肠 damp-heat pouring down into the large intestine

630. 寒痰 [hán tán]

631. dryness phlegm [zào tán]

632. 痰浊上扰 phlegm turbidity harassing the upper body

633. 痰蒙蔽心包 [tán zhuó méng bì xīn bāo]

634. phlegm turbidity obstructing the lung [tán zhuó zǔ fèi]

635. 水寒射肺 water-cold shooting into the lung

636. 食滞胃脘 [shí zhì wèi wǎn (guǎn)]

637. greater yáng (tài yáng) water amassment [tài yáng xù shuǐ]

638. 太阳热邪迫肺 greater yáng (tài yáng) heat evil distressing the lung

639. 热入血室 [rè rù xuè shì]

640. yáng brightness (yáng míng) channel heat [yáng míng jīng rè]

641. 阳明腑实 yáng brightness (yáng míng) bowel repletion

642. 太阴病 [tài yīn bìng]

643. reverting yīn (jué yīn) roundworm reversal [jué yīn huí jué]

644. 脾约 straitened spleen

645. 小结胸 [xiǎo jié xiōng]

646. lesser yáng (shào yáng) half-exterior half interior pattern [shào yáng bàn biǎo bàn lǐ]

647. 太阳蓄水 greater yáng (tài yáng) water amassment

648. 邪伤肺卫 [xié shāng fèi wèi]

649. dampness obstructing defense yáng [shī è wèi yǎng]

650. 湿阻气分 dampness obstructing the qì aspect

651. 热入气分 [rè rù qì fēn]

652. heat wearing true yīn [rè hào zhēn yīn]

653. 气营两燔 qì and construction both ablaze; dual blaze of qì and construction

654. 热炽毒盛 [rè chì dú shèng]

655. abnormal passage to the pericardium [nì chuán xīn bāo]

656. 阴虚风动 yīn vacuity stirring wind

657. 辨证施治 [biàn zhèng shī zhì]

658. identify patterns and determine treatment; determine treatment by patterns identified [*biàn zhèng lùn zhì*]

659. 同病异治 unlike treatment of like disease

660. 异病同治 [*yì bìng tóng zhì*]

661. act according to time, place, and person [*yīn shí yīn dì yīn rén zhì yí*]

662. 标本同治 treating the root and tip simultaneously

663. 反佐 [*fǎn zuǒ*]

664. straight treatment [*zhèng zhì*]

665. 从治 coacting treatment

666. 通因通用 [*tōng yīn tōng yòng*]

667. yáng disease is treated through yīn [*yáng bìng zhì yīn*]

668. 汗法 sweating

669. 发汗法 [*fā hàn fǎ*]

670. resolve the exterior; exterior resolution [*jiě biǎo*]

671. 辛凉解表 resolve the exterior with coolness and acridity; cool acrid exterior resolution

672. 助阳解表 [*zhù yáng jiě biǎo*]

673. enrich yīn and resolve the exterior [*zī yīn jiě biǎo*]

674. 透疹解表 outthrust papules and resolve the exterior

675. 疏表 [*shū biǎo*]

676. course wind [*shū fēng*]

677. 祛风 dispel wind

678. 祛风散寒 [*qū fēng sàn hán*]

679. outthrust the exterior [*tòu biǎo*]

680. 透邪 outthrust evils

681. 开鬼门 [*kāi guǐ mén*]

682. harmonize construction and defense; construction-defense harmonization [*tiáo hé yíng wèi*]

683. 涌吐 eject

684. 探吐 [*tàn tù*]

685. precipitation [*xià fǎ*]

686. 泻下 draining precipitation

687. 攻下 [*gōng xià*]

688. moist precipitation [*rùn xià*]

689. 峻下 drastic precipitation

690. 通泄阳明腑实 [*tōng xiè yáng míng fǔ shí*]

691. increase humor and precipitate with moistness; humor-increasing draining precipitation [*zēng yè xiè xià*]

692. 增水行舟 refloat the grounded ship

693. 急下存津 [*jí xià cún jīn*]

694. expel water [*zhú shuǐ*]

695. 去宛陈莝 eliminate stale water

696. 软坚除满 [*ruǎn jiān chú mǎn*]

697. harmonization [*hé fǎ*]

698. 和解表里 harmonize the exterior and interior

699. 调和肝胃 [*tiáo hé gān wèi*]

700. harmonize the liver [*hé gān*]

701. 和胃止痛 harmonize the stomach and relieve pain

702. 清法 [*qīng fǎ*]

703. clear repletion heat [*qīng shí rè*]

704. 清热泻火 clear heat and drain fire

705. 清热化湿 [*qīng rè huà shī*]

706. clear the heart [*qīng xīn*]

707. 清肝火 clear liver fire

708. 清肝泻肺 [qīng gān xiè fèi]

709. clear and discharge the lesser yáng [qīng xiè shào yáng]

710. 清金 clear metal

711. 清肠润燥 [qīng cháng rùn zào]

712. clear qì-aspect heat [qīng qì fēn rè]

713. 清营分热 clear construction-aspect heat

714. 气营两清 [qì yíng liǎng qīng]

715. cool the blood and resolve toxin [liáng xuè jiě dú]

716. 苦寒泄热 discharge heat with cold and bitterness

717. 甘温除（大）热 [gān wēn chú (dà) rè]

718. warming [wēn fǎ]

719. 祛寒法 dispelling cold

720. 温阳救逆 [wēn yáng jiù nì]

721. warm the center and dispel cold [wēn zhōng qū hán]

722. 理中 rectify the center

723. 温肝散寒 [wēn gān sàn hán]

724. warm and vitalize heart yáng [wen zhèn xīn yáng]

725. 温肺 warm the lung

726. 温肺化饮 [wēn fèi hào yǐn]

727. warm the kidney and supplement fire [wēn shèn bǔ huǒ]

728. 暖水脏 warm the water viscus

729. 温经散寒 [wēn jīng sàn hán]

730. warm and supplement the blood aspect [wēn bǔ xuè fēn]

731. 回阳救逆 return yáng and stem counterflow

732. 救阳 [jiù yáng]

733. supplementation [method] [bǔ fǎ]

734. 补养 supplement (and nourish); supplementation (and nourishing)

735. 养阴 [yǎng yīn]

736. enrich heart yīn [zī xīn yīn]

737. 滋补肝肾 enrich and supplement the liver and kidney

738. 救阴 [jiù yīn]

739. assist yáng [zhù yáng]

740. 壮阳 invigorate yáng

741. 温养 [wēn yǎng]

742. supplement spleen qì [bǔ pí qì]

743. 升提中气 upraise center qì

744. 益气生津 [yì qì shēng jīn]

745. supplement both qì and the blood [shuāng bǔ qì xuè]

746. 养血柔肝 nourish the blood and emolliate the liver

747. 甘寒生津 [gān hán shēng jīn]

748. boost qì and engender liquid [yì qì shēng jīn]

749. 滋水涵木 enrich water to moisten wood

750. 健脾 [jiàn pí]

751. bank up earth [péi tǔ]

752. 补火生土 supplement fire to engender earth

753. 补肾 [bǔ shèn]

754. combined treatment of lung and kidney [fèi shèn tóng zhì]

755. 引火归原 return fire to its source

756. 温补命门 [wēn bǔ mìng mén]

757. dispersion [xiāo fǎ]

758. 消导 abductive dispersion

759. 消食导滞 [xiāo shí dǎo zhì]

760. disperse food and transform stagnation [xiāo shí huà zhì]

761. 温中化食 warm the center and transform food

762. 消痞化积 [*xiāo pǐ huà jī*]

763. relieve glomus [*kāi pǐ*]

764. 开胃 open the stomach

765. 开胃进食 [*kāi wèi jìn shí*]

766. dispel phlegm [*qū tán*]

767. 宣肺化痰 diffuse the lung and transform phlegm

768. 清热化痰 [*qīng rè huà tán*]

769. dry dampness and transform phlegm [*zào shī huà tán*]

770. 治风化痰 control wind and transform phlegm

771. 消痰平喘 [*xiāo tán píng chuǎn*]

772. flush phlegm [*dí tán*]

773. 豁痰 sweep phlegm

774. 理气 [*lǐ qì*]

775. move qì [*xíng qì*]

776. 利气 disinhibit qì

777. 降气 [*jiàng qì*]

778. break qì [*pò qì*]

779. 开郁 open depression

780. 疏郁理气 [*shū yù lǐ qì*]

781. 疏肝 [*shū gān*]

782. course the liver and resolve depression [*shū gān jiě yù*]

783. 舒肝 soothe the liver

784. 宣肺 [*xuān fèi*]

785. diffuse and downbear lung qì [*xuān jiàng fèi qì*]

786. 辛开苦降 open with acridity and downbear with bitterness; acrid opening and bitter downbearing

787. 辛开苦泄 [*xīn kāi kǔ xiè*]

788. opening and discharging [*kāi xiè*]

789. 活血化瘀 quicken the blood and transform phlegm

790. 温化祛瘀 [*wēn huà qū yū*]

791. eliminate stasis and engender the new [*qù yū shēng xīn*]

792. 破瘀消癥 break stasis and disperse concretions

793. 逐瘀 [*zhú yū*]

794. break blood [*pò xuè*]

795. 止血 stanch bleeding

796. 补气摄血 [*bǔ qì shè xuè*]

797. return blood to the channels [*yǐn xuè guī jīng*]

798. 开窍 open the orifices; orifice opening

799. 宣窍 [*xuān qiào*]

800. warm opening [*wēn kāi*]

801. 清心开窍 clear the heart and open the orifices

802. 逐寒开窍 [*zhú hán kāi qiào*]

803. open the orifices and free the spirit [*kāi qiào tōng shén*]

804. 醒神 arouse the spirit

805. 开噤通关 [*kāi jìn tōng guān*]

806. quiet the spirit [*ān shén*]

807. 镇心 [*zhèn xīn*]

808. stabilize the mind [*dìng zhì*]

809. 宁神安魂 quiet the spirit and ethereal soul

810. 祛湿 [*qū shī*]

811. transform dampness [*huà shī*]

812. 芳香化湿 transform dampness with aroma

813. 辛香化浊 [*xīn xiāng huà zhuó*]

814. dry dampness and eliminate fullness [*zào shī chú mǎn*]

815. 利湿 disinhibit dampness

816. 清暑利湿 [*qīng shǔ lì shī*]

817. disinhibit dampness and abate jaundice [*lì shī tuì huáng*]

818. 宣通水道 free the waterways

819. 洁净腑 [*jié jìng fǔ*]

820. securing and astriction [*gù sè*]

821. 固摄 securing and containing

822. 敛汗固表 [*liàn hàn gù biǎo*]

823. astringe the intestines and check diarrhea [*sè cháng zhǐ xiè*]

824. 摄精 contain essence

825. 缩尿 [*suō niào*]

826. stem flooding and check discharge [*gù bēng zhǐ dài*]

827. 涩可固脱 astringency can stem desertion

828. 潜阳 [*qián yáng*]

829. subdue and settle [*qián zhèn*]

830. 熄风 extinguish wind

831. 平肝熄风 [*píng gān xī fēng*]

832. drain fire and extinguish wind [*xiè huǒ xī fēng*]

833. 养血祛风 nourish the blood and dispel wind

834. 伐肝 [*fā gān*]

835. resolve tetany [*jiě jìng*]

836. 调经 regulate menstruation

837. 通乳 [*tōng rǔ*]

838. supplement (and boost) the thoroughfare and controlling vessels [*bǔ yiè chōng rèn*]

839. 扶阳暖宫 support yáng and warm the palace

840. 清热安胎 [*qīng rè ān tāi*]

841. warm the palace and quiet the fetus [*nuǎn gōng ān tāi*]

842. 排脓托毒 expel pus and draw toxin

843. 拔脓 [*bá nóng*]

844. expel worms; worm expulsion [*qū chóng*]

845. 杀虫 kill worms

846. 安虫 [*ān chóng*]

847. cold and sweet [*gān hán*]

848. 微寒 slightly cold

849. 味苦性平 [*wèi kǔ xìng píng*]

850. balanced and sour [*suān píng*]

851. 性寒味苦有毒 cold in nature, bitter in flavor, and toxic

852. 甘微辛 [*gān wēi xīn*]

853. bitter and sweet [*kǔ gān*]

854. 酸温 warm and sour

855. 咸温 [*xián wēn*]

856. cool in nature and bitter in flavor [*xìng liáng wèi kǔ*]

857. 辛温无毒 warm, acrid, and non-toxic

858. 味厚 [*wèi hòu*]

859. mild flavor [*wèi bó*]

860. 升降浮沉 upbearing, downbearing, floating, and sinking

861. 升浮药 [*shēng fú yào*]

862. channel entry [*rù jīng*]

863. 炮制 processing of medicinals

864. 切片 [*qiē piān*]

865. grind to a powder [*wéi mò*]

866. 为粗末 grind to a rough powder

867. 磨成粉 [*mó chéng fěn*]

868. long-rise [*piǎo xǐ*]

869. 烧存性 nature-preservative burning

870. 制霜 [*zhì shuāng*]

871. stir-fry lightly; light stir-frying [*wēi chǎo*]

872. 炒黄 stir-fry until yellow

873. 水飞 [*shuǐ fēi*]

874. decocting pieces [*yǐn piàn*]

875. 膏药 plaster; medicinal paste
876. 药膏 [yào gāo]
877. elixir [dān]
878. 丸 pill
879. 散 [sǎn]
880. decoction [tāng]
881. 饮 beverage
882. 饮子 [yǐn zǐ]
883. take drenched [chōng fú]
884. 调服 take mixed (with fluid)
885. 顿服 [dùn fú]
886. take between meals [shí yuán fú]
887. 空腹服 take on an empty stomach
888. 调敷 [tiáo fū]
889. filiform needle [háo zhēn]
890. 三棱针 three-edged needle
891. 艾条 [ài tiáo]
892. number of cones [zhuàng shù]
893. 梅花针 plum-blossom needle
894. 七星针 [qī xīng zhēn]
895. insert the needle, needle insertion [jìn zhēn]
896. 捻针 needle
897. 留针 [liú zhēn]
898. remove the needle; needle removal [qǐ zhēn]
899. 迎随补泻 directional supplementation and drainage
900. 呼吸补泻 [hū xī bǔ xiè]
901. quick and slow supplementation and drainage [bǔ xiè]
902. 透天凉 heaven-penetrating cooling method
903. 烧山火 [shāo shān huǒ]
904. obtain qì [dé qì]
905. 艾炷灸 cone moxibustion
906. 艾条灸 [ài tiáo jiǔ]
907. indirect moxibustion [jiān jiē jiǔ]
908. 隔姜灸 moxibustion on ginger
909. 隔盐灸 [gé yán jiǔ]
910. natural moxibustion [tiān jiǔ]

附录2：中药名称
Appendix 2: Names of Chinese Medicinals

Medicinals are here presented in thematic order of functional class. For each entry, the Chinese name is followed by Pīnyīn and the English name; in final position is the Latin pharmaceutical name in parentheses.

It should be noted that some of the Latin names of medicinals have been revised to conform to the *Chinese Pharmacopoeia* (2000). As a result of this revision, certain English names of medicinals and formulas have also been changed.

解表药
Exterior-Resolving Medicinals

辛温解表药
Warm Acrid Exterior-Resolving Medicinals

麻黄 *má huáng*, ephedra (Ephedrae Herba)

桂枝 *guì zhī*, cinnamon twig (Cinnamomi Ramulus)

紫苏叶 *zǐ sū yè*, perilla leaf (Perillae Folium)

紫苏 *zǐ sū*, perilla (Perillae Folium, Caulis, et Calyx)

生姜 *shēng jiāng*, fresh ginger (Zingiberis Rhizoma Recens)

紫苏梗 *zǐ sū gěng*, perilla stem (Perillae Caulis)

香薷 *xiāng rú*, mosla (Moslae Herba)

姜皮 *jiāng pí*, ginger skin (Zingiberis Rhizomatis Cortex)

荆芥 *jīng jiè*, schizonepeta (Schizonepetae Herba)

防风 *fáng fēng*, saposhnikovia (Saposhnikoviae Radix)

羌活 *qiāng huó*, notopterygium (Notopterygii Rhizoma et Radix)

白芷 *bái zhǐ*, Dahurian angelica (Angelicae Dahuricae Radix)

藁本 *gǎo běn*, Chinese lovage (Ligustici Rhizoma)

苍耳子 *cāng ěr zǐ*, xanthium (Xanthii Fructus)

辛夷 *xīn yí*, magnolia flower (Magnoliae Flos)

葱白 *cōng bái*, scallion white (Allii Fistulosi Bulbus)

胡荽 *hú suī*, coriander (Coriandri Herba cum Radice)

柽柳 *chēng liǔ*, tamarisk (Tamaricis Cacumen)

辛凉解表药
Cool Acrid Exterior-Resolving Medicinals

薄荷 *bò hé*, mint (Menthae Herba)

牛蒡子 *niú bàng zǐ*, arctium (Arctii Fructus)

蝉蜕 *chán tuì*, cicada molting (Cicadae Periostracum)

淡豆豉 *dàn dòu chǐ*, fermented soybean (Sojae Semen Praeparatum)

大豆黄卷 *dà dòu huáng juǎn*, dried soybean sprout (Sojae Semen Germinatum)

桑叶 *sāng yè*, mulberry leaf (Mori Folium)

菊花 *jú huā*, chrysanthemum (Chrysanthemi Flos)

野菊花 *yě jú huā*, wild chrysanthemum flower (Chrysanthemi Indici Flos)

蔓荆子 *màn jīng zǐ*, vitex (Viticis Fructus)

葛根 *gé gēn*, pueraria (Puerariae Radix)

柴胡 *chái hú*, bupleurum (Bupleuri Radix)

升麻 *shēng má*, cimicifuga (Cimicifugae Rhizoma)

浮萍 *fú píng*, duckweed (Spirodelae Herba)

木贼 *mù zéi*, equisetum (Equiseti Hiemalis Herba)

清热药
Heat-Clearing Medicinals

清热泻火药
Heat-Clearing Fire-Draining Medicinals

石膏 *shí gāo*, gypsum (Gypsum Fibrosum)

生石膏 *shēng shí gāo*, crude gypsum (Gypsum Fibrosum Crudum)

知母 *zhī mǔ*, anemarrhena (Anemarrhenae Rhizoma)

芦根 *lú gēn*, phragmites (Phragmitis Rhizoma)

鲜芦根 *xiān lú gēn*, fresh phragmites (Phragmitis Rhizoma Recens)

天花粉 *tiān huā fěn*, trichosanthes root (Trichosanthis Radix)

山栀子 *shān zhī zǐ*, gardenia (Gardeniae Fructus)

夏枯草 *xià kū cǎo*, prunella (Prunellae Spica)

淡竹叶 *dàn zhú yè*, lophatherum (Lophatheri Herba)

寒水石 *hán shuǐ shí*, glauberite (Gypsum seu Calcitum)

鸭跖草 *yā zhí cǎo*, dayflower (Commelinae Herba)

密蒙花 *mì méng huā*, buddleia (Buddleja Flos)

青葙子 *qīng xiāng zǐ*, celosia (Celosiae Semen)

西瓜 *xī guā*, watermelon (Citrulli Fructus)

西瓜皮 *xī guā pí*, watermelon rind (Citrulli Exocarpium)

西瓜霜 *xī guā shuāng*, watermelon frost (Citrulli Praeparatio)

清热燥湿药
Heat-Clearing Dampness-Drying Medicinals

黄连 *huáng lián*, coptis (Coptidis Rhizoma)

黄芩 *huáng qín*, scutellaria (Scutellariae Radix)

黄柏 *huáng bǎi*, phellodendron (Phellodendri Cortex)

龙胆 *lóng dǎn*, gentian (Gentianae Radix)

苦参 *kǔ shēn*, flavescent sophora (Sophorae Flavescentis Radix)

马尾连 *mǎ wěi lián*, meadow rue (Thalictri Rhizoma et Radix)

十大功劳叶 *shí dà gōng láo yè*, mahonia (Mahoniae Folium)

清热凉血药
Heat-Clearing Blood-Cooling Medicinals

犀角 *xī jiǎo*, rhinoceros horn (Rhinocerotis Cornu)

水牛角 *shuǐ niú jiǎo*, water buffalo horn (Bubali Cornu)

干地黄 *gān dì huáng*, dried rehmannia (Rehmanniae Radix)

鲜地黄 *xiān dì huáng*, fresh rehmannia (Rehmanniae Radix Recens)

玄参 *xuán shēn*, scrophularia (Scrophulariae Radix)

牡丹皮 *mǔ dān pí*, moutan (Moutan Cortex)

赤芍药 *chì sháo yào*, red peony (Paeoniae Radix Rubra)

紫草 *zǐ cǎo*, arnebia/lithospermum (Arnebiae/Lithospermi Radix)

清热解毒
Heat-Clearing Toxin-Resolving Medicinals

金银花 *jīn yín huā*, lonicera (Lonicerae Flos)

忍冬藤 *rěn dōng téng*, lonicera stem (Lonicerae Caulis)

连翘 *lián qiào*, forsythia (Forsythiae Fructus)

蒲公英 *pú gōng yīng*, dandelion (Taraxaci Herba)

紫花地丁 *zǐ huā dì dīng*, violet (Violae Herba)

大青叶 *dà qīng yè*, isatis leaf (Isatidis Folium)

板蓝根 *bǎn lán gēn*, isatis root (Isatidis Radix)

南板蓝根 *nán bǎn lán gēn*, baphicacanthis (Baphicacanthis Cusiae Rhizoma et Radix)

青黛 *qīng dài*, indigo (Indigo Naturalis)

穿心莲 *chuān xīn lián*, andrographis (Andrographis Herba)

牛黄 *niú huáng*, bovine bezoar (Bovis Calculus)

蚤休 *zǎo xiū*, paris (Paridis Rhizoma)

半边莲 *bàn biān lián*, Chinese lobelia (Lobeliae Chinensis Herba)

拳参 *quán shēn*, bistort (Bistortae Rhizoma)

石指甲 *shí zhǐ jiǎ*, hanging stonecrop (Sedi Herba)

土茯苓 *tǔ fú líng*, smooth greenbrier root (Smilacis Glabrae Rhizoma)

鱼腥草 *yú xīng cǎo*, houttuynia (Houttuyniae Herba)

射干 *shè gān*, belamcanda (Belamcandae Rhizoma)

山豆根 *shān dòu gēn*, bushy sophora (Sophorae Tonkinensis Radix)

马勃 *mǎ bó*, puffball (Lasiosphaera seu Calvatia)

马齿苋 *mǎ chǐ xiàn*, purslane (Portulacae Herba)

白头翁 *bái tóu wēng*, pulsatilla (Pulsatillae Radix)

秦皮 *qín pí*, ash (Fraxini Cortex)

鸦胆子 *yā dǎn zǐ*, brucea (Bruceae Fructus)

大血藤 *dà xuè téng*, sargentodoxa (Sargentodoxae Caulis)

败酱草 *bài jiàng cǎo*, patrinia (Patriniae Herba)

墓头回 *mù tóu huí*, heterophyllous patrinia (Patriniae Heterophyllae Radix)

白花蛇舌草 *oldenlandia*, bái huā shé shé cǎo (Oldenlandiae Diffusae Herba)

熊胆 *xióng dǎn*, bear's gall (Ursi Fel)

白蔹 *bái liǎn*, ampelopsis (Ampelopsis Radix)

白鲜皮 *bái xiān pí*, dictamnus (Dictamni Cortex)

漏芦 *lòu lú*, rhaponticum (Rhapontici Radix)

禹州漏芦 *yǔ zhōu lòu lú*, echinops (Echinopsis Radix)

山慈姑 *shān cí gū*, cremastra/pleione (Cremastrae seu Pleiones Pseudobulbus)

天荞麦根 *tiān qiáo mài gēn*, wild buckwheat root (Fagopyri Cymosi Rhizoma et Radix)

冬青叶 *dōng qīng yè*, Chinese ilex leaf (Ilicis Chinensis Folium)

地锦草 *dì jǐn cǎo*, humifuse euphorbia (Euphorbiae Humifusae Herba)

白毛夏枯草 *bái máo xià kū cǎo*, bending bugle (Ajugae Decumbentis Herba)

鬼针草 *guǐ zhēn cǎo*, Spanish needles (Bidentis Bipinnatae Herba)

绿豆皮 *lü dòu pí*, mung bean seed-coat (Phaseoli Radiati Testa)

千里光 *qiān lǐ guāng*, climbing groundsel (Senecionis Scandentis Herba)

葎草 *lü cǎo*, Japanese hop (Humuli Scandentis Herba)

虎耳草 *hǔ ěr cǎo*, saxifrage (Saxifragae Herba)

地耳草 *dì ěr cǎo*, lesser hypericum (Hyperici Japonici Herba)

青叶胆 *qīng yè dǎn*, pretty swertia (Swertiae Pulchellae Herba)

鸡骨草 *jī gǔ cǎo*, prayer-beads (Abri Herba)

九节茶 *jiǔ jié chá*, sarcandra (Sarcandrae Ramulus et Folium)

半枝莲 *bàn zhī lián*, bearded scutellaria (Scutellariae Barbatae Herba)

天葵子 *tiān kuí zǐ*, semiaquilegia root (Semiaquilegiae Radix)

龙葵 *lóng kuí*, black nightshade (Solani Nigri Herba)

白毛藤 *bái máo téng*, climbing nightshade (Solani Lyrati Herba)

蛇莓 *shé méi*, snake strawberry (Duchesneae Herba)

凤尾草 *fèng wěi cǎo*, phoenix-tail fern (Pteridis Multifidi Herba)

白马骨 *bái mǎ gǔ*, serissa (Serissae Herba)

委陵菜 *wěi líng cài*, Chinese silverweed (Potentillae Chinensis Herba)

金莲花 *jīn lián huā*, globeflower (Trollii Flos)

挂金灯 *guà jīn dēng*, lantern plant calyx (Physalis Calyx seu Fructus)

蒟蒻 *jǔ ruò*, devil's tongue (Amorphophalli Tuber)

酸浆 *suān jiāng*, lantern plant (Physalis Alkekengi Herba)

金果榄 *jīn guǒ lǎn*, tinospora tuber (Tinosporae Radix)

青果 *qīng guǒ*, Chinese olive
(Canarii Fructus)

万年青根 *wàn nián qīng gēn*,
rohdea root (Rohdeae Rhizoma et
Radix)

藏青果 *zàng qīng guǒ*, unripe
chebule (Chebulae Fructus
Immaturus)

清虚热药
Vacuity-Heat–Clearing Medicinals

青蒿 *qīng hāo*, sweet wormwood
(Artemisiae Annuae Herba)

白薇 *bái wēi*, baiwei (Cynanchi
Atrati Radix)

地骨皮 *dì gǔ pí*, lycium bark
(Lycii Cortex)

银柴胡 *yín chái hú*, stellaria
(Stellariae Radix)

胡黄连 *hú huáng lián*, picrorhiza
(Picrorhizae Rhizoma)

泻下药
Draining Precipitation Medicinals

攻下药
Attacking precipitants

大黄 *dà huáng*, rhubarb (Rhei
Radix et Rhizoma)

生大黄 *shēng dà huáng*, raw
rhubarb (Rhei Radix et Rhizoma
Crudi)

芒硝 *máng xiāo*, mirabilite (Natrii
Sulfas)

玄明粉 *xuán míng fěn*, refined
mirabilite (Natrii Sulfas
Depuratus)

朴硝 *pò xiāo*, impure mirabilite
(Natrii Sulfas Non-Purus)

番泻叶 *fān xiè yè*, senna (Sennae
Folium)

芦荟 *lú huì*, aloe (Aloe)

巴豆 *bā dòu*, croton (Crotonis
Fructus)

巴豆霜 *bā dòu shuāng*, croton
frost (Crotonis Fructus
Pulveratus)

润下药
Moist Precipitants

火麻仁 *huǒ má rén*, hemp seed
(Cannabis Fructus)

郁李仁 *yù lǐ rén*, bush cherry
kernel (Pruni Semen)

逐水药
Water-Expelling Medicinals

甘遂 *gān suì*, kansui (Kansui
Radix)

续随子 *xù suí zǐ*, caper spurge seed
(Euphorbiae Semen)

大戟 *dà jǐ*, euphorbia/knoxia
(Euphorbiae seu Knoxiae Radix)

京大戟 *jīng dà jǐ*, Peking
euphorbia (Euphorbiae
Pekinensis Radix)

红大戟 *hóng dà jǐ*, knoxia
(Knoxiae Radix)

芫花 *yuán huā*, genkwa (Genkwa
Flos)

牵牛子 *qiān niú zǐ*, morning glory
(Pharbitidis Semen)

商陆 *shāng lù*, phytolacca
(Phytolaccae Radix)

续随子 *xù suí zǐ*, caper spurge seed
(Euphorbiae Semen)

祛风湿药
Wind-Damp–Dispelling
Medicinals

独活 *dú huó*, pubescent angelica
(Angelicae Pubescentis Radix)

威灵仙 *wēi líng xiān*, clematis (Clematidis Radix)

防己 *fáng jǐ*, fangji (Stephaniae Tetrandrae Radix)

(includes the following items)

木防己 *mù fáng jǐ*, woody fangji (Cocculi Radix)

粉防己 *fěn fáng jǐ*, mealy fangji (Stephaniae Tetrandrae Radix)

汉中防己 *hàn zhōng fáng jǐ*, northern fangji (Aristolochiae Heterophyllae Radix)

广防己 *guǎng fáng jǐ*, southern fangji (Aristolochiae Fangchi Radix)

秦艽 *qín jiāo*, large gentian (Gentianae Macrophyllae Radix)

豨莶 *xī xiān*, siegesbeckia (Siegesbeckiae Herba)

臭梧桐 *chòu wú tóng*, clerodendron (Clerodendri Folium)

木瓜 *mù guā*, chaenomeles (Chaenomelis Fructus)

络石藤 *luò shí téng*, star jasmine stem (Trachelospermi Caulis)

徐长卿 *xú cháng qīng*, paniculate cynanchum (Cynanchi Paniculati Radix)

桑枝 *sāng zhī*, mulberry twig (Mori Ramulus)

桑寄生 *sāng jì shēng*, mistletoe (Taxilli Herba)

五加皮 *wǔ jiā pí*, acanthopanax (Acanthopanacis Cortex)

香加皮 *xiāng jiā pí*, periploca (Periplocae Cortex)

狗骨 *gǒu gǔ*, dog's bone (Canis Os)

虎骨 *hǔ gǔ*, tiger bone (Tigris Os)

豹骨 *bào gǔ*, leopard's bone (Leopardi Os)

白花蛇 *bái huā shé*, krait/agkistrodon (Bungarus seu Agkistrodon)

蕲蛇 *qí shé*, agkistrodon (Agkistrodon)

海桐皮 *hǎi tóng pí*, erythrina (Erythrinae Cortex)

乌蛇 *wū shé*, black-striped snake (Zaocys)

蛇蜕 *shé tuì*, snake slough (Serpentis Periostracum)

原蚕沙 *yuán cán shā*, silkworm droppings (Bombycis Faeces)

海风藤 *hǎi fēng téng*, kadsura pepper stem (Piperis Kadsurae Caulis)

寻骨风 *xún gǔ fēng*, mollissima (Aristolochiae Mollissimae Herba)

千年健 *qiān nián jiàn*, homalomena (Homalomenae Rhizoma)

松节 *sōng jié*, knotty pine wood (Pini Lignum Nodi)

青风藤 *qīng fēng téng*, Orient vine (Sinomenii Caulis)

穿山龙 *chuān shān lóng*, Japanese dioscorea (Dioscoreae Nipponicae Rhizoma)

雷公藤 *léi gōng téng*, thunder god vine (Tripterygii Wilfordi Radix, Folium et Flos)

夏天无 *xià tiān wú*, bending corydalis (Corydalis Decumbentis Rhizoma)

伸筋草 *shēn jīn cǎo*, ground pine (Lycopodii Herba)

伸筋藤 *shēn jīn téng*, Chinese tinospora (Tinosporae Sinensis Caulis)

老鹳草 *lǎo guàn cǎo*, heron's-bill/cranesbill (Erodii seu Geranii Herba)

鹿衔草 *lù xián cǎo*, pyrola (Pyrolae Herba)

路路通 *lù lù tōng*, liquidambar fruit (Liquidambaris Fructus)

芳香化浊药
Aromatic Dampness-Transforming Medicinals

苍术 *cāng zhú*, atractylodes (Atractylodis Rhizoma)

厚朴 *hòu pò*, officinal magnolia bark (Magnoliae Officinalis Cortex)

厚朴花 *hòu pò huā*, officinal magnolia flower (Magnoliae Officinalis Flos)

藿香 *huò xiāng*, agastache (Agastaches Herba)

佩兰 *pèi lán*, eupatorium (Eupatorii Herba)

砂仁 *shā rén*, amomum (Amomi Fructus)

白豆蔻 *bái dòu kòu*, cardamom (Amomi Fructus Rotundus)

草豆蔻 *cǎo dòu kòu*, Katsumada's galangal seed (Alpiniae Katsumadai Semen)

草果 *cǎo guǒ*, tsaoko (Tsaoko Fructus)

石菖蒲 *shí chāng pú*, acorus (Acori Tatarinowii Rhizoma)

利水渗湿药
Water-Disinhibiting Dampness-Percolating Medicinals

茯苓 *fú líng*, poria (Poria)

茯苓皮 *fú líng pí*, poria skin (Poriae Cutis)

茯神 *fú shén*, root poria (Poria cum Pini Radice)

猪苓 *zhū líng*, polyporus (Polyporus)

泽泻 *zé xiè*, alisma (Alismatis Rhizoma)

薏苡仁 *yì yǐ rén*, coix (Coicis Semen)

薏苡根 *yì yǐ gēn*, coix root (Coicis Radix)

车前 *chē qián*, plantago (Plantaginis Herba)

车前子 *chē qián zǐ*, plantago seed (Plantaginis Semen)

滑石 *huá shí*, talcum (Talcum)

木通 *mù tōng*, trifoliate akebia (Akebiae Trifoliatae Caulis)

川木通 *chuān mù tōng*, Armand's clematis (Clematidis Armandii Caulis)

关木通 *guān mù tōng*, Manchurian Aristolochia (Aristolochiae Manshuriensis Caulis)

通草 *tōng cǎo*, rice-paper plant pith (Tetrapanacis Medulla)

小通草 *xiǎo tōng cǎo*, stachyurus/helwingia (Stachyuri seu Helwingiae Medulla)

灯心草 *dēng xīn cǎo*, juncus (Junci Medulla)

小金钱草 *xiǎo jīn qián cǎo*, dichondra (Dichondrae Herba)

金钱草 *jīn qián cǎo*, moneywort (Lysimachiae Herba)

海金沙 *hǎi jīn shā*, lygodium spore (Lygodii Spora)

石韦 *shí wéi*, pyrrosia (Pyrrosiae Folium)

地肤子 *dì fū zǐ*, kochia (Kochiae Fructus)

萹蓄 *biǎn xù*, knotgrass (Polygoni Avicularis Herba)

瞿麦 *qū mài*, dianthus (Dianthi Herba)

萆薢 *bì xiè*, fish poison yam (Dioscoreae Hypoglaucae seu Septemlobae Rhizoma)

粉萆薢 *fěn bì xiè*, hypoglaucus yam (Dioscorea Hypoglaucae Rhizoma)

绵萆薢 *mián bì xiè*, seven-lobed yam (Dioscorea Septemlobae Rhizoma)

茵陈蒿 *yīn chén hāo*, virgate wormwood (Artemisiae Scopariae Herba)

壶芦 *hú lú*, bottle gourd (Lagenariae Depressae Fructus)

冬瓜子 *dōng guā zǐ*, wax gourd seed (Benincasae Semen)

冬瓜皮 *dōng guā pí*, wax gourd rind (Benincasae Exocarpium)

赤小豆 *chì xiǎo dòu*, rice bean (Phaseoli Semen)

泽漆 *zé qī*, sun spurge (Euphorbiae Helioscopiae Herba)

玉米须 *yù mǐ xū*, corn silk (Mays Stylus)

冬葵子 *dōng kuí zǐ*, mallow seed (Malvae Semen)

蝼蛄 *lóu gū*, mole cricket (Gryllotalpa)

地耳草 *dì ěr cǎo*, lesser hypericum (Hyperici Japonici Herba)

虎杖 *hǔ zhàng*, bushy knotweed (Polygoni Cuspidati Rhizoma)

温里药
Interior-Warming Medicinals

附子 *fù zǐ*, aconite (Aconiti Radix Lateralis Praeparata)

白附片 *bái fù piàn*, white sliced aconite (Aconiti Radix Lateralis Alba Secta)

黑顺片 *hēi shùn piàn*, black sliced aconite (Aconiti Radix Lateralis Denigrata Secta)

熟附子 *shú fù zǐ*, cooked aconite (Aconiti Radix Lateralis Conquita)

咸附子 *xián fù zǐ*, salted aconite (Aconiti Radix Lateralis Salsa)

川乌头 *chuān wū tóu*, aconite root (Aconiti Radix)

草乌头 *cǎo wū tóu*, wild aconite (Aconiti Kusnezoffii Radix)

肉桂 *ròu guì*, cinnamon bark (Cinnamomi Cortex)

干姜 *gān jiāng*, dried ginger (Zingiberis Rhizoma)

炮姜 *pào jiāng*, blast-fried ginger (Zingiberis Rhizoma Praeparatum)

吴茱萸 *wú zhū yú*, evodia (Evodiae Fructus)

细辛 *xì xīn*, asarum (Asari Herba)

花椒 *huā jiāo*, zanthoxylum (Zanthoxyli Pericarpium)

高良姜 *gāo liáng jiāng*, lesser galangal (Alpiniae Officinarum Rhizoma)

椒目 *jiāo mù*, zanthoxylum seed (Zanthoxyli Semen)

丁香 *dīng xiāng*, clove (Caryophylli Flos)

红豆蔻 *hóng dòu kòu*, galangal fruit (Galangae Fructus)

母丁香 *mǔ dīng xiāng*, clove fruit (Caryophylli Fructus)

胡椒 *hú jiāo*, pepper (Piperis Fructus)

豆豉姜 *dòu chǐ jiāng*, litsea (Litseae Rhizoma et Radix)

荜茇 *bì bá*, long pepper (Piperis Longi Fructus)

荜澄茄 *bì chéng qié*, cubeb (Litseae Fructus)

茴香 *huí xiāng*, fennel (Foeniculi Fructus)

八角茴香 *bā jiǎo huí xiāng*, star anise (Anisi Stellati Fructus)

理气药

Qì-Rectifying Medicinals

陈皮 *chén pí*, tangerine peel (Citri Reticulatae Pericarpium)

橘白 *jú bái*, white tangerine peel (Citri Reticulatae Pericarpium Album)

橘红 *jú hóng*, red tangerine peel (Citri Reticulatae Exocarpium Rubrum)

橘核 *jú hé*, tangerine pip (Citri Reticulatae Semen)

橘络 *jú luò*, tangerine pith (Citri Fructus Fasciculus Vascularis)

橘叶 *jú yè*, tangerine leaf (Citri Reticulatae Folium)

化橘红 *huà jú hóng*, Huazhou pomelo rind (Citri Grandis Exocarpium Rubrum)

青皮 *qīng pí*, unripe tangerine peel (Citri Reticulatae Pericarpium Viride)

枳壳 *zhǐ qiào*, bitter orange (Aurantii Fructus)

枳实 *zhǐ shí*, unripe bitter orange (Aurantii Fructus Immaturus)

香橼 *xiāng yuán*, citron (Citri Fructus)

川楝子 *chuān liàn zǐ*, toosendan (Toosendan Fructus)

荔枝核 *lì zhī hé*, litchee pit (Litchi Semen)

香附子 *xiāng fù zǐ*, cyperus (Cyperi Rhizoma)

木香 *mù xiāng*, costusroot (Aucklandiae Radix)

广木香 *guǎng mù xiāng*, costusroot (Saussureae Radix)

川木香 *chuān mù xiāng*, common vladimiria (Vladimiriae Radix)

青木香 *qīng mù xiāng*, aristolochia root (Aristolochiae Radix)

乌药 *wū yào*, lindera (Linderae Radix)

薤白 *xiè bái*, Chinese chive (Allii Macrostemonis Bulbus)

檀香 *tán xiāng*, sandalwood (Santali Albi Lignum)

沉香 *chén xiāng*, aquilaria (Aquilariae Lignum Resinatum)

柿蒂 *shì dì*, persimmon calyx (Kaki Calyx)

甘松 *gān sōng*, nardostachys (Nardostachyos Radix et Rhizoma)

佛手柑 *fó shǒu gān*, Buddha's hand (Citri Sarcodactylis Fructus)

佛手花 *fó shǒu huā*, Buddha's hand flower (Citri Sarcodactylis Flos)

刀豆 *dāo dòu*, sword bean (Canavaliae Semen)

娑罗子 *suō luó zǐ*, horse chestnut (Aesculi Semen)

八月札 *bā yuè zhá*, akebia fruit (Akebiae Fructus)

玫瑰花 *méi guī huā*, rose (Rosae Rugosae Flos)

梅花 *méi huā*, mume flower (Mume Flos)

九香虫 *jiǔ xiāng chóng*, stinkbug (Aspongopus)

消食药
Food-Dispersing Medicinals

山楂 *shān zhā*, crataegus (Crataegi Fructus)

神曲 *shén qū*, medicated leaven (Massa Medicata Fermentata)

建神曲 *jiàn shén qū*, Fujian leaven (Massa Medicata Fermentata Fujianensis)

麦芽 *mài yá*, barley sprout (Hordei Fructus Germinatus)

稻芽 *dào yá*, rice sprout (Oryzae Fructus Germinatus)

谷芽 *gǔ yá*, millet sprout (Setariae Fructus Germinatus)

莱菔子 *lái fú zǐ*, radish seed (Raphani Semen)

鸡内金 *jī nèi jīn*, gizzard lining (Galli Gigeriae Endothelium Corneum)

驱虫药
Worm-Expelling Medicinals

使君子 *shǐ jūn zǐ*, quisqualis (Quisqualis Fructus)

苦楝皮 *kǔ liàn pí*, chinaberry bark (Meliae Cortex)

槟榔 *bīng láng*, areca (Arecae Semen)

大腹皮 *dà fù pí*, areca husk (Arecae Pericarpium)

南瓜子 *nán guā zǐ*, pumpkin seed (Cucurbitae Semen)

雷丸 *léi wán*, omphalia (Omphalia)

鹤虱 *hè shī*, carpesium seed (Carpesii Fructus)

南鹤虱 *nán hè shī*, wild carrot fruit (Carotae Fructus)

榧子 *fěi zǐ*, torreya (Torreyae Semen)

芜荑 *wú yí*, elm cake (Ulmi Fructus Praeparatio)

贯众 *guàn zhòng*, aspidium (Aspidii Rhizoma)

止血药
Blood-Stanching Medicinals

大蓟 *dà jì*, Japanese thistle (Cirsii Japonici Herba seu Radix)

小蓟 *xiǎo jì*, field thistle (Cirsii Herba)

地榆 *dì yú*, sanguisorba (Sanguisorbae Radix)

苎麻根 *zhù má gēn*, ramie (Boehmeriae Radix)

白茅根 *bái máo gēn*, imperata (Imperatae Rhizoma)

槐花 *huái huā*, sophora flower (Sophorae Flos)

槐角 *huái jiǎo*, sophora fruit (Sophorae Fructus)

侧柏叶 *cè bǎi yè*, arborvitae leaf (Platycladi Cacumen)

羊蹄根 *yáng tí gēn*, dock root (Rumicis Radix Recens)

紫珠 *zǐ zhū*, beauty-berry leaf (Callicarpae Formosanae Folium)

仙鶴草 *xiān hè cǎo*, agrimony (Agrimoniae Herba)

白及 *bái jí*, bletilla (Bletillae Rhizoma)

棕櫚皮 *zōng lü pí*, trachycarpus (Trachycarpi Petiolus)

百草霜 *bǎi cǎo shuāng*, weed soot (Herbarum Ustarum Fuligo)

藕節 *ǒu jié*, lotus root node (Nelumbinis Rhizomatis Nodus)

鐵莧 *tiě xiàn*, copperleaf (Acalyphae Herba)

三七 *sān qī*, notoginseng (Notoginseng Radix)

血余炭 *xuè yú tàn*, charred hair (Crinis Carbonisatus)

茜草根 *qiàn cǎo gēn*, madder (Rubiae Radix)

蒲黃 *pú huáng*, typha pollen (Typhae Pollen)

花蕊石 *huā ruǐ shí*, ophicalcite (Ophicalcitum)

卷柏 *juǎn bǎi*, selaginella (Selaginellae Herba)

伏龍肝 *fú lóng gān*, oven earth (Terra Flava Usta)

艾葉 *ài yè*, mugwort (Artemisiae Argyi Folium)

祛瘀活血藥
Stasis-Dispelling Blood-Quickening Medicinals

川芎 *chuān xiōng*, chuanxiong (Chuanxiong Rhizoma)

乳香 *rǔ xiāng*, frankincense (Olibanum)

没藥 *mò yào*, myrrh (Myrrha)

生没藥 *shēng mò yào*, raw myrrh (Myrrha Cruda)

延胡索 *yán hú suǒ*, corydalis (Corydalis Rhizoma)

郁金 *yù jīn*, curcuma (Curcumae Radix)

姜黃 *jiāng huáng*, turmeric (Curcumae Longae Rhizoma)

莪术 *é zhú*, zedoary (Curcumae Rhizoma)

三棱 *sān léng*, sparganium (Sparganii Rhizoma)

丹參 *dān shēn*, salvia (Salviae Miltiorrhizae Radix)

虎杖 *hǔ zhàng*, bushy knotweed (Polygoni Cuspidati Rhizoma)

益母草 *yì mǔ cǎo*, leonurus (Leonuri Herba)

茺蔚子 *chōng wèi zǐ*, leonurus fruit (Leonuri Fructus)

鸡血藤 *jī xuè téng*, spatholobus (Spatholobi Caulis)

桃仁 *táo rén*, peach kernel (Persicae Semen)

红花 *hóng huā*, carthamus (Carthami Flos)

藏红花 *zàng hóng huā*, saffron (Croci Stigma)

五灵脂 *wǔ líng zhī*, flying squirrel's droppings (Trogopteri Faeces)

牛膝 *niú xī*, achyranthes (Achyranthis Bidentatae Radix)

川牛膝 *chuān niú xī*, cyathula (Cyathulae Radix)

土牛膝 *tǔ niú xī*, native achyranthes (Achyranthis Radix)

穿山甲 *chuān shān jiǎ*, pangolin scales (Manitis Squama)

蟅虫 *zhè chóng*, ground beetle (Eupolyphaga seu Steleophaga)

水蛭 *shuǐ zhì*, leech (Hirudo)

虻虫 *méng chóng*, tabanus (Tabanus)

降真香 *jiàng zhēn xiāng*, dalbergia (Dalbergiae Odiferae Lignum)

泽兰 *zé lán*, lycopus (Lycopi Herba)

月季花 *yuè jì huā*, China tea rose (Rosae Chinensis Flos)

凌霄花 *líng xiāo huā*, campsis flower (Campsis Flos)

自然铜 *zì rán tóng*, pyrite (Pyritum)

王不留行 *wáng bù liú xíng*, vaccaria (Vaccariae Semen)

刘寄奴 *liú jì nú*, anomalous artemisia (Artemisiae Anomalae Herba)

苏木 *sū mù*, sappan (Sappan Lignum)

干漆 *gān qī*, lacquer (Toxicodendri Resina)

毛冬青 *máo dōng qīng*, hairy holly root (Ilicis Pubescentis Radix)

马鞭草 *mǎ biān cǎo*, verbena (Verbenae Herba)

积雪草 *jī xuě cǎo*, centella (Centellae Herb (cum Radice))

石见穿 *shí jiàn chuān*, Chinese sage (Salviae Chinensis Herba)

夜明砂 *yè míng shā*, bat's droppings (Verspertilionis Faeces)

鬼箭羽 *guǐ jiàn yǔ*, spindle tree wings (Euonymi Ramulus)

蜣螂 *qiāng láng*, dung beetle (Catharsius)

化痰止咳平喘药
Phlegm-Transforming, Cough-Suppressing, Panting-Calming Medicinals

化痰药
Phlegm-Transforming Medicinals

半夏 *bàn xià*, pinellia (Pinelliae Rhizoma)

法半夏 *fǎ bàn xià*, pro formula pinellia (Pinelliae Rhizoma Praeparatum)

姜半夏 *jiāng bàn xià*, ginger pinellia (Pinelliae Rhizoma cum Zingibere Praeparatum)

天南星 *tiān nán xīng*, arisaema (Arisaematis Rhizoma)

胆星 *dǎn xīng*, bile arisaema (Arisaema cum Bile)

白附子 *bái fù zǐ*, typhonium (Typhonii Rhizoma)

禹白附 *yǔ bái fù*, giant typhonium tuber (Typhonii Gigantei Tuber)

关白附 *guān bái fù*, Korean aconite (Aconiti Coreani Tuber)

白芥子 *bái jiè zǐ*, white mustard (Sinapis Alba Semen)

芥子 *jiè zǐ*, mustard seed (Sinapis Semen)

皂荚 *zào jiá*, gleditsia (Gleditsiae Fructus)

皂角刺 *zào jiǎo cì*, gleditsia thorn (Gleditsiae Spina)

桔梗 *jié gěng*, platycodon (Platycodonis Radix)

金沸草 *jīn fèi cǎo*, inula (Inulae Herba)

旋覆花 *xuán fù huā*, inula flower (Inulae Flos)

白前 *bái qián*, willowleaf swallowwort (Cynanchi Stauntonii Rhizoma)

前胡 *qián hú*, peucedanum (Peucedani Radix)

瓜蒌 *guā lóu*, trichosanthes (Trichosanthis Fructus)

瓜蒌子 *guā lóu zǐ*, trichosanthes seed (Trichosanthis Semen)

瓜蒌皮 *guā lóu pí*, trichosanthes rind (Trichosanthis Pericarpium)

贝母 *bèi mǔ*, fritillaria (Fritillariae Bulbus)

川贝母 *chuān bèi mǔ*, Sichuan fritillaria (Fritillariae Cirrhosae Bulbus)

浙贝母 *zhè bèi mǔ*, Zhejiang fritillaria (Fritillariae Thunbergii Bulbus)

竹茹 *zhú rú*, bamboo shavings (Bumbusae Caulis in Taenia)

天竹黄 *tiān zhú huáng*, bamboo sugar (Bambusae Concretio Silicea)

竹沥 *zhú lì*, dried bamboo sap (Bambusae Succus Exsiccatus)

海浮石 *hǎi fú shí*, costazia bone/pumice (Costaziae Os/Pumex)

海蛤壳 *hǎi gé qiào*, clamshell (Meretricis seu Cyclinae Concha)

礞石 *méng shí*, chlorite/mica (Chloriti seu Micae Lapis)

金礞石 *jīn méng shí*, mica (Micae Lapis Aureus)

青礞石 *qīng méng shí*, chlorite (Chloritae Lapis)

海藻 *hǎi zǎo*, sargassum (Sargassum)

昆布 *kūn bù*, kelp (Laminariae/Eckloniae Thallus)

海带 *hǎi dài*, eelgrass (Zosterae Marinae Herba)

黄药子 *huáng yào zǐ*, air potato (Dioscoreae Bulbiferae Rhizoma)

胖大海 *pàng dà hài*, sterculia (Sterculiae Lychnophorae Semen)

猪胆汁 *zhū dǎn zhī*, pig's bile (Suis Bilis)

蔊菜 *hān cài*, rorippa (Rorippae Herba seu Flos)

明党参 *míng dǎng shēn*, changium root (Changii Radix)

罗汉果 *luó hàn guǒ*, momordica (Momordicae Fructus)

荸荠 *bí qí*, water chestnut (Heleocharitis Cormus)

凤凰衣 *fèng huáng yī*, chicken's egg membrane (Galli Membrana Ovi)

止咳化痰药
Cough-Suppressing Panting-Calming Medicinals

杏仁 *xìng rén*, apricot kernel (Armeniacae Semen)

甜杏仁 *tián xìng rén*, sweet apricot kernel (Armeniacae Semen Dulce)

巴旦杏仁 *bā dàn xìng rén*, almond (Pruni Amygdali Semen)

百部 *bǎi bù*, stemona (Stemonae Radix)

紫菀 *zǐ wǎn*, aster (Asteris Radix)

款冬花 *kuǎn dōng huā*, coltsfoot (Farfarae Flos)

紫苏子 *zǐ sū zǐ*, perilla seed (Perillae Fructus)

桑白皮 *sāng bái pí*, mulberry root bark (Mori Cortex)

葶苈子 *tíng lì zǐ*, lepidium/descurainiae (Lepidii/Descurainiae Semen)

枇杷叶 *pí pá yè*, loquat leaf (Eriobotryae Folium)

马兜铃 *mǎ dōu líng*, aristolochia fruit (Aristolochiae Fructus)

紫金牛 *zǐ jīn niú*, Japanese ardisia (Ardisiae Japonicae Herba)

白果 *bái guǒ*, ginkgo (Ginkgo Semen)

洋金花 *yáng jīn huā*, datura flower (Daturae Flos)

华山参 *huá shān shēn*, physochlaina (Physochlainae Radix)

钟乳石 *zhōng rǔ shí*, stalactite (Stalactitum)

钟乳粉 *zhōng rǔ fěn*, powdered stalactite (Stalactitum Pulveratum)

满山红 *mǎn shān hóng*, Daurian rhododendron (Rhododendri Daurici Folium)

鹅管石 *é guǎn shí*, goose throat stone (Balanophyllia seu Stalactitum)

安神药
Spirit-Quieting Medicinals

重镇安神药
Heavy settling spirit-quieting medicinals

朱砂 *zhū shā*, cinnabar (Cinnabaris)

磁石 *cí shí*, loadstone (Magnetitum)

龙骨 *lóng gǔ*, dragon bone (Mastodi Ossis Fossilia)

龙齿 *lóng chǐ*, dragon tooth (Mastodi Dentis Fossilia)

牡蛎 *mǔ lì*, oyster shell (Ostreae Concha)

琥珀 *hǔ pò*, amber (Succinum)

珍珠母 *zhēn zhū mǔ*, mother-of-pearl (Concha Margaritifera)

珍珠 *zhēn zhū*, pearl (Margarita)

紫石英 *zǐ shí yīng*, fluorite (Fluoritum)

养心安神药
Heart-nourishing spirit-quieting medicinals

酸枣仁 *suān zǎo rén*, spiny jujube (Ziziphi Spinosi Semen)

柏子仁 *bǎi zǐ rén*, arborvitae seed (Platycladi Semen)

远志 *yuǎn zhì*, polygala (Polygalae Radix)

茯神 *fú shén*, root poria (Poria cum Pini Radice)

夜交藤 *yè jiāo téng*, flowery knotweed stem (Polygoni Multiflori Caulis)

龙眼肉 *lóng yǎn ròu*, longan flesh (Longan Arillus)

莲子 *lián zǐ*, lotus seed (Nelumbinis Semen)

莲子心 *lián zǐ xīn*, lotus plumule (Nelumbinis Plumula)

五味子 *wǔ wèi zǐ*, schisandra (Schisandrae Fructus)

合欢皮 *hé huān pí*, silk tree bark (Albizziae Cortex)

合欢花 *hé huān huā*, silk tree flower (Albizziae Flos)

夜合花 *yè hé huā*, dwarf magnolia (Magnoliae Coco Flos)

灵芝 *líng zhī*, ganoderma (Ganoderma)

平肝熄风药
Liver-Calming Wind-Extinguishing Medicinals

羚羊角 *líng yáng jiǎo*, antelope horn (Saigae Tataricae Cornu)

山羊角 *shān yáng jiǎo*, goral horn (Naemorhedi Goral Cornu)

石决明 *shí jué míng*, abalone shell (Haliotidis Concha)

牡蛎 *mǔ lì*, oyster shell (Ostreae Concha)

生牡蛎 *shēng mǔ lì*, crude oyster shell (Ostreae Concha Cruda)

珍珠 *zhēn zhū*, pearl (Margarita)

珍珠母 *zhēn zhū mǔ*, mother-of-pearl (Concha Margaritifera)

玳瑁 *dài mào*, hawksbill shell (Eretmochelydis Carapax)

紫贝 *zǐ bèi*, purple cowrie (Mauritiae, Erosariae, seu Cypraeae Testa)

代赭石 *dài zhě shí*, hematite (Haematitum)

钩藤 *gōu téng*, uncaria (Uncariae Ramulus cum Uncis)

天麻 *tiān má*, gastrodia (Gastrodiae Rhizoma)

决明子 *jué míng zǐ*, fetid cassia (Cassiae Semen)

刺蒺藜 *cì jí lí*, tribulus (Tribuli Fructus)

黑大豆 *hēi dà dòu*, black soybean (Sojae Semen Atrum)

全蝎 *quán xiē*, scorpion (Scorpio)

蜈蚣 *wú gōng*, centipede (Scolopendra)

白僵蚕 *bái jiāng cán*, silkworm (Bombyx Batryticatus)

地龙 *dì lóng*, earthworm (Pheretima)

铁落 *tiě luò*, iron flakes (Ferri Frusta)

开窍药
Orifice-Opening Medicinals

麝香 *shè xiāng*, musk (Moschus)

冰片 *bīng piàn*, borneol (Borneolum)

安息香 *ān xī xiāng*, benzoin (Benzoinum)

苏合香 *sū hé xiāng*, storax (Styrax)

石菖蒲 *shí chāng pú*, acorus (Acori Tatarinowii Rhizoma)

补益药
Supplementing Medicinals

补气药
Qì-Supplementing Medicinals

人参 *rén shēn*, ginseng (Ginseng Radix)

红参 *hóng shēn*, red ginseng (Ginseng Radix Rubra)

高丽参 *gāo lì shēn*, Korean ginseng (Ginseng Radix Coreensis)

西洋参 *xī yáng shēn*, American ginseng (Panacis Quinquefolii Radix)

党参 *dǎng shēn*, codonopsis (Codonopsis Radix)

太子参 *tài zǐ shēn*, pseudostellaria (Pseudostellariae Radix)

黄芪 *huáng qí*, astragalus (Astragali Radix)

红芪 *hóng qí*, hedysarum (Hedysari Radix)

白术 *bái zhú*, white atractylodes (Atractylodis Macrocephalae Rhizoma)

山药 *shān yào*, dioscorea (Dioscoreae Rhizoma)

扁豆 *biǎn dòu*, lablab (Lablab Semen Album)

甘草 *gān cǎo*, licorice (Glycyrrhizae Radix)

大枣 *dà zǎo*, jujube (Jujubae Fructus)

饴糖 *yí táng*, malt sugar (Maltosum)

蜜 *mì*, honey (Mel)

补阳药
Yáng-Supplementing Medicinals

鹿茸 *lù róng*, velvet deerhorn (Cervi Cornu Pantotrichum)

鹿角 *lù jiǎo*, deerhorn (Cervi Cornu)

鹿角胶 *lù jiǎo jiāo*, deerhorn glue (Cervi Cornus Gelatinum)

鹿角霜 *lù jiǎo shuāng*, degelatinated deerhorn (Cervi Cornu Degelatinatum)

牡狗阴茎 *mǔ gǒu yīn jīng*, dog's penis (Canis Penis)

紫河车 *zǐ hé chē*, placenta (Hominis Placenta)

蛤蚧 *gé jiè*, gecko (Gecko)

冬虫夏草 *dōng chóng xià cǎo*, cordyceps (Cordyceps)

胡桃仁 *hú táo rén*, walnut (Juglandis Semen)

肉苁蓉 *ròu cōng róng*, cistanche (Cistanches Herba)

锁阳 *suǒ yáng*, cynomorium (Cynomorii Herba)

巴戟天 *bā jǐ tiān*, morinda (Morindae Officinalis Radix)

淫羊藿 *yín yáng huò*, epimedium (Epimedii Herba)

仙茅 *xiān máo*, curculigo (Curculiginis Rhizoma)

杜仲 *dù zhòng*, eucommia (Eucommiae Cortex)

续断 *xù duàn*, dipsacus (Dipsaci Radix)

狗脊 *gǒu jǐ*, cibotium (Cibotii Rhizoma)

骨碎补 *gǔ suì bǔ*, drynaria (Drynariae Rhizoma)

补骨脂 *bǔ gǔ zhī*, psoralea (Psoraleae Fructus)

益智仁 *yì zhì rén*, alpinia (Alpiniae Oxyphyllae Fructus)

沙苑子 *shā yuàn zǐ*, complanate astragalus seed (Astragali Complanati Semen)

菟丝子 *tù sī zǐ*, cuscuta (Cuscutae Semen)

韭菜 *jiǔ cài*, Chinese leek (Allii Tuberosi Folium)

韭子 *jiǔ zǐ*, Chinese leek seed (Allii Tuberosi Semen)

胡芦巴 *hú lú bā*, fenugreek (Trigonellae Semen)

阳起石 *yáng qǐ shí*, actinolite (Actinolitum)

海马 *hǎi mǎ*, seahorse (Hippocampus)

海龙 *hǎi lóng*, pipe-fish (Sygnathus)

补血药
Blood-Supplementing Medicinals

当归 *dāng guī*, Chinese angelica (Angelicae Sinensis Radix)

熟地黄 *shú dì huáng*, cooked rehmannia (Rehmanniae Radix Praeparata)

何首乌 *hé shǒu wū*, flowery knotweed (Polygoni Multiflori Radix)

夜交藤 *yè jiāo téng*, flowery knotweed stem (Polygoni Multiflori Caulis)

白芍药 *bái sháo yào*, white peony (Paeoniae Radix Alba)

阿胶 *ē jiāo*, ass hide glue (Asini Corii Colla)

龙眼肉 *lóng yǎn ròu*, longan flesh (Longan Arillus)

鸡血藤 *jī xuè téng*, spatholobus (Spatholobi Caulis)

补阴药
Yīn-Supplementing Medicinals

沙参 *shā shēn*, adenophora/glehnia (Adenophorae seu Glehniae Radix)

北沙参 *běi shā shēn*, glehnia (Glehniae Radix)

南沙参 *nán shā shēn*, adenophora (Adenophorae Radix)

麦门冬 *mài mén dōng*, ophiopogon (Ophiopogonis Radix)

天门冬 *tiān mén dōng*, asparagus (Asparagi Radix)

石斛 *shí hú*, dendrobium (Dendrobii Herba)

玉竹 *yù zhú*, Solomon's seal (Polygonati Odorati Rhizoma)

黄精 *huáng jīng*, polygonatum (Polygonati Rhizoma)

百合 *bǎi hé*, lily bulb (Lilii Bulbus)

枸杞子 *gǒu qǐ zǐ*, lycium berry (Lycii Fructus)

蕤仁 *ruí rén*, prinsepia (Prinsepiae Nux)

楮实子 *chǔ shí zǐ*, broussonetia (Broussonetiae Fructus)

桑椹 *sāng shèn*, mulberry (Mori Fructus)

墨旱莲 *mò hàn lián*, eclipta (Ecliptae Herba)

女贞子 *nǚ zhēn zǐ*, ligustrum (Ligustri Lucidi Fructus)

龟版 *guī bǎn*, tortoise shell (Testudinis Carapax et Plastrum)

龟版胶 *guī bǎn jiāo*, tortoise shell glue (Testudinis Carapacis et Pastri Gelatinum)

鳖甲 *biē jiǎ*, turtle shell (Trionycis Carapax)

鳖甲胶 *biē jiǎ jiāo*, turtle shell glue (Trionycis Caparacis Gelatinum)

黑脂麻 *hēi zhī má*, black sesame (Sesami Semen Nigrum)

收涩药
Astringent Medicinals

五味子 *wǔ wèi zǐ*, schisandra (Schisandrae Fructus)

乌梅 *wū méi*, mume (Mume Fructus)

五倍子 *wǔ bèi zǐ*, sumac gallnut (Galla Chinensis)

浮小麦 *fú xiǎo mài*, light wheat (Tritici Fructus Levis)

麻黄根 *má huáng gēn*, ephedra root (Ephedrae Radix)

糯稻根须 *nuò dào gēn xū*, glutinous rice root (Oryzae Glutinosae Radix)

石榴皮 *shí liú pí*, pomegranate rind (Granati Pericarpium)

诃子 *hē zǐ*, chebule (Chebulae Fructus)

肉豆蔻 *ròu dòu kòu*, nutmeg (Myristicae Semen)

赤石脂 *chì shí zhī*, halloysite (Halloysitum Rubrum)

禹余粮 *yǔ yú liáng*, limonite (Limonitum)

罂粟壳 *yīng sù qiào*, poppy husk (Papaveris Pericarpium)

莲肉 *lián ròu*, lotus seed (Nelumbinis Semen)

莲房 *lián fáng*, lotus receptacle (Nelumbinis Receptaculum)

莲须 *lián xū*, lotus stamen (Nelumbinis Stamen)

芡实 *qiàn shí*, euryale (Euryales Semen)

山茱萸 *shān zhū yú*, cornus (Corni Fructus)

金樱子 *jīn yīng zǐ*, Cherokee rose fruit (Rosae Laevigatae Fructus)

覆盆子 *fù pén zǐ*, rubus (Rubi Fructus)

桑螵蛸 *sāng piāo xiāo*, mantis egg-case (Mantidis Oötheca)

海螵蛸 *hǎi piāo xiāo*, cuttlefish bone (Sepiae Endoconcha)

刺猬皮 *cì wèi pí*, hedgehog's pelt (Erinacei Pellis)

涌吐药
Ejection Medicinals

瓜蒂 *guā dì*, melon stalk (Melonis Pedicellus)

常山 *cháng shān*, dichroa (Dichroae Radix)

蜀漆 *shǔ qī*, dichroa leaf (Dichroae Folium)

胆矾 *dǎn fán*, chalcanthite (Chalcanthitum)

藜芦 *lí lú*, veratrum (Veratri Nigri Radix et Rhizoma)

人参芦 *rén shēn lú*, ginseng top (Ginseng Rhizoma)

皂荚 *zào jiá*, gleditsia (Gleditsiae Fructus)

外用药
Medicinals for External Use

硫黄 *liú huáng*, sulfur (Sulphur)

雄黄 *xióng huáng*, realgar (Realgar)

雌黄 *cī huáng*, orpiment (Auripigmentum)

砒石 *pī shí*, arsenic (Arsenicum)

轻粉 *qīng fěn*, calomel (Calomelas)

升丹 *shēng dān*, upborne elixir (Sublimatum Triplex)

铅丹 *qiān dān*, minium (Minium)

密陀僧 *mì tuó sēng*, litharge (Lithargyrum)

炉甘石 *lú gān shí*, calamine (Calamina)

硼砂 *péng shā*, borax (Borax)

白矾 *bái fán*, alum (Alumen)

绿矾 *lü fán*, melanterite (Melanteritum)

石灰 *shí huī*, limestone (Calx)

硝石 *xiāo shí*, niter (Nitrum)

硇砂 *náo shā*, sal ammoniac (Sal Ammoniacum)

毛茛 *máo gèn*, Japanese ranunculus (Ranunculi Japonici Herba et Radix)

大蒜 *dà suàn*, garlic (Allii Sativi Bulbus)

斑蝥 *bān máo*, mylabris (Mylabris)

蟾酥 *chán sū*, toad venom (Bufonis Venenum)

马钱子 *mǎ qián zǐ*, nux vomica (Strychni Semen)

马钱子粉 *mǎ qián zǐ fěn*, powdered nux vomica (Strychni Semen Pulveratum)

木鳖子 *mù biē zǐ*, momordica (Momordicae Semen)

蛇床子 *shé chuáng zǐ*, cnidium seed (Cnidii Fructus)

露蜂房 *lù fēng fáng*, hornet's nest (Vespae Nidus)

木芙蓉花 *mù fú róng huā*, cotton rose (Hibisci Mutabilis Flos)

木芙蓉叶 *mù fú róng yè*, cotton rose leaf (Hibisci Mutabilis Folium)

大风子 *dà fēng zǐ*, hydnocarpus (Hydnocarpi Semen)

木槿皮 *mù jǐn pí*, rose-of-Sharon root bark (Hibisci Syriaci Radicis Cortex)

土荆皮 *tǔ jīng pí*, golden larch bark (Pseudolaricis Cortex)

木槿花 *mù jǐn huā*, rose-of-Sharon (Hibisci Syriaci Flos)

丝瓜络 *sī guā luò*, loofah (Luffae Fructus Retinervus)

狼毒 *láng dú*, Chinese wolfsbane (Stellerae seu Euphorbiae Radix)

血竭 *xuè jié*, dragon's blood (Daemonoropis Resina)

樟脑 *zhāng nǎo*, camphor (Camphora)

松香 *sōng xiāng*, rosin (Pini Resina)

孩儿茶 *hái ér chá*, cutch (Catechu)

瓦楞子 *wǎ léng zǐ*, ark shell (Arcae Concha)

壁虎 *bì hǔ*, house lizard (Gecko Swinhoana)

象皮 *xiàng pí*, elephant's hide (Elephantis Corium)

虫白腊 *chóng bái là*, insect wax (Cera Chinensis)

蜂腊 *fēng là*, yellow wax (Cera Flava)

附录3：方剂名称
Appendix 3: Chinese Formula Names

解表剂
Exterior-Resolving Formulas

辛温解表
Resolve the exterior with warmth and acridity

葱豉汤 *cōng chǐ tāng*, Scallion and Fermented Soybean Decoction

大羌活汤 *dà qiāng huó tāng*, Major Notopterygium Decoction

大青龙汤 *dà qīng lóng tāng*, Major Green-Blue Dragon Decoction

葛根汤 *gé gēn tāng*, Pueraria Decoction

桂枝加葛根汤 *guì zhī jiā gé gēn tāng*, Cinnamon Twig Decoction Plus Pueraria

桂枝加厚朴杏仁汤 *guì zhī jiā hòu pò xìng rén tāng*, Cinnamon Twig Decoction Plus Official Magnolia Bark and Apricot Kernel

桂枝加芍药汤 *guì zhī jiā sháo yào tāng*, Cinnamon Twig Decoction Plus Peony

桂枝汤 *guì zhī tāng*, Cinnamon Twig Decoction

活人葱豉汤 *huó rén cōng chǐ tāng*, Book of Life Scallion and Fermented Soybean Decoction

活人香薷散 *huó rén xiāng rú yǐn*, Book of Life Renewal Mosla Powder

加味香苏散 *jiā wèi xiāng sū sǎn*, Supplemented Cyperus and Perilla Powder

荆防败毒散 *jīng fáng bài dú sǎn*, Schizonepeta and Saposhnikovia Toxin-Vanquishing Powder

荆防汤 *jīng fáng tāng*, Schizonepeta and Saposhnikovia Decoction

九味羌活汤 *jiǔ wèi qiāng huó tāng*, Nine-Ingredient Notopterygium Decoction

连须葱白汤 *lián xū cōng bái tāng*, Scallion with Root Decoction

六味香薷饮 *liù wèi xiāng rú yǐn*, Six-Ingredient Mosla Beverage

麻黄加术汤 *má huáng jiā zhú tāng*, Ephedra Decoction Plus White Atractylodes

麻黄汤 *má huáng tāng*, Ephedra Decoction

麻杏薏甘汤 *má xìng yì gān tāng*, Ephedra, Apricot Kernel, Coix, and Licorice Decoction

三拗汤 *sān ào tāng*, Rough and Ready Three Decoction

三物香薷饮 *sān wù xiāng rú yǐn*, Three-Agent Mosla Powder

神术散 *shén zhú sǎn*, Wondrous Atractylodes Powder

四味香薷饮 *sì wèi xiāng rú yǐn*, Four-Ingredient Mosla Beverage

五物香薷饮 *wǔ wù xiāng rú yǐn*, Five Agents Mosla Beverage

香薷散 *xiāng rú sǎn*, Mosla Powder

香薷汤 *xiāng rú tāng*, Mosla Decoction

香苏散 *xiāng sū sǎn*, Cyperus and Perilla Powder

阳旦汤 *yáng dàn*, Yáng Dawn Decoction

辛凉解表
Resolve the exterior with coolness and acridity

柴葛解肌汤 *chái gé jiě jī tāng*, Bupleurum and Pueraria Flesh-Resolving Decoction

葱豉桔梗汤 *cōng chǐ jié gěng tāng*, Scallion, Fermented Soybean, and Platycodon Decoction

浮萍黄芩汤 *fú píng huáng qín tāng*, Duckweed and Scutellaria Decoction

干葛解肌汤 *gān gé jiě jī tāng*, Pueraria Flesh-Resolving Decoction

感冒二方 *gǎn mào èr fāng*, Common Cold Formula 2

加味麻杏石甘汤 *jiā wèi má xìng shí gān tāng*, Supplemented Ephedra, Apricot Kernel, Gypsum, and Licorice Decoction

麻杏甘石汤 *má xìng gān shí tāng*, Ephedra, Apricot Kernel, Licorice, and Gypsum Decoction, also called Ephedra, Apricot Kernel, Gypsum, and Licorice Decoction (*má xìng shí gān tāng*), and Ephedra, Apricot Kernel, Gypsum, and Licorice Decoction (*má huáng xìng rén shí gāo gān cǎo tāng*)

羌蓝汤 *qiāng lán tāng*, Notopterygium and Isatis Root Decoction

桑菊饮 *sāng jú yǐn*, Mulberry Leaf and Chrysanthemum Beverage

升麻葛根汤 *shēng má gé gēn tāng*, Cimicifuga and Pueraria Decoction

铁笛丸 *tiě dí wán*, Iron Flute Pill

响声破笛丸 *xiǎng shēng pò dí wán*, Broken Flute Pill

新加香薷饮 *xīn jiā xiāng rú yǐn*, Newly Supplemented Mosla Beverage

宣毒发表汤 *xuān dú fā biǎo tāng*, Toxin-Diffusing Exterior-Effusing Decoction

银翘马勃散 *yín qiào mǎ bó sǎn*, Lonicera, Forsythia, and Puffball Powder

银翘散 *yín qiào sǎn*, Lonicera and Forsythia Powder

银翘汤 *yín qiào tāng*, Lonicera and Forsythia Decoction

越婢汤 *yuè bì tāng*, Spleen-Effusing Decoction

竹叶柳蒡汤 *zhú yè liǔ bàng tāng*, Lophatherum, Tamarisk, and Arctium Decoction

滋阴解表
Enrich yīn and resolve the exterior

归葛汤 *guī gé tāng*, Chinese Angelica and Pueraria Decoction

加减葳蕤汤 *jiā jiǎn wēi ruí tāng*, Solomon's Seal Variant Decoction

葱白七味饮 *cōng bái qī wèi yǐn*, Scallion White Seven-Ingredient Beverage (nourishes the blood and resolves the exterior)

助阳解表
Assist yáng and resolve the exterior

麻黄附子甘草汤 *má huáng fù zǐ gān cǎo tāng*, Ephedra, Aconite, and Licorice Decoction

麻黄附子细辛汤 *má huáng fù zǐ xì xīn tāng*, Ephedra, Aconite, and Asarum Decoction

再造散 *zài zào sǎn*, Renewal Powder

益气解表
Boost qì and resolve the exterior

仓廪散 *cāng lǐn sǎn*, Old Rice Granary Powder

人参败毒散 *rén shēn bài dú sǎn*, Ginseng Toxin-Vanquishing Powder

参苏饮 *shēn sū yǐn*, Ginseng and Perilla Beverage

十味香薷饮 *shí wèi xiāng rú yǐn*, Ten-Ingredient Mosla Beverage

表里双解
Resolve both exterior and interior

大柴胡汤 *dà chái hú tāng*, Major Bupleurum Decoction

防风通圣散 *fáng fēng tōng shèng sǎn*, Saposhnikovia Sage-Inspired Powder

桂枝加大黄汤 *guì zhī jiā dà huáng tāng*, Cinnamon Twig Decoction Plus Rhubarb

厚朴七物汤 *hòu pò qī wù tāng*, Officinal Magnolia Bark Seven Agents Decoction

三黄石膏汤 *sān huáng shí gāo tāng*, Three Yellows and Gypsum Decoction

石膏汤 *shí gāo tāng*, Gypsum Decoction

五积散 *wǔ jī sǎn*, Five Accumulations Powder

清热剂
Heat-Clearing Formulas

清气分热
Clear qì-aspect heat

白虎加地黄汤 *bái hǔ jiā dì huáng tāng*, White Tiger Decoction Plus Rehmannia

白虎加桂枝汤 *bái hǔ jiā guì zhī tāng*, White Tiger Decoction Plus Cinnamon Twig

白虎加人参汤 *bái hǔ jiā rén shēn tāng*, White Tiger Decoction Plus Ginseng

白虎汤 *bái hǔ tāng*, White Tiger Decoction

镇逆白虎汤 *zhèn nì bái hǔ tāng*, Counterflow-Settling White Tiger Decoction

栀子豉汤 *zhī zǐ chǐ tāng*, Gardenia and Fermented Soybean Decoction

栀子甘草豉汤 *zhī zǐ gān cǎo chǐ tāng*, Gardenia, Licorice, and Fermented Soybean Decoction

栀子厚朴汤 *zhī zǐ hòu pò tāng*, Gardenia and Officinal Magnolia Bark Decoction

栀子生姜豉汤 *zhī zǐ shēng jiāng chǐ tāng*, Gardenia, Fresh Ginger, and Fermented Soybean Decoction

竹叶石膏汤 *zhú yè shí gāo tāng*, Lophatherum and Gypsum Decoction

清营凉血
Clear construction and cool the blood

加减玉女煎 *jiā jiǎn yù nü jiān*, Jade Lady Variant Brew

荆芩四物汤 *jīng qín sì wù tāng*, Schizonepeta and Scutellaria Four Agents Decoction

芩连四物汤 *qín lián sì wù tāng*, Scutellaria and Coptis Four Agents Decoction

清宫汤 *qīng gōng tāng*, Palace-Clearing Decoction

清营汤 *qīng yíng tāng*, Construction-Clearing Decoction

三黄四物汤 *sān huáng sì wù tāng*, Three Yellows Four Agents Decoction

四物加黄芩黄连汤 *sì wù jiā huáng qín huáng lián tāng*, Four Agents Decoction Plus Scutellaria and Coptis

犀地清络饮 *xī dì qīng luò yǐn*, Rhinoceros Horn and Rehmannia Network-Clearing Beverage

犀角地黄汤 *xī jiǎo dì huáng tāng*, Rhinoceros Horn and Rehmannia Decoction

先期汤 *xiān qí tāng*, Premature Periods Decoction

瘀血灌眼睛方 *yū xuè guàn yǎn jīng fāng*, Eye Stasis Formula

气营两清
Clear both qì and construction

黑膏（方）*hēi gāo* (*fāng*), Black Paste (Formula)

化斑汤 *huà bān tāng*, Macule-Transforming Decoction

清瘟败毒饮 *qīng wēn bài dú yǐn*, Scourge-Clearing Toxin-Vanquishing Beverage

清热解暑
Clear heat and resolve summerheat

碧玉散 *bì yù sǎn*, Jasper Jade Powder

桂苓甘露饮 *guì líng gān lù yǐn*, Cinnamon and Poria Sweet Dew Beverage

鸡苏散 *jī sū sǎn*, Mint Powder

李氏清暑益气汤 *lǐ shì qīng shǔ yì qì tāng*, Lǐ's Summerheat-Clearing Qì-Boosting Decoction

六一散 *liù yī sǎn*, Six-to-One Powder

清络饮 *qīng luò yǐn*, Network-Clearing Beverage

清暑益气汤 *qīng shǔ yì qì tāng*, Summerheat-Clearing Qì-Boosting Decoction

王氏清暑益气汤 *wáng shì qīng shǔ yì qì tāng*, Wang's Summerheat-Clearing Qì-Boosting Decoction

益元散 *yì yuán sǎn*, Origin-Boosting Powder

清热解毒
Clear heat and resolve toxin

板蓝大青汤 *bǎn lán dà qīng tāng*, Isatis Root and Leaf Decoction

感冒退热冲剂 *gǎn mào tuì rè chōng jì*, Common Cold Fever-Abating Granules

化斑解毒汤 *huà bān jiě dú tāng*, Macule-Transforming Toxin-Resolving Decoction

黄连解毒汤 *huáng lián jiě dú tāng*, Coptis Toxin-Resolving Decoction

解热散血汤 *jiě rè sàn xuè tāng*, Heat-Resolving Blood-Dissipating Decoction

抗白喉合剂 *kàng bái hóu hé jì*, Diphtheria Mixture

普济消毒饮 *pǔ jì xiāo dú yǐn*, Universal Aid Toxin-Dispersing Beverage

普济消毒饮去升麻柴胡黄芩黄连方 *pǔ jì xiāo dú yǐn qù shēng má chái hú huáng qín huáng lián*, Universal Aid Toxin-Dispersing Beverage Minus Cimicifuga, Bupleurum, Scutellaria, & Coptis

清解片 *qīng jiě piàn*, Clearing Resolution Tablet

宣明丸 *xuān míng wán*, Brightness Pill

玄参解毒汤 *xuán shēn jiě dú tāng*, Scrophularia Toxin-Resolving Decoction

玄参升麻汤 *xuán shēn shēng má tāng*, Scrophularia and Cimicifuga Decoction

银黄片 *yín huáng piàn*, Lonicera and Scutellaria Tablet

治乙脑方 *zhì yǐ nǎo fāng*, Encephalitis Formula

清宁丸 *qīng níng wán*, Clear and Quiet Pill

清脏腑热
Clear bowel and visceral heat

白头翁汤 *bái tóu wēng tāng*, Pulsatilla Decoction

柴胡清肝散 *chái hú qīng gān sǎn*, Bupleurum Liver-Clearing Powder

当归龙荟丸 *dāng guī lóng huì wán*, Chinese Angelica, Gentian, and Aloe Pill

导赤散 *dǎo chì sǎn*, Red-Abducting Powder

耳聋丸 *ěr lóng wán*, Deafness Pill

甘草栀子汤 *gān cǎo zhī zǐ tāng*, Licorice and Gardenia Decoction

甘露饮 *gān lù yǐn*, Sweet Dew Beverage

葛根黄芩黄连汤 *gé gēn huáng qín huáng lián tāng*, Pueraria, Scutellaria, and Coptis Decoction

黄连羊肝丸 *huáng lián yáng gān wán*, Coptis and Goat's Liver Pill

黄芩汤 *huáng qín tāng*, Scutellaria Decoction

加味白头翁汤 *jiā wèi bái tóu wēng tāng*, Supplemented Pulsatilla Decoction

菌痢草药方 *jùn lì cǎo yào fāng*, Bacillary Dysentery Herbal Formula

连附六一汤 *lián fù liù yī tāng*, Coptis and Aconite Six-to-One Decoction

凉膈连翘散 *liáng gé lián qiào sǎn*, Diaphragm-Cooling Forsythia Powder

凉膈散 *liáng gé sǎn*, Diaphragm-Cooling Powder

龙胆泻肝汤 *lóng dǎn xiè gān tāng*, Gentian Liver-Draining Decoction

清肺饮子 *qīng fèi yǐn zǐ*, Lung-Clearing Drink

清胃散 *qīng wèi sǎn*, Stomach-Clearing Powder

清心莲子饮 qīng xīn lián zǐ yǐn, Heart-Clearing Lotus Seed Beverage

清眩饮 qīng xuàn yǐn, Dizziness-Clearing Beverage

清胰二号 qīng yí èr hào, Pancreas-Clearing Formula No. 2

清胰一号 qīng yí yī hào, Pancreas-Clearing Formula No. 1

芍药汤 sháo yào tāng, Peony Decoction

退热散 tuì rè sǎn, Heat-Abating Powder

犀角散 xī jiǎo sǎn, Rhinoceros Horn Powder

香连丸 xiāng lián wán, Costusroot and Coptis Pill

泻白散 xiè bái sǎn, White-Draining Powder

泻肝安神丸 xiè gān ān shén wán, Liver-Draining Spirit-Quieting Pill

泻黄散 xiè huáng sǎn, Yellow-Draining Powder

泻脾散 xiè pí sǎn, Spleen-Draining Powder

泻青丸 xiè qīng wán, Green-Blue–Draining Pill

泻心汤 xiè xīn tāng, Heart-Draining Decoction

玉女煎 yù nü jiān, Jade Lady Brew

知母饮 zhī mǔ yǐn, Anemarrhena Beverage

栀子柏皮汤 zhī zǐ bǎi pí tāng, Gardenia and Phellodendron Decoction

竹叶汤 zhú yè tāng, Lophatherum Decoction

左金丸 zuǒ jīn wán, Left-Running Metal Pill

清虚热
Clear vacuity heat

当归六黄汤 dāng guī liù huáng tāng, Chinese Angelica Six Yellows Decoction

地骨皮饮 dì gǔ pí yǐn, Lycium Root Bark Beverage

两地汤 liǎng dì tāng, Rehmannia and Lycium Root Bark Decoction

秦艽鳖甲散 qín jiāo biē jiǎ sǎn, Large Gentian and Turtle Shell Powder

秦艽扶羸汤 qín jiāo fú léi tāng, Large Gentian Emaciation Decoction

清骨散 qīng gǔ sǎn, Bone-Clearing Powder

青蒿鳖甲汤 qīng hāo biē jiǎ tāng, Sweet Wormwood and Turtle Shell Decoction

清经汤（散）qīng jīng tāng (sǎn), Channel-Clearing (Menses-Clearing) Decoction (Powder)

知柏地黄丸 zhī bǎi dì huáng wán, Anemarrhena, Phellodendron, and Rehmannia Pill

滋阴降火汤 zī yīn jiàng huǒ tāng, Yīn-Enriching Fire-Downbearing Decoction

泻下剂
Precipitant Formulas

寒下
Cold precipitation

白虎承气汤 bái hǔ chéng qì tāng, White Tiger Qì-Coordinating Decoction

大承气汤 dà chéng qì tāng, Major Qì-Coordinating Decoction

大陷胸汤 *dà xiàn xiōng tāng*, Major Chest Bind Decoction

大陷胸丸 *dà xiàn xiōng wán*, Major Chest Bind Pill

导赤承气汤 *dǎo chì chéng qì tāng*, Red-Abducting Qì-Coordinating Decoction

复方大承气汤 *fù fāng dà chéng qì tāng*, Compound Formula Major Qì-Coordinating Decoction

厚朴三物汤 *hòu pò sān wù tāng*, Official Magnolia Bark Three Agents Decoction

三一承气汤 *sān yī chéng qì tāng*, Three-in-One Qì-Coordinating Decoction

调胃承气汤 *tiáo wèi chéng qì tāng*, Stomach-Regulating Qì-Coordinating Decoction

小承气汤 *xiǎo chéng qì tāng*, Minor Qì-Coordinating Decoction

宣白承气汤 *xuān bái chéng qì tāng*, White-Diffusing Qì-Coordinating Decoction

温下
Warm precipitation

半硫丸 *bàn liú wán*, Pinellia and Sulfur Pill

大黄附子汤 *dà huáng fù zǐ tāng*, Rhubarb and Aconite Decoction

三物白散 *sān wù bái sǎn*, Three Agents White Powder

三物备急丸 *sān wù bèi jí wán*, Three Agents Emergency Pill

三物小白散 *sān wù xiǎo bái sǎn*, Three Agents Little White Powder

温脾汤 *wēn pí tāng*, Spleen-Warming Decoction

润下
Moist precipitation

更衣丸 *gēng yī wán*, Toilette Pill

济川煎 *jì chuān jiān*, Ferry Brew

麻子仁丸 *má zǐ rén wán*, Cannabis Fruit Pill

润肠汤 *rùn cháng tāng*, Intestine-Moistening Decoction

润肠丸 *rùn cháng wán*, Intestine-Moistening Pill

五仁汤 *wǔ rén tāng*, Five Kernels Decoction

五仁丸 *wǔ rén wán*, Five Kernels Pill

攻补兼施
Simultaneous supplementation and attack

承气养营汤 *chéng qì yǎng yíng tāng*, Qì-Coordinating Construction-Nourishing Decoction

黄龙汤 *huáng lóng tāng*, Yellow Dragon Decoction

新加黄龙汤 *xīn jiā huáng lóng tāng*, Newly Supplemented Yellow Dragon Decoction

玉烛散 *yù zhú sǎn*, Jade Candle Powder

增液承气汤 *zēng yè chéng qì tāng*, Humor-Increasing Qì-Coordinating Decoction

逐水
Expel water

己椒苈黄丸 *jǐ jiāo lì huáng wán*, Fangji, Zanthoxylum, Lepidium/Descurainiae, and Rhubarb Pill

莱朴通结汤 *lái pò tōng jié tāng*, Radish Seed and Official

Magnolia Bark Bind-Freeing Decoction

三花神佑丸 *sān huā shén yòu wán*, Three Flowers Spirit Protection Pill

十枣汤 *shí zǎo tāng*, Ten Jujubes Decoction

续随子丸 *xù suí zǐ wán*, Caper Spurge Seed Pill

禹功散 *yǔ gōng sǎn*, Water Controller Yu Powder

舟车丸 *zhōu chē (jū) wán*, Boats and Carts Pill

子龙丸 *zǐ lóng wán*, Young Dragon Pill

和解剂
Harmonizing Formulas

和解少阳
Harmonize lesser yáng

柴胡枳桔汤 *chái hú zhǐ jié tāng*, Bupleurum Decoction Plus Bitter Orange and Platycodon

小柴胡汤 *xiǎo chái hú tāng*, Minor Bupleurum Decoction

柴胡桂枝干姜汤 *chái hú guì zhī gān jiāng tāng*, Bupleurum, Cinnamon Twig, and Dried Ginger Decoction

调和肝脾
Harmonize the liver and stomach

柴胡疏肝散 *chái hú shū gān sǎn*, Bupleurum Liver-Coursing Powder

柴芍六君子汤 *chái sháo liù jūn zǐ tāng*, Bupleurum and Peony Six Gentlemen Decoction

丹栀逍遥散 *dān zhī xiāo yáo sǎn*, Moutan and Gardenia Free Wanderer Powder

黑逍遥散 *hēi xiāo yáo sǎn*, Black Free Wanderer Powder

四逆散 *sì nì sǎn*, Counterflow Cold Powder

痛泻要方 *tòng xiè yào fāng*, Pain and Diarrhea Formula

戊己丸 *wù jǐ wán*, Fifth and Sixth Heavenly Stem Pill

逍遥散 *xiāo yáo sǎn*, Free Wanderer Powder

调和胃肠
Harmonize the stomach and intestines

半夏泻心汤 *bàn xià xiè xīn tāng*, Pinellia Heart-Draining Decoction

甘草泻心汤 *gān cǎo xiè xīn tāng*, Licorice Heart-Draining Decoction

黄连汤 *huáng lián tāng*, Coptis Decoction

生姜泻心汤 *shēng jiāng xiè xīn tāng*, Fresh Ginger Heart-Draining Decoction

失笑丸 *shī xiào wán*, Sudden Smile Pill

治疟
Control malaria

柴胡达原饮 *chái hú dá yuán yǐn*, Bupleurum Membrane-Source–Opening Beverage

达原饮 *dá yuán yǐn*, Membrane-Source–Opening Beverage

截疟七宝饮 *jié nüè qī bǎo yǐn*, Malaria-Interrupting Seven-Jewel Beverage

七宝散 *qī bǎo sǎn*, Seven-Jewel Powder

清脾饮 *qīng pí yǐn*,
Spleen-Clearing Beverage

祛湿剂
Dampness-Dispelling Formulas

燥湿和胃
Dry dampness and harmonize the stomach

不换金正气散 *bù huàn jīn zhèng qì sǎn*, Priceless Qì-Righting Powder

柴平汤 *chái píng tāng*, Bupleurum Stomach-Calming Decoction

二加减正气散 *èr jiā jiǎn zhèng qì sǎn*, Second Variant Qì-Righting Powder

葛花解醒汤 *gé huā jiě chéng tāng*, Pueraria Flower Liquor-Resolving Decoction

藿香正气散 *huò xiāng zhèng qì sǎn*, Agastache Qì-Righting Powder

六和汤 *liù hé tāng*, Six Harmonizations Decoction

平胃散 *píng wèi sǎn*, Stomach-Calming Powder

神术散 *shén zhú sǎn*, Wondrous Atractylodes Powder

暑湿正气丸 *shǔ shī zhèng qì wán*, Summerheat-Damp Qì-Righting Pill

四加减正气散 *sì jiā jiǎn zhèng qì sǎn*, Fourth Variant Qì-Righting Powder

缩脾饮 *suō pí yǐn*, Amomum Splenic Beverage

胃苓汤 *wèi líng tāng*, Stomach-Calming Poria Five Decoction

五加减正气散 *wǔ jiā jiǎn zhèng qì sǎn*, Fifth Variant Qì-Righting Powder

许学士神术散 *xǔ xué shì shén zhú sǎn*, Xǔ's Wondrous Atractylodes Powder

一加减正气散 *yī jiā jiǎn zhèng qì sǎn*, First Variant Qì-Righting Powder

醉乡玉屑 *zuì xiāng yù xiè*, Enchanted Land Jade Shavings

清热祛湿
Clear heat and dispel dampness

八正散 *bā zhèng sǎn*, Eight Corrections Powder

萆薢渗湿汤 *bì xiè shèn shī tāng*, Fish Poison Yam Dampness-Percolating Decoction

蚕矢汤 *cán shǐ tāng*, Silkworm Droppings Decoction

胆道排石汤 *dǎn dào pái shí tāng*, Biliary Calculus Decoction

当归拈痛汤 *dāng guī niān tòng tāng*, Chinese Angelica Pain-Assuaging Decoction

二妙散（丸）*èr miào sǎn (wán)*, Mysterious Two Powder (Pill)

茯苓皮汤 *fú líng pí tāng*, Poria Skin Decoction

附子泻心汤 *fù zǐ xiè xīn tāng*, Aconite Heart-Draining Decoction

肝胆管结石方 *gān dǎn guǎn jié shí fāng*, Hepatolith Formula

甘露消毒丹 *gān lù xiāo dú dān*, Sweet Dew Toxin-Dispersing Elixir

蒿芩清胆汤 *hāo qín qīng dǎn tāng*, Sweet Wormwood and

Scutellaria Gallbladder-Clearing Decoction

琥珀散 *hǔ pò sǎn*, Amber Powder

化石散 *huà shí sǎn*, Stone-Transforming Powder

化阴煎 *huà yīn jiān*, Yīn-Forming Brew

黄疸茵陈冲剂 *huáng dǎn yīn chén chōng jì*, Jaundice Virgate Wormwood Granules

黄芩滑石汤 *huáng qín huá shí tāng*, Scutellaria and Talcum Decoction

藿朴夏苓汤 *huò pò xià líng tāng*, Agastache, Official Magnolia Bark, Pinellia, and Poria Decoction

加减木防己汤 *jiā jiǎn mù fáng jǐ táng*, Woody Fangji Variant Decoction

利胆排石片 *lì dǎn pái shí piàn*, Gallbladder-Disinhibiting Stone-Expelling Tablet

利胆退黄汤 *lì dǎn tuì huáng tāng*, Gallbladder-Disinhibiting Jaundice-Abating Decoction

连朴饮 *lián pò yǐn*, Coptis and Officinal Magnolia Bark Beverage

木通散 *mù tōng sǎn*, Trifoliate Akebia Powder

排石汤 *pái shí tāng*, Stone-Expelling Decoction

清胆利湿汤 *qīng dǎn lì shī tāng*, Gallbladder-Clearing Dampness-Disinhibiting Decoction

清肝渗湿汤 *qīng gān shèn shī tāng*, Liver-Clearing Dampness-Percolating Decoction

青麟丸 *qīng lín wán*, Green-Blue Unicorn Pill

清宁丸 *qīng níng wán*, Clear and Quiet Pill

三加减正气散 *sān jiā jiǎn zhèng qì sǎn*, Third Variant Qì-Righting Powder

三金汤 *sān jīn tāng*, Golden Three Decoction

三妙散 *sān miǎo sǎn*, Mysterious Three Powder

三妙丸 *sān miào wán*, Mysterious Three Pill

三仁汤 *sān rén tāng*, Three Kernels Decoction

石苇散 *shí wéi sǎn*, Pyrrosia Powder

四妙丸 *sì miào wán*, Mysterious Four Pill

五淋散 *wǔ lín sǎn*, Five Stranguries Powder

五痿汤 *wǔ wěi tāng*, Five Wiltings Decoction

消白饮 *xiāo bái yǐn*, Whiteness-Dispersing Beverage

泻湿汤 *xiè shī tāng*, Dampness-Draining Decoction

薏苡竹叶散 *yì yǐ zhú yè sǎn*, Coix and Lophatherum Powder

茵陈蒿汤 *yīn chén hāo tāng*, Virgate Wormwood Decoction

茵陈五苓散 *yīn chén wǔ líng sǎn*, Virgate Wormwood and Poria Five Powder

中满分消丸 *zhōng mǎn fēn xiāo wán*, Center Fullness Separating and Dispersing Pill

滋肾丸 *zī shèn wán*, Kidney-Enriching Pill

利水渗湿
Disinhibit water and percolate dampness

白术散 *bái zhú sǎn*, White Atractylodes Powder

春泽汤 *chūn zé tāng*, Spring Pond Decoction

导水茯苓汤 *dǎo shuǐ fú líng tāng*, Water-Abducting Poria Decoction

防己茯苓汤 *fáng jǐ fú líng tāng*, Fangji and Poria Decoction

防己黄芪汤 *fáng jǐ huáng qí tāng*, Fangji and Astragalus Decoction

廓清饮 *kuò qīng yǐn*, Thorough Clearing Beverage

牡蛎泽泻散 *mǔ lì zé xiè sǎn*, Oyster Shell and Alisma Powder

木防己汤 *mù fáng jǐ tāng*, Woody Fangji Decoction

四苓散 *sì líng sǎn*, Poria Four Powder

五苓散 *wǔ líng sǎn*, Poria Five Powder

五皮散（饮）*wǔ pí sǎn (yǐn)*, Five-Peel Powder (Beverage)

猪苓汤 *zhū líng tāng*, Polyporus Decoction

温化水湿
Warm and transform water-damp

萆薢分清饮 *bì xiè fēn qīng yǐn*, Fish Poison Yam Clear-Turbid Separation Beverage

茯苓甘草汤 *fú líng gān cǎo tāng*, Poria and Licorice Decoction

甘草干姜茯苓白术汤 *gān cǎo gān jiāng fú líng bái zhú tāng*, Licorice, Dried Ginger, Poria, and White Atractylodes Decoction

鸡鸣散 *jī míng sǎn*, Cockcrow Powder

理苓汤 *lǐ líng tāng*, Rectifying Poria Decoction

苓桂术甘汤 *líng guì zhú gān tāng*, Poria, Cinnamon Twig, White Atractylodes, and Licorice Decoction

肾着汤 *shèn zhuó tāng*, Kidney Fixity Decoction

实脾饮 *shí pí yǐn*, Spleen-Firming Beverage

真武汤 *zhēn wǔ tāng*, True Warrior Decoction

术附汤 *zhú fù tāng*, White Atractylodes and Aconite Decoction

胡芦巴散 *hú lú bā sǎn*, Fenugreek Powder

葫芦巴丸 *hú lú bā wán*, Fenugreek Pill

木瓜牛膝丸 *mù guā niú xī wán*, Chaenomeles and Achyranthes Pill

定痛丸 *dìng tòng wán*, Pain-Relieving Pill

祛风胜湿
Dispel wind and overcome dampness

白薇丸 *bái wēi wán*, Black Sallowwort Pill

白术附子汤 *bái zhú fù zǐ tāng*, White Atractylodes and Aconite Decoction

百一蠲痹汤 *bǎi yī juān bì tāng*, Hundred and One Formulas Impediment-Alleviating Decoction

豹骨木瓜酒 *bào gǔ mù guā jiǔ*, Leopard's Bone and Chaenomelis Wine

程氏蠲痹汤 *chéng shì juàn bì tāng*, Cheng's Impediment-Alleviating Decoction

除湿蠲痹汤 *chú shī juān bì tāng*, Dampness-Eliminating Impediment-Alleviating Decoction

除湿汤 *chú shī tāng*, Damp-Eliminating Decoction

大活络丹 *dà huó luò dān*, Major Network-Quickening Elixir

防己汤 *fáng jǐ tāng*, Fangji Decoction

风湿豨桐片 *fēng shī xī tóng piàn*, Siegesbeckia and Clerodendron Wind-Damp Tablet

甘草附子汤 *gān cǎo fù zǐ tāng*, Licorice and Aconite Decoction

桂枝附子汤 *guì zhī fù zǐ tāng*, Cinnamon Twig and Aconite Decoction

桂枝加术附汤 *guì zhī jiā zhú fù tāng*, Cinnamon Twig Decoction Plus White Atractylodes and Aconite

国公酒 *guó gōng jiǔ*, Statesman Wine

海桐皮酒 *hǎi tóng pí jiǔ*, Erythrina Wine

活络丹 *huó luò dān*, Network-Quickening Elixir

蠲痹汤 *juān bì tāng*, Impediment-Alleviating Decoction

羌活除湿汤 *qiāng huó chú shī tāng*, Notopterygium Dampness-Eliminating Decoction

羌活胜湿汤 *qiāng huó shèng shī tāng*, Notopterygium Dampness-Overcoming Decoction

三痹汤 *sān bì tāng*, Three Impediment Decoction

桑枝虎杖汤 *sāng zhī hǔ zhàng tāng*, Mulberry Twig and Bushy Knotweed Decoction

上中下通用痛风方 *shàng zhōng xià tōng yòng tòng fēng fāng*, Upper, Middle, and Lower Body General-Use Wind Pain Formula

史国公浸酒方 *shǐ guó gōng jìn jiǔ fāng*, Statesman Shi's Wine-Steeped Formula

五痹汤 *wǔ bì tāng*, Five Impediments Decoction

豨桐丸 *xī tóng wán*, Siegesbeckia and Clerodendron Pill

小活络丹 *xiǎo huó luò dān*, Minor Network-Quickening Elixir

薏苡仁汤 *yì yǐ rén tāng*, Coix Decoction

独活寄生汤 *dú huó jì shēng tāng*, Pubescent Angelica and Mistletoe Decoction

舒筋汤 *shū jīn tāng*, Sinew-Soothing Decoction

润燥剂
Dryness-Moistening Formulas

轻宣润燥
Moisten dryness by light diffusion

翘荷汤 *qiào hé tāng*, Forsythia and Mint Decoction

清燥救肺汤 *qīng zào jiù fèi tāng*, Dryness-Clearing Lung-Rescuing Decoction

桑杏汤 *sāng xìng tāng*, Mulberry Leaf and Apricot Kernel Decoction

杏苏散 *xìng sū sǎn*, Apricot Kernel and Perilla Powder

滋阴润燥
Enrich yīn and moisten dryness

百合固金汤 *bǎi hé gù jīn tāng*, Lily Bulb Metal-Securing Decoction

百花膏 *bǎi huā gāo*, Lily Bulb and Coltsfoot Paste

补肺阿胶汤 *bǔ fèi ē jiāo tāng*, Ass Hide Glue Decoction

阿胶散 *ē jiāo sǎn*, Ass Hide Glue Powder

阿胶汤 *ē jiāo tāng*, Ass Hide Glue Decoction

黄芪汤 *huáng qí tāng*, Astragalus Decoction

活血润燥生津散 *huó xuè rùn zào shēng jīn sǎn*, Blood-Quickening Dryness-Moistening Liquid-Engendering Powder

连梅汤 *lián méi tāng*, Coptis and Mume Decoction

麦门冬汤 *mài mén dōng tāng*, Ophiopogon Decoction

清咽养营汤 *qīng yān yǎng yíng tāng*, Throat-Clearing Construction-Nourishing Decoction

琼玉膏 *qióng yù gāo*, Fine Jade Paste

润燥安胎汤 *rùn zào ān tāi tāng*, Dryness-Moistening Fetus-Quieting Decoction

沙参麦冬汤 *shā shēn mài dōng tāng*, Adenophora/Glehnia and Ophiopogon Decoction

四阴汤 *sì yīn tāng*, Four-Yīn Decoction

五汁饮 *wǔ zhī yǐn*, Five Juices Beverage

消渴方 *xiāo kě fāng*, Dispersion-Thirst Formula

养胃汤 *yǎng wèi tāng*, Stomach-Nourishing Decoction

养阴清肺汤 *yǎng yīn qīng fèi tāng*, Yīn-Nourishing Lung-Clearing Decoction

益胃汤 *yì wèi tāng*, Stomach-Boosting Decoction

玉液汤 *yù yè tāng*, Jade Humor Decoction

增液汤 *zēng yè tāng*, Humor-Increasing Decoction

温里剂
Interior-Warming Formulas

温中散寒
Warm the center and dispel cold

大建中汤 *dà jiàn zhōng tāng*, Major Center-Fortifying Decoction

当归建中汤 *dāng guī jiàn zhōng tāng*, Chinese Angelica Center-Fortifying Decoction

丁桂散 *dīng guì sǎn*, Clove and Cinnamon Powder

丁萸理中汤 *dīng yú lǐ zhōng tāng*, Clove and Evodia Center-Rectifying Decoction

附桂理中丸 *fù guì lǐ zhōng wán*, Aconite and Cinnamon Center-Rectifying Pill

附子粳米汤 *fù zǐ gěng mǐ tāng*, Aconite and Rice Decoction

附子理中丸 *fù zǐ lǐ zhōng wán*, Aconite Center-Rectifying Pill

甘草干姜汤 *gān cǎo gān jiāng tāng*, Licorice and Dried Ginger Decoction

桂附理中汤 *guì fù lǐ zhōng tāng*, Cinnamon and Aconite Center-Rectifying Decoction

桂枝加桂汤 *guì zhī jiā guì tāng*, Cinnamon Twig Decoction Plus Extra Cinnamon

桂枝人参汤 *guì zhī rén shēn tāng*, Cinnamon Twig and Ginseng Decoction

厚朴温中汤 *hòu pò wēn zhōng tāng*, Officinal Magnolia Bark Center-Warming Decoction

黄芪建中汤 *huáng qí jiàn zhōng tāng*, Astragalus Center-Fortifying Decoction

九痛丸 *jiǔ tòng wán*, Nine Pains Pill

理阴煎 *lǐ yīn jiān*, Yīn-Rectifying Brew

理中汤 *lǐ zhōng tāng*, Center-Rectifying Decoction

理中丸 *lǐ zhōng wán*, Center-Rectifying Pill

人参汤 *rén shēn tāng*, Ginseng Decoction

胃关煎 *wèi guān jiān*, Stomach Gate Brew

温经汤 *wēn jīng tāng*, Channel-Warming (Menses-Warming) Decoction

吴茱萸加附子汤 *wú zhū yú jiā fù zǐ tāng*, Evodia Decoction with Aconite Decoction

吴茱萸汤 *wú zhū yú tāng*, Evodia Decoction

小建中汤 *xiǎo jiàn zhōng tāng*, Minor Center-Fortifying Decoction

茵陈四逆汤 *yīn chén sì nì tāng*, Virgate Wormwood Counterflow Cold Decoction

茵陈术附汤 *yīn chén zhú fù tāng*, Virgate Wormwood, Atractylodes, and Aconite Decoction

枳实理中丸 *zhǐ shí lǐ zhōng wán*, Unripe Bitter Orange Center-Rectifying Pill

治中汤 *zhì zhōng tāng*, Center-Ordering Decoction

逐寒荡惊汤 *zhú hán dàng jīng tāng*, Cold-Dispelling Fright-Assuaging Decoction

回阳救逆
Return yáng and stem counterflow

白通加猪胆汁汤 *bái tōng jiā zhū dǎn zhī tāng*, Scallion Yáng-Freeing Decoction Plus Pig's Bile

白通汤 *bái tōng tāng*, Scallion Yáng-Freeing Decoction

大顺散 *dà shùn sǎn*, Great Rectifying Powder

独参汤 *dú shēn tāng*, Pure Ginseng Decoction

茯苓四逆汤 *fú líng sì nì tāng*, Poria Counterflow Cold Decoction

黑锡丹 *hēi xí dān*, Galenite Elixir

回阳返本汤 *huí yáng fǎn běn tāng*, Yáng-Returning Root-Reviving Decoction

回阳救急汤 *huí yáng jiù jí tāng*, Yáng-Returning Emergency Decoction

浆水散 *jiāng shuǐ sǎn*, Millet Water Powder

芪附汤 *qí fù tāng*, Astragalus and Aconite Decoction

参附龙牡汤 *shēn fù lóng mǔ tāng*, Ginseng, Aconite, Dragon Bone, and Oyster Shell Decoction

参附汤 *shēn fù tāng*, Ginseng and Aconite Decoction

四逆加人参汤 *sì nì jiā rén shēn tāng*, Counterflow Cold Decoction Plus Ginseng

四逆汤 *sì nì tāng*, Counterflow Cold Decoction

通脉四逆汤 *tōng mài sì nì tāng*, Vessel-Freeing Counterflow Cold Decoction

益元汤 *yì yuán tāng*, Origin-Boosting Decoction

正阳散 *zhèng yáng sǎn*, Yáng-Righting Powder

温经散寒
Warm the channels and dissipate cold

当归四逆加吴茱萸生姜汤 *dāng guī sì nì jiā wú zhū yú shēng jiāng tāng*, Chinese Angelica Counterflow Cold Decoction Plus Evodia and Fresh Ginger

当归四逆汤 *dāng guī sì nì tāng*, Chinese Angelica Counterflow Cold Decoction

黄芪桂枝五物汤 *huáng qí guì zhī wǔ wù tāng*, Astragalus and Cinnamon Twig Five Agents Decoction

乌头桂枝汤 *wū tóu guì zhī tāng*, Aconite Main Tuber and Cinnamon Twig Decoction

乌头汤 *wū tóu tāng*, Aconite Main Tuber Decoction

理气剂
Qì-Rectifying Formulas

行气
Move qì

半夏厚朴汤 *bàn xià hòu pò tāng*, Pinellia and Official Magnolia Bark Decoction

肠粘连缓解汤 *cháng zhān lián huǎn jiě tāng*, Intestinal Adhesion Decoction

催生饮 *cuī shēng yǐn*, Birth-Hastening Beverage

导气汤 *dǎo qì tāng*, Qì-Abducting Decoction

栝楼薤白白酒汤 *guā lóu xiè bái bái jiǔ tāng*, Trichosanthes, Chinese Chive, and White Liquor Decoction

栝楼薤白半夏汤 *guā lóu xiè bái bàn xià tāng*, Trichosanthes, Chinese Chive, and Pinellia Decoction

栝楼枳实汤 *guā lóu zhǐ shí tāng*, Trichosanthes and Unripe Bitter Orange Decoction

厚朴生姜半夏甘草人参汤 *hòu pò shēng jiāng bàn xià gān cǎo rén shēn tāng*, Official Magnolia Bark, Fresh Ginger, Pinellia, Licorice, and Ginseng Decoction

化肝煎 *huà gān jiān*, Liver-Transforming Brew

济生橘核丸 *jì shēng jú hé wán*, Life Saver Tangerine Pip Pill

加味乌药汤 *jiā wèi wū yào tāng*, Supplemented Lindera Decoction

金铃子散 *jīn líng zǐ sǎn*, Toosendan Powder

橘核丸 *jú hé wán*, Tangerine Pip Pill

良附丸 *liáng fù wán*, Lesser Galangal and Cyperus Pill

六磨汤 *liù mò tāng*, Six Milled Ingredients Decoction

木香顺气散 *mù xiāng shùn qì sǎn*, Costusroot Qì-Normalizing Powder

木香顺气丸 *mù xiāng shùn qì wán*, Costusroot Qì-Normalizing Pill

暖肝煎 *nuǎn gān jiān*, Liver-Warming Brew

排气饮 *pái qì yǐn*, Qì-Discharging Beverage

启膈散 *qǐ gé sǎn*, Diaphragm-Arousing Powder

清胆行气汤 *qīng dǎn xíng qì tāng*, Gallbladder-Clearing Qì-Moving Decoction

三层茴香丸 *sān céng huí xiāng wán*, Three-Option Anise Pill

十香丸 *shí xiāng wán*, Ten Fragrances Pill

疏肝解郁汤 *shū gān jiě yù tāng*, Liver-Coursing Depression-Resolving Decoction

舒肝丸 *shū gān wán*, Liver-Soothing Pill

舒气散 *shū qì sǎn*, Qì-Smoothing Powder

四磨饮 *sì mò yǐn*, Four Milled Ingredients Beverage

四七汤 *sì qī tāng*, Four-Seven Decoction

天台乌药散 *tiān tái wū yào sǎn*, Tiantai Lindera Powder

调肝散 *tiáo gān sǎn*, Liver-Regulating Powder

通经活络汤 *tōng jīng huó luò tāng*, Channel-Freeing Network-Quickening Decoction

乌药散 *wū yào sǎn*, Lindera Powder

乌药汤 *wū yào tāng*, Lindera Decoction

五磨饮子 *wǔ mò yǐn zǐ*, Five Milled Ingredients Drink

香朴丸 *xiāng pò wán*, Costusroot and Officinal Magnolia Bark Pill

香砂平胃丸 *xiāng shā píng wèi wán*, Costusroot and Amomum Stomach-Calming Pill

越鞠丸 *yuè jú wán*, Depression-Overcoming Pill

正气天香散 *zhèng qì tiān xiāng sǎn*, Qì-Righting Lindera and Cyperus Powder

枳壳散 *zhǐ qiào sǎn*, Bitter Orange Powder

枳实薤白桂枝汤 *zhǐ shí xiè bái guì zhī tāng*, Unripe Bitter Orange, Chinese Chive, and Cinnamon Twig Decoction

紫苏安胎饮 *zǐ sū ān tāi yǐn*, Perilla Leaf Fetus-Quieting Beverage

降逆止呕
Downbear counterflow and check vomiting

大半夏汤 *dà bàn xià tāng*, Major Pinellia Decoction

丁香柿蒂汤 *dīng xiāng shì dì tāng*, Clove and Persimmon Decoction

干姜人参半夏丸 *gān jiāng rén shén bàn xià wán*, Dried Ginger, Ginseng, and Pinellia Pill

济生橘皮竹茹汤 *jì shēng jú pí zhú rú tāng*, Life Saver Tangerine

Peel and Bamboo Shavings
Decoction

橘皮竹茹汤 *jú pí zhú rú tāng*,
Tangerine Peel and Bamboo
Shavings Decoction

茅葛汤 *máo gé tāng*, Imperata and
Pueraria Decoction

芩连橘茹汤 *qíng lián jú rú tāng*,
Scutellaria, Coptis, Tangerine
Peel, and Bamboo Shavings
Decoction

柿蒂汤 *shì dì tāng*, Persimmon
Decoction

柿钱散 *shì qián sǎn*, Gingerless
Clove and Persimmon Powder

小半夏汤 *xiǎo bàn xià tāng*,
Minor Pinellia Decoction

旋覆花代赭石汤 *xuán fù huā dài
zhě shí tāng*, Inula and Hematite
Decoction

竹茹汤 *zhú rú tāng*, Bamboo
Shavings Decoction

降气平喘
Downbear qì and calm panting

定喘汤 *dìng chuǎn tāng*,
Panting-Stabilizing Decoction

九味理中汤 *jiǔ wèi lǐ zhōng tāng*,
Nine-Ingredient
Center-Rectifying Decoction

参赭镇气汤 *shēn zhě zhèn qì
tnag1*, Codonopsis and Hematite
Qì-Settling Decoction

苏子降气汤 *sū zǐ jiàng qì tāng*,
Perilla Seed Qì-Downbearing
Decoction

消导化积剂
Abductive Dispersion and Accumulation-Transforming Formulas

消食导滞
Disperse food and abduct stagnation

保赤散 *bǎo chì sǎn*,
Infant-Safeguarding Red Powder

保和丸 *bǎo hé wán*,
Harmony-Preserving Pill

大安丸 *dà ān wán*, Great
Tranquility Pill

健脾丸 *jiàn pí wán*,
Spleen-Fortifying Pill

橘半枳术丸 *jú bàn zhǐ zhú wán*,
Tangerine Peel, Pinellia, Unripe
Bitter Orange, and White
Atractylodes Pill

木香槟榔丸 *mù xiāng bīng láng
wán*, Costusroot and Areca Pill

木香导滞丸 *mù xiāng dǎo zhì
wán*, Costusroot
Stagnation-Abducting Pill

启脾散 *qǐ pí sǎn*, Spleen-Arousing
Pill

曲麦枳术丸 *qū mài zhǐ zhú wán*,
Medicated Leaven, Barley
Sprout, Unripe Bitter Orange, and
White Atractylodes Pill

曲蘗枳术丸 *qū niè zhǐ zhú wán*,
Medicated Leaven, Barley
Sprout, Unripe Bitter Orange, and
White Atractylodes Pill

人参启脾丸 *rén shēn qǐ pí wán*,
Ginseng Spleen-Arousing Pill

三黄枳术丸 *sān huáng zhǐ zhú
wán*, Three Yellows Bitter Orange
and White Atractylodes Pill

三消饮 *sān xiāo yǐn*, Three
Dispersers Beverage

香砂枳术丸 *xiāng shā zhǐ zhú
wán*, Costusroot, Amomum,

Unripe Bitter Orange, and White Atractylodes Pill

消痞阿魏丸 *xiāo pǐ ē wèi wán*, Glomus-Dispersing Asafetida Pill

小温中丸 *xiǎo wēn zhōng wán*, Minor Center-Warming Pill

楂曲平胃散 *zhā qū píng wèi sǎn*, Crataegus and Medicated Leaven Stomach-Calming Powder

枳实导滞丸 *zhǐ shí dǎo zhì wán*, Unripe Bitter Orange Stagnation-Abducting Pill

枳实消痞丸 *zhǐ shí xiāo pǐ wán*, Unripe Bitter Orange and Glomus-Dispersing Pill

枳术丸 *zhǐ zhú wán*, Unripe Bitter Orange and White Atractylodes Pill

消瘿瘰痰核
Disperse goiter, scrofula, and phlegm nodes

攻消和解软坚汤 *gōng xiāo hé jiě ruǎn jiān tāng*, Offensive Dispersion Harmonizing and Softening Decoction

海藻玉壶汤 *hǎi zǎo yù hú tāng*, Sargassum Jade Flask Decoction

内消瘰疬丸 *nèi xiāo luǒ lì wán*, Scrofula Internal Dispersion Pill

芩连二陈汤 *qín lián èr chén tāng*, Scutellaria and Coptis Two Matured Ingredients Decoction

芩连二母丸 *qín lián èr mǔ wán*, Scutellaria, Coptis, Anemarrhena, and Fritillaria Pill

散肿溃坚汤 *sàn zhǒng kuì jiān tāng*, Swelling-Dispersing Hardness-Breaking Decoction

四海舒郁丸 *sì hǎi shū yù wán*, Four Seas Depression-Soothing Pill

犀黄丸 *xī huáng wán*, Rhinoceros Bezoar Pill

夏枯草膏 *xià kū cǎo gāo*, Prunella Paste

夏枯草汤 *xià kū cǎo tāng*, Prunella Decoction

香贝养营汤 *xiāng bèi yǎng yíng tāng*, Cyperus and Fritillaria Construction-Nourishing Decoction

消瘰丸 *xiāo luǒ wán*, Scrofula-Dispersing Pill

消瘿汤 *xiāo yǐng tāng*, Goiter-Dispersing Decoction

小金丹 *xiǎo jīn dān*, Minor Golden Elixir

消癥瘕积聚
Disperse concretions, conglomerations, accumulations and gatherings

鳖甲煎丸 *biē jiǎ jiān wán*, Turtle Shell Decocted Pill

鳖甲饮子 *biē jiǎ yǐn zǐ*, Turtle Shell Drink

桂枝茯苓丸 *guì zhī fú líng wán*, Cinnamon Twig and Poria Pill

牡丹皮散 *mǔ dān pí sǎn*, Moutan Powder

三棱汤 *sān léng tāng*, Sparganium Decoction

硝石矾石散 *xiāo shí fǎn shí sǎn*, Niter and Alum Powder

驱虫剂
Worm-Expelling Formulas

百部灌肠剂 *bǎi bù guàn cháng jì*, Stemona Enema

布袋丸 *bù dài wán*, Cloth Bag Pill

伐木丸 *fā mù wán*,
Wood-Quelling Pill

肥儿丸 *féi ér wán*, Chubby Child
Pill

榧子贯众汤 *fěi zǐ guàn zhòng
tāng*, Torreya and Aspidium
Decoction

甘草粉蜜汤 *gān cǎo fěn mì tāng*,
Licorice, Processed Galenite, and
Honey Decoction

化虫丸 *huà chóng wán*,
Worm-Transforming Pill

理中安蛔散 *lǐ zhōng ān huí sǎn*,
Center-Rectifying
Roundworm-Quieting Powder

连梅安蛔汤 *lián méi ān huí tāng*,
Picrorhiza and Mume
Roundworm-Quieting Decoction

驱蛔汤二号 *qū huí tāng èr hào*,
Roundworm-Expelling Decoction
No. 2

驱绦汤 *qū tāo tāng*,
Tapeworm-Expelling Decoction

使君子大黄粉 *shǐ jūn zǐ dà huáng
fěn*, Quisqualis and Rhubarb
Powder

使君子散 *shǐ jūn zǐ sǎn*,
Quisqualis Powder

万应丸 *wàn yìng wán*, Myriad
Applications Pill

乌梅丸 *wū méi wán*, Mume Pill

枣矾丸 *zǎo fán wán*, Jujube and
Melanterite Pill

治腹内虫方 *zhì fù nèi chóng fāng*,
Abdominal Worm Formula

追虫丸 *zhuī chóng wán*,
Worm-Expelling Pill

理血剂
Blood-Rectifying Formulas

See "Supplement the blood" under
Supplementing Formulas

祛瘀活血
Dispel stasis and quicken the blood

八厘散 *bā lí sǎn*, Eight Pinches
Powder

补阳还五汤 *bǔ yáng huán wǔ
tāng*, Yáng-Supplementing
Five-Returning Decoction

柴胡细辛汤 *chái hú xì xīn tāng*,
Bupleurum and Asarum
Decoction

大黄蟅虫丸 *dà huáng zhè chóng
wán*, Rhubarb and Ground Beetle
Pill

代抵当丸 *dài dǐ dàng wán*,
Substitute Dead-On Pill

丹参饮 *dān shēn yǐn*, Salvia
Beverage

当归活血汤 *dāng guī huó xuè
tāng*, Chinese Angelica
Blood-Quickening Decoction

抵当汤 *dǐ dàng tāng*, Dead-On
Decoction

抵当丸 *dǐ dàng wán*, Dead-On Pill

夺命丹 *duó mìng dān*,
Life-Clutching Elixir

复元活血汤 *fù yuán huó xuè tāng*,
Origin-Restorative
Blood-Quickening Decoction

膈下逐瘀汤 *gé xià zhú yū tāng*,
Infradiaphragmatic
Stasis-Expelling Decoction

宫外孕二号方 *gōng wài yùn èr
hào fāng*, Ectopic Pregnancy
Formula No. II

冠心二号 *guàn xīn èr hào*,
Coronary No. 2

过期饮 *guò qī yǐn*, Overdue Beverage

活络效灵丹 *huó luò xiào líng dān*, Network-Quickening Efficacious Elixir

接骨丹 *jiē gǔ dān*, Bone-Joining Elixir

救母丹 *jiù mǔ dān*, Mother's Rescue Elixir

七厘散 *qī lí sǎn*, Seven Pinches Powder

三黄宝腊丸 *sān huáng bǎo là wán*, Three Yellow Jewels Wax Pill

三黄腊丸 *sān huáng là wán*, Three Yellows Wax Pill

散结定疼汤 *sàn jié dìng téng tāng*, Bind-Dissipating Pain-Relieving Decoction

少腹逐瘀汤 *shào fù zhú yū tāng*, Lesser Abdomen Stasis-Expelling Decoction

身痛逐瘀汤 *shēn tòng zhú yū tāng*, Generalized Pain Stasis-Expelling Decoction

生化汤 *shēng huà tāng*, Engendering Transformation Decoction

失笑散 *shī xiào sǎn*, Sudden Smile Powder

手拈散 *shǒu niān sǎn*, Instant Relief Powder

舒筋活血片 *shū jīn huó xuè piàn*, Sinew-Soothing Blood-Quickening Tablet

四藤汤 *sì téng tāng*, Four Stems Decoction

桃核承气汤 *táo hé chéng qì tāng*, Peach Kernel Qì-Coordinating Decoction

桃红四物汤 *táo hóng sì wù tāng*, Peach Kernel and Carthamus Four Agents Decoction

桃仁承气汤 *táo rén chéng qì tāng*, Peach Kernel Qì-Coordinating Decoction

通窍活血汤 *tōng qiào huó xuè tāng*, Orifice-Freeing Blood-Quickening Decoction

通瘀煎 *tōng yū jiān*, Stasis-Freeing Brew

下瘀血汤 *xià yū xuè tāng*, Stasis-Precipitating Decoction

血府逐瘀汤 *xuè fǔ zhú yū tāng*, House of Blood Stasis-Expelling Decoction

延胡索汤 *yán hú suǒ tāng*, Corydalis Decoction

益母胜金丹 *yì mǔ shèng jīn dān*, Leonurus (Motherwort) Metal-Overcoming Elixir

止血
Stanch bleeding

白及合剂 *bái jí hé jì*, Bletilla Mixture

白及枇杷丸 *bái jí pí pá wán*, Bletilla and Loquat Pill

柏叶汤 *bǎi yè tāng*, Arborvitae Leaf Decoction

花蕊石散 *huā ruǐ shí sǎn*, Ophicalcite Powder

槐花散 *huái huā sǎn*, Sophora Flower Powder

槐角丸 *huái jiǎo wán*, Sophora Fruit Pill

黄土汤 *huáng tǔ tāng*, Yellow Earth Decoction

咳血方 *ké xuè fāng*, Blood Cough Formula

凉血地黄汤 *liáng xuè dì huáng tāng*, Blood-Cooling Rehmannia Decoction

宁血汤 *níng xuè tāng*, Blood-Quieting Decoction

十灰散（丸）*shí huī sǎn (wán)*, Ten Cinders Powder (Pill)

四生丸 *sì shēng wán*, Four Fresh Agents Pill

小蓟饮子 *xiǎo jì yǐn zǐ*, Field Thistle Drink

脏连丸 *zàng lián wán*, Pig's Intestines and Coptis Pill

止血粉 *zhǐ xuè fěn*, Blood-Stanching Powder

止血汤 *zhǐ xuè tāng*, Blood-Stanching Decoction

猪脏丸 *zhū zàng wán*, Pig's Intestine Pill

祛痰剂
Phlegm-Dispelling Formulas

燥湿化痰
Dry dampness and transform phlegm

半夏茯苓汤 *bàn xià fú líng tāng*, Pinellia and Poria Decoction

导痰汤 *dǎo tán tāng*, Phlegm-Abducting Decoction

二陈汤 *èr chén tāng*, Two Matured Ingredients Decoction

金水六君煎 *jīn shuǐ liù jūn jiān*, Six Gentlemen Metal and Water Brew

六安煎 *liù ān jiān*, Six Quietings Brew

平陈汤 *píng chén tāng*, Calming Matured Ingredients Decoction

温胆汤 *wēn dǎn tāng*, Gallbladder-Warming Decoction

香砂二陈汤 *xiāng shā èr chén tāng*, Costusroot and Amomum Two Matured Ingredients Decoction

指迷茯苓丸 *zhǐ mí fú líng wán*, Pathfinder Poria Pill

宣肺化痰
Diffuse the lung and transform phlegm

华盖散 *huá gài sǎn*, Florid Canopy Powder

金沸草散 *jīn fèi cǎo sǎn*, Inula Powder

伤风咳嗽吞剂 *shāng fēng ké sòu tūn jì*, Wind-Damage Cough Swill-Down Pill

通宣理肺丸 *tōng xuān lǐ fèi wán*, Diffusing-Freeing Lung-Rectifying Pill

止嗽散 *zhǐ sòu sǎn*, Cough-Stopping Powder

清热化痰
Clear heat and transform phlegm

柴胡陷胸汤 *chái hú xiàn xiōng tāng*, Bupleurum Chest Bind Decoction

黛蛤散 *dài gé sǎn*, Indigo and Clamshell Powder

二母散 *èr mǔ sǎn*, Anemarrhena and Fritillaria Powder

甘桔汤 *gān jié tāng*, Licorice and Platycodon Decoction

滚痰丸 *gǔn tán wán*, Phlegm-Rolling Pill

桔梗汤 *jié gěng tāng*, Platycodon Decoction

鸬鹚涎丸 *lú cí xián wán*, Cormorant Drool Pill

礞石滚痰丸 *méng shí gǔn tán wán*, Chlorite/Mica Phlegm-Rolling Pill

气管炎片 *qì guǎn yán piàn*, Bronchitis Tablet

芩部丹 *qín bù dān*, Scutellaria, Stemona, and Salvia Elixir

清肺化痰丸 *qīng fèi huà tán wán*, Lung-Clearing Phlegm-Transforming Pill

清肺汤 *qīng fèi tāng*, Lung-Clearing Decoction

清金化痰汤 *qīng jīn huà tán tāng*, Metal-Clearing Phlegm-Transforming Decoction

清气化痰丸 *qīng qì huà tán wán*, Qì-Clearing Phlegm-Transforming Pill

桑白皮汤 *sāng bái pí tāng*, Mulberry Root Bark Decoction

葶苈大枣泻肺汤 *tíng lì dà zǎo xiè fèi tāng*, Lepidium/Descurainiae and Jujube Lung-Draining Decoction

小陷胸汤 *xiǎo xiàn xiōng tāng*, Minor Chest Bind Decoction

雪羹汤 *xuě gēng tāng*, Snow Soup Decoction

止嗽化痰定喘丸 *zhǐ sòu huà tán dìng chuǎn wán*, Cough-Suppressing Phlegm-Transforming Panting-Stabilizing Pill

竹沥达痰丸 *zhú lì dá tán wán*, Bamboo Sap Phlegm-Outthrusting Pill

温肺化饮（痰）
Warm the lung and transform rheum (phlegm)

冷哮丸 *lěng xiāo wán*, Cold Wheezing Pill

理中化痰丸 *lǐ zhōng huà tán wán*, Center-Rectifying Phlegm-Transforming Pill

苓甘五味姜辛汤 *líng gān wǔ wèi jiāng xīn tāng*, Poria, Licorice, Schisandra, Ginger, and Asarum Decoction

射干麻黄汤 *shè gān má huáng tāng*, Belamcanda and Ephedra Decoction

痰饮丸 *tán yǐn wán*, Phlegm-Rheum Pill

温肺止流丹 *wēn fèi zhǐ liú dān*, Lung-Warming Nose-Drying Elixir

小青龙加石膏汤 *xiǎo qīng lóng jiā shí gāo tāng*, Minor Green-Blue Dragon Decoction Plus Gypsum

小青龙汤 *xiǎo qīng lóng tāng*, Minor Green-Blue Dragon Decoction

越婢加半夏汤 *yuè bì jiā bàn xià tāng*, Spleen-Effusing Decoction Plus Pinellia

润肺化痰
Moisten the lung and transform phlegm

贝母栝蒌散 *bèi mǔ guā lóu sǎn*, Fritillaria and Trichosanthes Powder

润肺散 *rùn fèi sǎn*, Lung-Moistening Powder

紫菀汤 *zǐ wǎn tāng*, Aster Decoction

治风化痰
Control wind and transform phlegm

半夏白术天麻汤 *bàn xià bái zhú tiān má tāng*, Pinellia, White Atractylodes, and Gastrodia Decoction

不换金丹 *bù huàn jīn dān*, Priceless Elixir

大醒风汤 *dà xǐng fēng tāng*, Major Wind Arousal Decoction

钩藤散 *gōu téng sǎn*, Uncaria Powder

青州白丸子 *qīng zhōu bái wán zǐ*, Qīngzhōu White Pill

三生饮 *sān shēng yǐn*, Three Raw Agents Beverage

天南星丸 *tiān nán xīng wán*, Arisaema Pill

星香汤 *xīng xiāng tāng*, Arisaema and Costusroot Decoction

顺气化痰
Normalize qì and transform phlegm

三子养亲汤 *sān zǐ yǎng qīn tāng*, Three-Seed Filial Devotion Decoction

顺气导痰汤 *shùn qì dǎo tán tāng*, Qì-Normalizing Phlegm-Abducting Decoction

顺气消食化痰丸 *shùn qì xiāo shí huà tán wán*, Qì-Normalizing Food-Dispersing Phlegm-Transforming Pill

安神剂
Spirit-Quieting Formulas

重镇安神
Quiet the spirit with heavy settlers

柴胡加龙骨牡蛎汤 *chái hú jiā lóng gǔ mǔ lì tāng*, Bupleurum Decoction Plus Dragon Bone and Oyster Shell

磁朱丸 *cí zhū wán*, Loadstone and Cinnabar Pill

桂枝加龙骨牡蛎汤 *guì zhī jiā lóng gǔ mǔ lì tāng*, Cinnamon Twig Decoction Plus Dragon Bone and Oyster Shell

桂枝救逆汤 *guì zhī jiù nì tāng*, Cinnamon Twig Counterflow-Stemming Decoction

琥珀安神汤 *hǔ pò ān shén tāng*, Amber Spirit-Quieting Decoction

孔圣枕中丹 *kǒng shèng zhěn zhōng dān*, Sagacious Confucius' Pillow Elixir

孔子枕中散 *kǒng zǐ zhěn zhōng sǎn*, Confucius' Pillow Powder

神曲丸 *shén qū wán*, Medicated Leaven Pill

生铁落饮 *shēng tiě luò yǐn*, Iron Flakes Beverage

远志丸 *yuǎn zhì wán*, Polygala Pill

珍珠母丸 *zhēn zhū mǔ wán*, Mother-of-Pearl Pill

枕中丹 *zhěn zhōng dān*, Pillow Elixir

朱砂安神丸 *zhū shā ān shén wán*, Cinnabar Spirit-Quieting Pill

养心安神
Nourish the heart and quiet the spirit

安神定志丸 *ān shén dìng zhì wán*, Spirit-Quieting Mind-Stabilizing Pill

安神丸 *ān shén wán*, Spirit-Quieting Pill

柏子养心丸 *bǎi zǐ yǎng xīn wán*,
Arborvitae Seed
Heart-Nourishing Pill

定志丸 *dìng zhì wán*,
Mind-Stabilizing Pill

阿胶黄连汤 *ē jiāo huáng lián
tāng*, Ass Hide Glue and Coptis
Decoction

甘草小麦大枣汤 *gān cǎo xiǎo
mài dà zǎo tāng*, Licorice, Wheat,
and Jujube Decoction

甘麦大枣汤 *gān mài dà zǎo tāng*,
Licorice, Wheat, and Jujube
Decoction

黄连阿胶汤 *huáng lián ē jiāo
tāng*, Coptis and Ass Hide Glue
Decoction

加味定志丸 *jiā wèi dìng zhì wán*,
Supplemented Mind-Stabilizing
Pill

交泰丸 *jiāo tài wán*, Peaceful
Interaction Pill

妙香散 *miào xiāng sǎn*,
Mysterious Fragrance Powder

人参滋补片 *rén shēn zī bǔ piàn*,
Enriching Ginseng Tablet

三才封髓丹 *sān cái fēng suǐ dān*,
Heaven, Human, and Earth
Marrow-Retaining Elixir

酸枣仁汤 *suān zǎo rén tāng*,
Spiny Jujube Decoction

天王补心丹 *tiān wáng bǔ xīn dān*,
Celestial Emperor
Heart-Supplementing Elixir

养心汤 *yǎng xīn tāng*,
Heart-Nourishing Decoction

滋补片 *zī bǔ piàn*, Enriching
Supplementation Tablet

其他安神剂
Other spirit-quieting formulas

半夏秫米汤 *bàn xià shú mǐ tāng*,
Pinellia and Broomcorn Millet
Decoction

半夏汤 *bàn xià tāng*, Pinellia
Decoction

黄连温胆汤 *huáng lián wēn dǎn
tāng*, Coptis
Gallbladder-Warming Decoction

加味温胆汤 *jiā wèi wēn dǎn tāng*,
Supplemented
Gallbladder-Warming Decoction

十味温胆汤 *shí wèi wēn dǎn tāng*,
Ten-Ingredient
Gallbladder-Warming Decoction

十一味温胆汤 *shí yī wèi wēn dǎn
tāng*, Eleven-Ingredient
Gallbladder-Warming Decoction

祛风剂
Wind-Dispelling Formulas

疏散外风
Course and dissipate external wind

苍耳散 *cāng ěr sǎn*, Xanthium
Powder

苍耳子散 *cāng ěr zǐ sǎn*,
Xanthium Powder

除风益损汤 *chú fēng yì sǔn tāng*,
Wind-Eliminating Boosting
Decoction

川芎茶调散 *chuān xiōng chá tiáo
sǎn*, Tea-Blended Chuanxiong
Powder

大秦艽汤 *dà qín jiāo tāng*, Large
Gentian Decoction

侯氏黑散 *hóu shì hēi sǎn*, Hou's
Black Powder

藿胆丸 *huò dǎn wán*, Agastache
and Pig's Bile Pill

菊花茶调散 *jú huā chá tiáo sǎn*, Tea-Blended Chrysanthemum Powder

决明子散 *jué míng zǐ sǎn*, Fetid Cassia Powder

明目上清丸 *míng mù shàng qīng wán*, Eye Brightener Clear-Raising Pill

清上蠲痛汤 *qīng shàng juān tòng tāng*, Upper-Body-Clearing Pain-Alleviating Decoction

驱风散热饮子 *qū fēng sàn rè yǐn zǐ*, Wind-Expelling Heat-Dissipating Drink

石决明散 *shí jué míng sǎn*, Abalone Shell Powder

疏风养血汤 *shū fēng yǎng xuè tāng*, Wind-Coursing Blood-Nourishing Decoction

洗心散 *xǐ xīn sǎn*, Heart-Washing Powder

消风散 *xiāo fēng sǎn*, Wind-Dispersing Powder

消风养血汤 *xiāo fēng yǎng xuè tāng*, Wind-Dispersing Blood-Nourishing Decoction

小续命汤 *xiǎo xù mìng tāng*, Minor Life-Prolonging Decoction

辛夷散 *xīn yí sǎn*, Officinal Magnolia Flower Powder

修肝汤 *xiū gān tāng*, Liver-Repairing Decoction

平熄内风
Calm and extinguish internal wind

大定风珠 *dà dìng fēng zhū*, Major Wind-Stabilizing Pill

地黄饮子 *dì huáng yǐn zǐ*, Rehmannia Drink

阿胶鸡子黄汤 *ē jiāo jī zǐ huáng tāng*, Ass Hide Glue and Egg Yolk Decoction

钩藤汤 *gōu téng tāng*, Uncaria Decoction

建瓴汤 *jiàn líng tāng*, Sweeping Down Decoction

羚角钩藤汤 *líng jiǎo gōu téng tāng*, Antelope Horn and Uncaria Decoction

羚羊角汤 *líng yáng jiǎo tāng*, Antelope Horn Decoction

三甲复脉汤 *sān jiǎ fù mài tāng*, Triple-Armored Pulse-Restorative Decoction

天麻钩藤饮 *tiān má gōu téng yǐn*, Gastrodia and Uncaria Beverage

镇肝熄风汤 *zhèn gān xī fēng tāng*, Liver-Settling Wind-Extinguishing Decoction

祛风解痉
Dispel wind and resolve tetany

撮风散 *cuò fēng sǎn*, Pursing Wind Powder

钩藤饮 *gōu téng yǐn*, Uncaria Beverage

羚羊角散 *líng yáng jiǎo sǎn*, Antelope Horn Powder

牵正散 *qiān zhèng sǎn*, Pull Aright Powder

五虎追风散 *wǔ hǔ zhuī fēng sǎn*, Five-Tigers-Chasing-the-Wind Powder

玉真散 *yù zhēn sǎn*, True Jade Powder

止痉散 *zhǐ jìng sǎn*, Tetany-Relieving Powder

开窍剂
Orifice-Opening Formulas

清热开窍
Clear heat and open the orifices

安宫牛黄丸 *ān gōng niú huáng wán*, Peaceful Palace Bovine Bezoar Pill

抱龙丸 *bào lóng wán*, Dragon-Embracing Pill

琥珀抱龙丸 *hǔ pò bào lóng wán*, Amber Dragon-Embracing Pill

凉惊丸 *liáng jīng wán*, Fright-Cooling Pill

牛黄抱龙丸 *niú huáng bào lóng wán*, Bovine Bezoar Dragon-Embracing Pill

牛黄清心丸 *niú huáng qīng xīn wán*, Bovine Bezoar Heart-Clearing Pill

神犀丹 *shén xī dān*, Spirit-Like Rhinoceros Horn Elixir

小儿回春丹 *xiǎo ér huí chūn dān*, Children's Return-of-Spring Elixir

行军散 *xíng jūn sǎn*, Troop-Marching Powder

醒脑静 *xǐng nǎo jìng*, Xingnaojing

至宝丹 *zhì bǎo dān*, Supreme Jewel Elixir

紫雪丹 *zǐ xuě dān*, Purple Snow Elixir

逐寒开窍
Expel cold and open the orifices

冠心苏合丸 *guān xīn sū hé wán*, Coronary Storax Pill

红灵丹 *hóng líng dān*, Red Spirit Elixir

苏合香丸 *sū hé xiāng wán*, Storax Pill

通关散 *tōng guān sǎn*, Gate-Freeing Powder

卧龙丹 *wò lóng dān*, Sleeping Dragon Elixir

武侯行军散 *wǔ hóu xíng jūn sǎn*, Warlord's Troop-Marching Powder

玉枢丹 *yù shū dān*, Jade Pivot Elixir

诸葛行军散 *zhū gě xíng jūn sǎn*, Zhuge's Troop-Marching Powder

紫金粉 *zǐ jīn fěn*, Purple Gold Powder

化痰开窍
Transform phlegm and open the orifices

涤痰汤 *dí tán tāng*, Phlegm-Flushing Decoction

癫狂丸 *diān kuáng wán*, Mania and Withdrawal Pill

定痫丸 *dìng xián wán*, Fit-Settling Pill

回春丹 *huí chūn dān*, Return-of-Spring Elixir

补益剂
Supplementing Formulas

补气
Supplement qì

保元汤 *bǎo yuán tāng*, Origin-Preserving Decoction

补肺汤 *bǔ fèi tāng*, Lung-Supplementing Decoction

补中益气汤 *bǔ zhōng yì qì tāng*, Center-Supplementing Qì-Boosting Decoction

举元煎 *jǔ yuán jiān*, Origin-Lifting Brew

六君子汤 *liù jūn zǐ tāng*, Six Gentlemen Decoction

六神散 *liù shén sǎn*, Wondrous Six Powder

七味白术散 *qī wèi bái zhú sǎn*, Seven-Ingredient White Atractylodes Powder

人参蛤蚧散 *rén shēn gé jiè sǎn*, Ginseng and Gecko Powder

人参胡桃汤 *rén shēn hú táo tāng*, Ginseng and Walnut Decoction

人参健脾丸 *rén shēn jiàn pí wán*, Ginseng Spleen-Fortifying Pill

参蚧散 *shēn jiè sǎn*, Ginseng with Gecko Powder

参苓白术散 *shēn líng bái zhú sǎn*, Ginseng, Poria, and White Atractylodes Powder

升陷汤 *shēng xiàn tāng*, Fall-Upbearing Decoction

升阳益胃汤 *shēng yáng yì wèi tāng*, Yáng-Upbearing Stomach-Boosting Decoction

顺气和中汤 *shùn qì hé zhōng tāng*, Qì-Normalizing Center-Harmonizing Decoction

四君子汤 *sì jūn zǐ tāng*, Four Gentlemen Decoction

香砂六君子汤 *xiāng shā liù jūn zǐ tāng*, Costusroot and Amomum Six Gentlemen Decoction

香砂六君子丸 *xiāng shā liù jūn zǐ wán*, Costusroot and Amomum Six Gentlemen Pill

异功散 *yì gōng sǎn*, Special Achievement Powder

益气聪明汤 *yì qì cōng míng tāng*, Qì-Boosting Sharp and Bright Decoction

资生丸 *zī shēng wán*, Life-Promoting Pill

补血
Supplement the blood

艾附暖宫丸 *ài fù nuǎn gōng wán*, Mugwort and Cyperus Palace-Warming Pill

安胎和气饮 *ān tāi hé qì yǐn*, Fetus-Quieting Qì-Harmonizing Beverage

补肝汤 *bǔ gān tāng*, Liver-Supplementing Decoction

补荣汤 *bǔ róng tāng*, Construction-Supplementing Decoction

大营煎 *dà yíng jiān*, Major Construction Brew

当归芍药散 *dāng guī sháo yào sǎn*, Chinese Angelica and Peony Powder

当归生姜羊肉汤 *dāng guī shēng jiāng yáng ròu tāng*, Chinese Angelica, Fresh Ginger, and Goat Meat Decoction

阿胶四物汤 *ē jiāo sì wù tāng*, Ass Hide Glue Four Agents Decoction

复脉汤 *fù mài tāng*, Pulse-Restorative Decoction

归芍地黄汤 *guī sháo dì huáng tāng*, Chinese Angelica, Peony, and Rehmannia Decoction

加减复脉汤 *jiā jiǎn fù mài tāng*, Pulse-Restorative Variant Decoction

加味当归芍药散 *jiā wèi dāng guī sháo yào sǎn*, Supplemented Chinese Angelica and Peony Powder

四物汤 *sì wù tāng*, Four Agents Decoction

四物汤加味方 *sì wù tāng jiā wèi fāng*, Supplemented Four Agents Decoction Formula

送子丹 *sòng zǐ dān*, Child-Delivering Elixir

下乳天浆饮 *xià rǔ tiān jiāng yǐn*, Celestial Fluid Lactation-Promoting Beverage

小营煎 *xiǎo yíng jiān*, Minor Construction Brew

炙甘草汤 *zhì gān cǎo tāng*, Honey-Fried Licorice Decoction

苎根汤 *zhù gēn tāng*, Ramie (Boehmeria) Decoction

滋燥养营汤 *zī zào yǎng yíng tāng*, Dryness-Enriching Construction-Nourishing Decoction

气血双补
Supplement both qì and the blood

安胎饮 *ān tāi yǐn*, Fetus-Quieting Beverage

八珍汤 *bā zhēn tāng*, Eight-Gem Decoction

八珍益母丸 *bā zhēn yì mǔ wán*, Eight-Gem Leonurus (Motherwort) Pill

保产无忧方 *bǎo chǎn wú yōu fāng*, Carefree Pregnancy Formula

肠宁汤 *cháng níng tāng*, Abdomen-Quieting Decoction

当归补血汤 *dāng guī bǔ xuè tāng*, Chinese Angelica Blood-Supplementing Decoction

当归羊肉汤 *dāng guī yáng ròu tāng*, Chinese Angelica and Goat Meat Decoction

归脾汤 *guī pí tāng*, Spleen-Returning Decoction

归瑱建中汤 *guī qí jiàn zhōng tāng*, Chinese Angelica and Astragalus Center-Fortifying Decoction

归芍六君丸 *guī sháo liù jūn wán*, Chinese Angelica and Peony Six Gentlemen Pill

何人饮 *hé rén yǐn*, Flowery Knotweed and Ginseng Beverage

人参养荣汤（丸）*rén shēn yǎng róng tāng* (*wán*), Ginseng Construction-Nourishing Decoction (Pill)

圣愈汤 *shèng yù tāng*, Sagacious Cure Decoction

十全大补汤 *shí quán dà bǔ tāng*, Perfect Major Supplementation Decoction

薯蓣丸 *shǔ yù wán*, Dioscorea Pill

泰山磐石散 *tài shān pán shí sǎn*, Rock of Taishan Fetus-Quieting Powder

通乳丹 *tōng rǔ dān*, Lactation Elixir

乌鸡白凤丸 *wū jī bái fèng wán*, Black Chicken and White Phoenix Pill

转胎方 *zhuǎn tāi fāng*, Fetus-Turning Formula

补阳
Supplement yáng

八味地黄丸 *bā wèi dì huáng wán*, Eight-Ingredient Rehmannia Pill

斑龙丸 *bān lóng wán*, Striped Dragon Pill

补肾固冲丸 *bǔ shèn gù chōng wán*, Kidney-Supplementing Thoroughfare-Securing Pill

二仙汤 *èr xiān tāng*, Two Immortals Decoction

骨质增生丸 *gǔ zhí zēng shēng wán*, Hyperosteogeny Pill

龟鹿二仙胶 *guī lù èr xiān jiāo*, Tortoise Shell and Deerhorn Two Immortals Glue

桂附八味丸 *guì fù bā wèi wán*, Cinnamon Bark and Aconite Eight-Ingredient Pill

桂枝甘草汤 *guì zhī gān cǎo tāng*, Cinnamon Twig and Licorice Decoction

河车八味丸 *hé chē bā wèi wán*, Eight-Ingredient Placenta Pill

化水种子汤 *huà shuǐ zhòng zǐ tāng*, Water-Transforming Seed-Planting Decoction

济生肾气丸 *jì shēng shèn qì wán*, Life Saver Kidney Qì Pill

加味金刚丸 *jiā wèi jīn gāng wán*, Supplemented Metal Strength Pill

加味肾气丸 *jiā wèi shèn qì wán*, Supplemented Kidney Qì Pill

健腰丸 *jiàn yāo wán*, Lumbus-Fortifying Pill

内补丸 *nèi bǔ wán*, Internal Supplementation Pill

全鹿丸 *quán lù wán*, Whole Deer Pill

肾气丸 *shèn qì wán*, Kidney Qì Pill

十补丸 *shí bǔ wán*, Ten Supplements Pill

右归丸 *yòu guī wán*, Right-Restoring [Life Gate] Pill

右归饮 *yòu guī yǐn*, Right-Restoring [Life Gate] Beverage

援土固胎汤 *yuán tǔ gù tāi tāng*, Earth-Rescuing Fetus-Securing Decoction

赞育丹 *zàn yù dān*, Procreation Elixir

补阴
Supplement yīn

八仙长寿丸 *bā xiān cháng shòu wán*, Eight Immortals Longevity Pill

补肾壮筋汤 *bǔ shèn zhuàng jīn tāng*, Kidney-Supplementing Sinew-Strengthening Decoction

大补阴丸 *dà bǔ yīn wán*, Major Yīn Supplementation Pill

大造丸 *dà zào wán*, Great Creation Pill

地黄丸 *dì huáng wán*, Rehmannia Pill

地黄饮子 *dì huáng yǐn zǐ*, Rehmannia Drink

都气丸 *dū qì wán*, Metropolis Qì Pill

耳聋左慈丸 *ěr lóng zuǒ cí wán*, Deafness Left-Benefiting Loadstone Pill

二甲复脉汤 *èr jiǎ fù mài tāng*, Double-Armored Pulse-Restorative Decoction

二至丸 *èr zhì wán*, Double Supreme Pill

还少丹 *huán shào dān*, Rejuvenation Elixir

健步虎潜丸 *jiàn bù hǔ qián wán*, Steady Gait Hidden Tiger Pill

六味地黄丸 *liù wèi dì huáng wán*, Six-Ingredient Rehmannia Pill

麦味地黄丸 *mài wèi dì huáng wán*, Ophiopogon and Rehmannia Pill

明目地黄丸 *míng mù dì huáng wán*, Eye Brightener Rehmannia Pill

七宝美髯丹 *qī bǎo měi rán dān*, Seven-Jewel Beard-Blackening Elixir

杞菊地黄汤 *qǐ jú dì huáng tāng*, Lycium Berry, Chrysanthemum, and Rehmannia Decoction

杞菊地黄丸 *qǐ jú dì huáng wán*, Lycium Berry, Chrysanthemum, and Rehmannia Pill

桑椹子膏 *sāng shèn zǐ gāo*, Mulberry Paste

石斛明目丸 *shí hú míng mù wán*, Dendrobium Eye Brightener Pill

石斛夜光丸 *shí hú yè guāng wán*, Dendrobium Night Vision Pill

寿胎丸 *shòu tāi wán*, Fetal Longevity Pill

文武膏 *wén wǔ tāng*, Mulberry Paste

五子补肾丸 *wǔ zǐ bǔ shèn wán*, Five-Seed Kidney-Supplementing Pill

五子衍宗丸 *wǔ zǐ yǎn zōng wán*, Five-Seed Progeny Pill

一贯煎 *yī guàn jiān*, All-the-Way-Through Brew

一甲复脉汤 *yī jiǎ fù mài tāng*, Single-Armored Pulse-Restorative Decoction

月华丸 *yuè huá wán*, Moonlight Pill

驻景丸加减方 *zhù jǐng wán jiā jiǎn fāng*, Long Vistas Pill Variant Formula

滋水清肝饮 *zǐ shuǐ qīng gān yǐn*, Water-Enriching Liver-Clearing Beverage

滋阴大补丸 *zī yīn dà bǔ wán*, Yīn-Enriching Major Supplementation Pill

左归丸 *zuǒ guī wán*, Left-Restoring [Kidney Yīn] Pill

左归饮 *zuǒ guī yǐn*, Left-Restoring [Kidney Yīn] Beverage

滋阴益气
Enrich yīn and boost qì

人参固本丸 *rén shēn gù běn wán*, Ginseng Root-Securing Pill

人参黄芪散 *rén shēn huáng qí sǎn*, Ginseng and Astragalus Powder

三才汤 *sān cái tāng*, Heaven, Human, and Earth Decoction

生脉散 *shēng mài sǎn*, Pulse-Engendering Powder

所以载丸 *suǒ yǐ zài wán*, Wherewithal-to-Bear Pill

固涩剂
Securing and Astringing Formulas

敛汗固表
Constrain sweat and secure the exterior

柏子仁丸 *bǎi zǐ rén wán*, Arborvitae Seed Pill

牡蛎散 *mǔ lì sǎn*, Oyster Shell Powder

玉屏风散 *yù píng fēng sǎn*, Jade Wind-Barrier Powder

止汗散 *zhǐ hàn sǎn*, Perspiration-Checking Powder

涩肠固脱
Astringe the intestines and stem desertion

赤石脂禹余粮汤 *chì shí zhī yǔ yú liáng tāng*, Halloysite and Limonite Decoction

纯阳真人养脏汤 *chún yáng zhēn rén yǎng zàng tāng*, Pure Yáng True Man Viscus-Nourishing Decoction

大桃花汤 *dà táo huā tāng*, Major Peach Blossom Decoction

地榆丸 *dì yú wán*, Sanguisorba Pill

二神丸 *èr shén wán*, Two Spirits Pill

脾肾双补丸 *pí shèn shuāng bǔ wán*, Spleen-Kidney Supplementation Pill

四神丸 *sì shén wán*, Four Spirits Pill

桃花汤 *táo huā tāng*, Peach Blossom Decoction

益黄散 *yì huáng sǎn*, Yellow-Boosting Powder

真人养脏汤 *zhēn rén yǎng zàng tāng*, True Man Viscus-Nourishing Decoction

驻车丸 *zhù chē wán*, Carriage-Halting Pill

涩精止遗
Astringe essence and check semininal emission and enuresis

茯菟丹 *fú tù dān*, Poria and Cuscuta Elixir

膏淋汤 *gāo lín tāng*, Unctuous Strangury Decoction

巩堤丸 *gǒng tí wán*, Dyke-Strengthening Pill

固脬汤 *gù pāo tāng*, Bladder-Securing Decoction

固真丸 *gù zhēn wán*, True-Securing Pill

既济丸 *jì jì wán*, Immediate Aid Pill

金锁固精丸 *jīn suǒ gù jīng wán*, Golden Lock Essence-Securing Pill

秘元煎 *mì yuán jiān*, Origin-Securing Brew

桑螵蛸散 *sāng piāo xiāo sǎn*, Mantis Egg-Case Powder

水陆二仙丹 *shuǐ lù èr xiān dān*, Land and Water Two Immortals Elixir

松石猪肚丸 *sōng shí zhū dǔ wán*, Song-Shi Pig's Stomach Pill

缩泉丸 *suō quán wán*, Stream-Reducing Pill

菟丝子丸 *tù sī zǐ wán*, Cuscuta Seed Pill

威喜丸 *wēi xǐ wán*, Powerful Happiness Pill

猪肚丸 *zhū dǔ wán*, Pig's Stomach Pill

固崩止带
Stem flooding and check discharge

白带片 *bái dài piàn*, White Discharge Tablet

崩证极验方 *bēng zhèng jí yàn fāng*, Well-Tried Flooding Formula

侧柏樗皮丸 *cè bǎi shū pí wán*, Arborvitae Leaf and Toona Bark Pill

地榆散 *dì yú sǎn*, Sanguisorba Powder

丁香胶艾汤 *dīng xiāng jiāo ài tāng*, Clove, Ass Hide Glue, and Mugwort Decoction

断下汤 *duàn xià tāng*, Precipitation-Checking Decoction

固本止崩汤 *gù běn zhǐ bēng tāng*, Root-Securing Flood-Stanching Decoction

固冲汤 *gù chōng tāng*, Thoroughfare-Securing Decoction

固经丸 gù jīng wán,
Menses-Securing Pill

加味黄土汤 jiā wèi huáng tǔ tāng,
Supplemented Yellow Earth
Decoction

胶艾汤 jiāo ài tāng, Ass Hide
Glue and Mugwort Decoction

鹿角菟丝丸 lù jiǎo tù sī wán,
Deerhorn and Cuscuta Pill

清带汤 qīng dài tāng,
Discharge-Clearing Decoction

清热固经汤 qīng rè gù jīng tāng,
Heat-Clearing Channel-Securing
(Menses-Securing) Decoction

清热止崩汤 qīng rè zhǐ bēng tāng,
Heat-Clearing Uterine Bleeding
Decoction

完带汤 wán dài tāng,
Discharge-Ceasing Decoction

易黄汤 yì huáng tāng,
Transforming Yellow Decoction

愈带丸 yù dài wán,
Discharge-Curing Pill

止带片 zhǐ dài piàn,
Discharge-Checking Tablet

滋肾固冲汤 zī shèn gù chōng
tāng, Kidney-Enriching
Thoroughfare-Securing
Decoction

敛肺止咳
Constrain the lung and suppress
cough

定喘散 dìng chuǎn sǎn,
Panting-Stabilizing Powder

九仙丹 jiǔ xiān dān, Nine
Immortals Elixir

九仙散 jiǔ xiān sǎn, Nine
Immortals Powder

五味子汤 wǔ wèi zǐ tāng,
Schisandra Decoction

一服散 yī fú sǎn, One Dose
Powder

涌吐剂
Ejection Formulas

实证
Repletion patterns

二圣散 èr shèng sǎn, Sagacious
Two Powder

瓜蒂散 guā dì sǎn, Melon Stalk
Powder

急救稀涎散 jí jiù xī xián sǎn,
Emergency Drool-Thinning
Powder

三圣散 sān shèng sǎn, Sagacious
Three Powder

稀涎散 xī xián sǎn,
Drool-Thinning Powder

盐汤探吐方 yán tāng tàn tù fāng,
Mechanical Ejection Brine

虚证
Vacuity patterns

参芦饮 shēn lú yǐn, Ginseng Tops
Beverage

痈疡剂
Oral Formulas for
Welling-Abscesses and Sores

内痈
Internal welling-abscess

赤小豆当归散 chì xiǎo dòu dāng
guī sǎn, Rice Bean and Chinese
Angelica Powder

大黄牡丹皮汤 dà huáng mǔ dān
pí tāng, Rhubarb and Moutan
Decoction

锦红片 jǐn hóng piàn, Red
Brocade Tablet

阑尾化瘀汤 lán wěi huà yū tāng,
Appendix Stasis-Transforming
Decoction

阑尾清化汤 *lán wěi qīng huà tāng*, Appendix Clearing and Transforming Decoction

阑尾清解汤 *lán wěi qīng jiě tāng*, Appendix-Clearing and Resolving Decoction

清肠饮 *qīng cháng yǐn*, Intestine-Clearing Beverage

苇茎汤 *wěi jīng tāng*, Phragmites Stem Decoction

薏苡附子败酱散 *yì yǐ fù zǐ bài jiàng sǎn*, Coix, Aconite, and Patrinia Powder

治脓胸方 *zhì nóng xiōng fāng*, Pyothorax Formula

外疡阳证
External sores—yáng patterns

疮毒丸 *chuāng dú wán*, Sore-Toxin Pill

代刀散 *dài dāo sǎn*, Spare-the-Knife Powder

瓜蒌牛蒡汤 *guā lóu niú bàng tāng*, Trichosanthes and Arctium Decoction

连翘金贝煎 *lián qiào jīn bèi jiān*, Forsythia, Lonicera, and Bolbostemma Brew

六神丸 *liù shén wán*, Six Spirits Pill

内疏黄连汤 *nèi shū huáng lián tāng*, Internal Coursing Coptis Decoction

牛黄醒消丸 *niú huáng xǐng xiāo wán*, Bovine Bezoar Awake to Relief Pill

四妙汤 *sì miào tāng*, Mysterious Four Decoction

四妙勇安汤 *sì miào yǒng ān tāng*, Mysterious Four Resting Hero Decoction

透脓散 *tòu nóng sǎn*, Pus-Outthrusting Powder

托里定痛汤 *tuō lǐ dìng tòng tāng*, Internal Expression and Pain-Relieving Decoction

托里透脓汤 *tuō lǐ tòu nóng tāng*, Internal Expression Pus-Expelling Decoction

托里消毒散 *tuō lǐ xiāo dú sǎn*, Internal Expression Toxin-Dispersing Powder

外科蟾酥丸 *wài kē chán sū wán*, External Medicine Toad Venom Pill

五宝散 *wǔ bǎo sǎn*, Five-Jewel Powder

五神汤 *wǔ shén tāng*, Five Spirits Decoction

五味消毒饮 *wǔ wèi xiāo dú yǐn*, Five-Ingredient Toxin-Dispersing Beverage

仙方活命饮 *xiān fāng huó mìng yǐn*, Immortal Formula Life-Giving Beverage

消疮饮 *xiāo chuāng yǐn*, Sore-Healing Beverage

消痔饮 *xiāo zhì yǐn*, Hemorrhoid-Dispersing Beverage

心悟透脓散 *xīn wù tòu nóng sǎn*, Medical Insights Pus-Outthrusting Powder

醒消丸 *xǐng xiāo wán*, Awake to Dispersion Pill

外疡阴证
External sores—yīn patterns

万灵丹 *wàn líng dān*, Unlimited Efficacy Elixir

阳和汤 *yáng hé tāng*, Harmonious Yáng Decoction

外用剂
Formulas for External Use

内科外用剂
Internal medicine formulas for external use

甘遂散 *gān suì sǎn*, Kansui Powder

瓜蒂神妙散 *guā dì shén miào sǎn*, Melon Stalk Wonder Powder

瓜丁散 *guā dīng sǎn*, Melon Pedicel Powder

坎离砂 *kǎn lí shā*, Fire and Water Hexagram Granules

硫葱敷剂 *liú cōng fū jì*, Sulfur and Scallion Topical Application

暖脐膏 *nuǎn qí gāo*, Navel-Warming Paste

哮喘敷治方 *xiāo chuǎn fù zhì fāng*, Wheezing and Panting External Application Formula

眼耳喉鼻科外用剂
Eye, ear, nose, and throat formulas for external use

八宝眼药 *bā bǎo yǎn yào*, Eight-Jewel Eye Medication

白敬宇眼药 *bái jìng yǔ yǎn yào*, Bai Jing-Yu's Eye Medication

白氏眼药 *bái shì yǎn yào*, Bai's Eye Medication

冰硼散 *bīng péng sǎn*, Borneol and Borax Powder

光明丹 *guāng míng dān*, Bright and Glorious Elixir

磨障灵光膏 *mó zhàng líng guāng gāo*, Obstruction-Abrading Spirit Light Paste

砒枣散 *pī zǎo sǎn*, Arsenic and Jujube Powder

青黛散 *qīng dài sǎn*, Indigo Powder

锡类散 *xí lèi sǎn*, Tin-Like Powder

珠黄散 *zhū huáng sǎn*, Pearl and Bezoar Powder

嗜鼻碧云散 *xiù bí bì yún sǎn*, Nasal Insufflation Jasper Clouds Powder

外科外用剂
External medicine formulas for external use

八宝丹 *bā bǎo dān*, Eight-Jewel Elixir

白斑二号药膏 *bái bān èr hào yào gāo*, Leukoplakia No. 3 Medicinal Paste

白斑洗剂 *bái bān xǐ jì*, Leukoplakia Wash

白斑一号药膏 *bái bān yī hào yào gāo*, Leukoplakia No. 1 Medicinal Paste

白降丹 *bái jiàng dān*, White Downborne Elixir

避火丹 *bì huǒ dān*, Fire-Repelling Elixir

颠倒散 *diān dǎo sǎn*, Reversal Powder

复方黄连膏 *fù fāng huáng lián gāo*, Compound Formula Coptis Paste

桂麝散 *guì shè sǎn*, Cinnamon Twig and Musk Powder

黑虎丹 *hēi hǔ dān*, Black Tiger Elixir

红升丹 *hóng shēng dān*, Red Upborne Elixir

黄芩汤洗方 *huáng qín tāng xǐ fāng*, Scutellaria Decoction Wash Formula

回阳玉龙膏 *huí yáng yù lóng gāo*, Yáng-Returning Jade Dragon Paste

夹纸膏 *jiā zhǐ gāo*, Paper Plaster

金黄散 *jīn huáng sǎn*, Golden Yellow Powder

九一丹 *jiǔ yī dān*, Nine-to-One Elixir

枯痔散 *kū zhì sǎn*, Alum Hemorrhoid-Desiccating Powder

苦参汤 *kǔ shēn tāng*, Flavescent Sophora Decoction

千捶膏 *qiān chuí gāo*, Thoroughly Pounded Paste

清凉膏 *qīng liáng gāo*, Cool Clearing Paste

如意金黄散 *rú yì jīn huáng sǎn*, Agreeable Golden Yellow Powder

三黄洗剂 *sān huáng xǐ jì*, Three Yellows Wash Preparation

三品一条枪 *sān pǐn yī tiáo qiāng*, Three-Shot Gun

蛇床子散 *shé chuáng zǐ sǎn*, Cnidium Seed Powder

生肌散 *shēng jī sǎn*, Flesh-Engendering Powder

生肌玉红膏 *shēng jī yù hóng gāo*, Flesh-Engendering Jade and Red Paste

五倍子散 *wǔ bèi zǐ sǎn*, Sumac Gallnut Powder

五五丹 *wǔ wǔ dān*, Five-to-Five Elixir

阳和解凝膏 *yáng hé jiě níng gāo*, Harmonious Yáng Decongealing Plaster

羊蹄根散 *yáng tí gēn sǎn*, Curled Dock Root Powder

一扫光 *yī sǎo guāng*, Gone-in-One-Sweep

玉红膏 *yù hóng gāo*, Jade and Red Paste

玉露散 *yù lù sǎn*, Jade Dew Powder

熨风散 *yùn fēng sǎn*, Wind-Smoothing Powder

伤科外用剂
External injuries formulas for external use

八仙逍遥汤 *bā xiān xiāo yáo tāng*, Eight Immortals Free Wanderer Decoction

定痛膏 *dìng tòng gāo*, Pain-Relieving Paste

狗皮膏 *gǒu pí gāo*, Dog Skin Plaster

海桐皮汤 *hǎi tóng pí tāng*, Erythrina Decoction

如圣金刀散 *rú shèng jīn dāo sǎn*, Sagacious Incised Wound Powder

散瘀和伤汤 *sàn yū hé shāng tāng*, Stasis-Dissipating Injury Decoction

伤湿止痛膏 *shāng shī zhǐ tòng gāo*, Dampness Damage Pain-Relieving Plaster

舒筋活血洗方 *shū jīn huó xuè xǐ fāng*, Sinew-Soothing Blood-Quickening Wash Formula

桃花散 *táo huā sǎn*, Peach Blossom Powder

陀僧膏 *tuó sēng gāo*, Litharge Paste

外敷接骨散 *wài fū jiē gǔ sǎn*, Topical Bone-Joining Powder

万应膏 *wàn yìng gāo*, Myriad Applications Paste

五黄散 *wǔ huáng sǎn*, Five Yellows Powder

正骨烫药 *zhèng gǔ tàng yào*, Bone-Righting Hot Pack

止血散 *zhǐ xuè sǎn*,
Blood-Stanching Powder

紫荆皮散 *zǐ jīng pí sǎn*, Cercis
Powder

紫云膏 *zǐ yún gāo*, Purple Clouds
Plaster

妇科外用剂

Gynecological formulas for external use

霉滴净丸 *méi dī jīng wán*,
Trichomonas Cleansing Pill

蛇床子冲洗剂 *shé chuáng zǐ
chōng xǐ jì*, Cnidium Seed Rinse

治癌剂

Cancer Formulas

黄药子酒 *huáng yào zǐ jiǔ*, Air
Potato Wine

开关散 *kāi guān sǎn*,
Gate-Opening Powder

龙虎三胆散 *lóng hǔ sān dǎn sǎn*,
Earthworm, House Lizard, and
Three Gallbladders Powder

食道癌二号方 *shí dào ái èr hào
fāng*, Esophageal Cancer No. 2
Formula

食道癌一号方 *shí dào ái yī hào
fāng*, Esophageal Cancer No. 1
Formula

调元肾气丸 *tiáo yuán shèn qì
wán*, Origin-Regulating Kidney
Qì Pill

信枣散 *xìn zǎo sǎn*,
Arsenic-Jujube Powder

附录4：经穴名称
Appendix 4: Names of Channel Points

肺经
Lung Channel

中府 *zhōng fǔ* Central Treasury, LU-1
云门 *yún mén* Cloud Gate, LU-2
天府 *tiān fǔ* Celestial Storehouse, LU-3
侠白 *xiá bái* Guarding White, LU-4
尺泽 *chǐ zé* Cubit Marsh, LU-5
孔最 *kǒng zuì* Collection Hole, LU-6
列缺 *liè quē* Broken Sequence, LU-7
经渠 *jīng qú* Channel Ditch, LU-8
太渊 *tài yuān* Great Abyss, LU-9
鱼际 *yú jì* Fish Border, LU-10
少商 *shào shāng* Lesser Shang, LU-11

大肠经
Large Intestine Channel

商阳 *shāng yáng* Shang Yáng, LI-1
二间 *èr jiān* Second Space, LI-2
三间 *sān jiān* Third Space, LI-3
合谷 *hé gǔ* Union Valley, LI-4
阳溪 *yáng xī* Yáng Ravine, LI-5
偏历 *piān lì* Veering Passageway, LI-6
温溜 *wēn liù* Warm Dwelling, LI-7
下廉 *xià lián* Lower Ridge, LI-8
上廉 *shàng lián* Upper Ridge, LI-9
手三里 *shǒu sān lǐ* Arm Three Li, LI-10
曲池 *qū chí* Pool at the Bend, LI-11
肘髎 *zhǒu liáo* Elbow Bone-Hole, LI-12
手五里 *shǒu wǔ lǐ* Arm Five Li, LI-13
臂臑 *bì nào* Upper Arm, LI-14
肩髃 *jiān yú* Shoulder Bone, LI-15
巨骨 *jù gǔ* Great Bone, LI-16
天鼎 *tiān dǐng* Celestial Tripod, LI-17
扶突 *fú tú* Protuberance Assistant, LI-18
禾髎 *hé liáo* Grain Bone-Hole, LI-19
迎香 *yíng xiāng* Welcome Fragrance, LI-20

胃经
Stomach Channel

承泣 *chéng qì* Tear Container, ST-1
四白 *sì bái* Four Whites, ST-2
巨髎 *jù liáo* Great Bone-Hole, ST-3
地仓 *dì cāng* Earth Granary, ST-4
大迎 *dà yíng* Great Reception, ST-5
颊车 *jiá chē* Cheek Carriage, ST-6
下关 *xià guān* Below the Joint, ST-7
头维 *tóu wéi* Head Corner, ST-8
人迎 *rén yíng* Man's Prognosis, ST-9
水突 *shuǐ tú* Water Prominence, ST-10
气舍 *qì shè* Qì Abode, ST-11
缺盆 *quē pén* Empty Basin, ST-12
气户 *qì hù* Qì Door, ST-13
库房 *kù fáng* Storeroom, ST-14
屋翳 *wū yì* Roof, ST-15
膺窗 *yīng chuāng* Breast Window, ST-16
乳中 *rǔ zhōng* Breast Center, ST-17
乳根 *rǔ gēn* Breast Root, ST-18
不容 *bù róng* Not Contained, ST-19
承满 *chéng mǎn* Assuming Fullness, ST-20
梁门 *liáng mén* Beam Gate, ST-21
关门 *guān mén* Pass Gate, ST-22
太乙 *tài yǐ* Supreme Unity, ST-23
滑肉门 *huá ròu mén* Slippery Flesh Gate, ST-24
天枢 *tiān shū* Celestial Pivot, ST-25
外陵 *wài líng* Outer Mound, ST-26
大巨 *dà jù* Great Gigantic, ST-27
水道 *shuǐ dào* Waterway, ST-28
归来 *guī lái* Return, ST-29
气冲 *qì chōng* Qì Thoroughfare, ST-30
髀关 *bì guān* Thigh Joint, ST-31
伏兔 *fú tù* Crouching Rabbit, ST-32

阴市 *yīn shì* Yīn Market, ST-33

梁丘 *liáng qiū* Beam Hill, ST-34

犊鼻 *dú bí* Calf's Nose, ST-35

足三里 *zú sān lǐ* Leg Three Li, ST-36

上巨虚 *shàng jù xū* Upper Great Hollow, ST-37

条口 *tiáo kǒu* Ribbon Opening, ST-38

下巨虚 *xià jù xū* Lower Great Hollow, ST-39

丰隆 *fēng lóng* Bountiful Bulge, ST-40

解溪 *jiě xī* Ravine Divide, ST-41

冲阳 *chōng yáng* Surging Yáng, ST-42

陷谷 *xiàn gǔ* Sunken Valley, ST-43

内庭 *nèi tíng* Inner Court, ST-44

厉兑 *lì duì* Severe Mouth, ST-45

脾经
Spleen Channel

隐白 *yǐn bái* Hidden White, SP-1

大都 *dà dū* Great Metropolis, SP-2

太白 *tài bái* Supreme White, SP-3

公孙 *gōng sūn* Yellow Emperor, SP-4

商丘 *shāng qiū* Shang Hill, SP-5

三阴交 *sān yīn jiāo* Three Yīn Intersection, SP-6

漏谷 *lòu gǔ* Leaking Valley, SP-7

地机 *dì jī* Earth's Crux, SP-8

阴陵泉 *yīn líng quán* Yīn Mound Spring, SP-9

血海 *xuè hǎi* Sea of Blood, SP-10

箕门 *jī mén* Winnower Gate, SP-11

冲门 *chōng mén* Surging Gate, SP-12

府舍 *fǔ shè* Bowel Abode, SP-13

腹结 *fù jié* Abdominal Bind, SP-14

大横 *dà héng* Great Horizontal, SP-15

腹哀 *fù āi* Abdominal Lament, SP-16

食窦 *shí dòu* Food Hole, SP-17

天溪 *tiān xī* Celestial Ravine, SP-18

胸乡 *xiōng xiāng* Chest Village, SP-19

周荣 *zhōu róng* All-Round Flourishing, SP-20

大包 *dà bāo* Great Embracement, SP-21

心经
Heart Channel

极泉 *jí quán* Highest Spring, HT-1

青灵 *qīng líng* Green-Blue Spirit, HT-2

少海 *shào hǎi* Lesser Sea, HT-3

灵道 *líng dào* Spirit Pathway, HT-4

通里 *tōng lǐ* Connecting Li, HT-5

阴郄 *yīn xī* Yīn Cleft, HT-6

神门 *shén mén* Spirit Gate, HT-7

少府 *shào fǔ* Lesser House, HT-8

少冲 *shào chōng* Lesser Surge, HT-9

小肠经
Small Intestine Channel

少泽 *shào zé* Lesser Marsh, SI-1

前谷 *qián gǔ* Front Valley, SI-2

后溪 *hòu xī* Back Ravine, SI-3

腕骨 *wàn gǔ* Wrist Bone, SI-4

阳谷 *yáng gǔ* Yáng Valley, SI-5

养老 *yǎng lǎo* Nursing the Aged, SI-6

支正 *zhī zhèng* Branch to the Correct, SI-7

小海 *xiǎo hǎi* Small Sea, SI-8

肩贞 *jiān zhēn* True Shoulder, SI-9

臑俞 *nào shū* Upper Arm Transport, SI-10

天宗 *tiān zōng* Celestial Gathering, SI-11

秉风 *bǐng fēng* Grasping the Wind, SI-12

曲垣 *qū yuán* Crooked Wall, SI-13

肩外俞 *jiān wài shū* Outer Shoulder Transport, SI-14

肩中俞 *jiān zhōng shū* Central Shoulder Transport, SI-15

天窗 *tiān chuāng* Celestial Window, SI-16

天容 *tiān róng* Celestial Countenance, SI-17

颧髎 *quán liáo* Cheek Bone-Hole, SI-18

听宫 *tīng gōng* Auditory Palace, SI-19

膀胱经
Bladder Channel

睛明 *jīng míng* Bright Eyes, BL-1

攒竹 *zǎn zhú* Bamboo Gathering, BL-2

眉冲 *méi chōng* Eyebrow Ascension, BL-3

曲差 *qū chā* Deviating Turn, BL-4

五处 *wǔ chù* Fifth Place, BL-5

承光 *chéng guāng* Light Guard, BL-6

通天 *tōng tiān* Celestial Connection, BL-7

络却 *luò què* Declining Connection, BL-8

玉枕 *yù zhěn* Jade Pillow, BL-9

天柱 *tiān zhù* Celestial Pillar, BL-10

大杼 *dà zhù* Great Shuttle, BL-11

风门 *fēng mén* Wind Gate, BL-12

肺俞 *fèi shū* Lung Transport, BL-13

厥阴俞 *jué yīn shū* Reverting Yīn
Transport, BL-14

心俞 *xīn shū* Heart Transport, BL-15

督俞 *dū shū* Governing Transport, BL-16

膈俞 *gé shū* Diaphragm Transport, BL-17

肝俞 *gān shū* Liver Transport, BL-18

胆俞 *dǎn shū* Gallbladder Transport, BL-19

脾俞 *pí shū* Spleen Transport, BL-20

胃俞 *wèi shū* Stomach Transport, BL-21

三焦俞 *sān jiāo shū* Triple Burner
Transport, BL-22

肾俞 *shèn shū* Kidney Transport, BL-23

气海俞 *qì hǎi shū* Sea-of-Qì Transport,
BL-24

大肠俞 *dà cháng shū* Large Intestine
Transport, BL-25

关元俞 *guān yuán shū* Pass Head
Transport, BL-26

小肠俞 *xiǎo cháng shū* Small Intestine
Transport, BL-27

膀胱俞 *páng guāng shū* Bladder Transport,
BL-28

中膂俞 *zhōng lü shū* Central Backbone
Transport, BL-29

白环俞 *bái huán shū* White Ring
Transport, BL-30

上髎 *shàng liáo* Upper Bone-Hole, BL-31

次髎 *cì liáo* Second Bone-Hole, BL-32

中髎 *zhōng liáo* Central Bone-Hole, BL-33

下髎 *xià liáo* Lower Bone-Hole, BL-34

会阳 *huì yáng* Meeting of Yáng, BL-35

承扶 *chéng fú* Support, BL-36

殷门 *yīn mén* Gate of Abundance,
BL-37 (BL-51)

浮郄 *fú xī* Superficial Cleft, BL-38

委阳 *wěi yáng* Bend Yáng, BL-39 (BL-53)

委中 *wěi zhōng* Bend Center, BL-40

附分 *fù fēn* Attached Branch, BL-41

魄户 *pò hù* Corporeal Soul Door,
BL-42 (BL-37)

膏肓俞 *gāo huāng shū* Gao Huang
Transport, BL-43

神堂 *shén táng* Spirit Hall, BL-44

谚譆 *yī xǐ* Yi Xi, BL-45

膈关 *gé guān* Diaphragm Pass,
BL-46 (BL-41)

魂门 *hún mén* Hun Gate, BL-47 (BL-42)

阳纲 *yáng gāng* Yáng Headrope,
BL-48 (BL-43)

意舍 *yì shè* Mentation Abode, BL-49

胃仓 *wèi cāng* Stomach Granary,
BL-50 (BL-45)

肓门 *huāng mén* Huang Gate,
BL-51 (BL-46)

志室 *zhì shì* Will Chamber, BL-52 (BL-47)

胞肓 *bāo huāng* Bladder Huang, BL-53

秩边 *zhì biān* Sequential Limit, BL-54

合阳 *hé yáng* Yáng Union, BL-55

承筋 *chéng jīn* Sinew Support, BL-56

承山 *chéng shān* Mountain Support, BL-57

飞扬 *fēi yáng* Taking Flight, BL-58

跗阳 *fù yáng* Instep Yáng, BL-59

昆仑 *kūn lún* Kunlun Mountains, BL-60

仆参 *pú cān* Subservient Visitor, BL-61

申脉 *shēn mài* Extending Vessel, BL-62

金门 *jīn mén* Metal Gate, BL-63

京骨 *jīng gǔ* Capital Bone, BL-64

束骨 *shù gǔ* Bundle Bone, BL-65

通谷 (足) *tōng gǔ (zú)* Valley Passage,
BL-66

至阴 *zhì yīn* Reaching Yīn, BL-67

肾经
Kidney Channel

涌泉 *yǒng quán* Gushing Spring, KI-1
然谷 *rán gǔ* Blazing Valley, KI-2
太溪 *tài xī* Great Ravine, KI-3
大钟 *dà zhōng* Large Goblet, KI-4
水泉 *shuǐ quán* Water Spring, KI-5
照海 *zhào hǎi* Shining Sea, KI-6
复溜 *fù liū* Recover Flow, KI-7
交信 *jiāo xìn* Intersection Reach, KI-8
筑宾 *zhú bīn* Guest House, KI-9
阴谷 *yīn gǔ* Yīn Valley, KI-10
横骨 *héng gǔ* Pubic Bone, KI-11
大赫 *dà hè* Great Manifestation, KI-12
气穴 *qì xué* Qì Point, KI-13
四满 *sì mǎn* Fourfold Fullness, KI-14
中注 *zhōng zhù* Central Flow, KI-15
肓俞 *huāng shū* Huang Transport, KI-16
商曲 *shāng qū* Shang Bend, KI-17
石关 *shí guān* Stone Pass, KI-18
阴都 *yīn dū* Yīn Metropolis, KI-19
通谷（腹）*tōng gǔ (fù)* Open Valley, KI-20
幽门 *yōu mén* Dark Gate, KI-21
步廊 *bù láng* Corridor Walk, KI-22
神封 *shén fēng* Spirit Seal, KI-23
灵墟 *líng xū* Spirit Ruins, KI-24
神藏 *shén cáng* Spirit Storehouse, KI-25
彧中 *yù zhōng* Lively Center, KI-26
俞府 *shū fǔ* Transport House, KI-27

心包经
Pericardium Channel

天池 *tiān chí* Celestial Pool, PC-1
天泉 *tiān quán* Celestial Spring, PC-2
曲泽 *qū zé* Marsh at the Bend, PC-3
郄门 *xī mén* Cleft Gate, PC-4
间使 *jiān shǐ* Intermediary Courier, PC-5
内关 *nèi guān* Inner Pass, PC-6

大陵 *dà líng* Great Mound, PC-7
劳宫 *láo gōng* Palace of Toil, PC-8
中冲 *zhōng chōng* Central Hub, PC-9

三焦经
Triple Burner Channel

关冲 *guān chōng* Passage Hub, TB-1
液门 *yè mén* Humor Gate, TB-2
腋门 *yè mén* Armpit Gate, TB-2
中渚 *zhōng zhǔ* Central Islet, TB-3
阳池 *yáng chí* Yáng Pool, TB-4
外关 *wài guān* Outer Pass, TB-5
支沟 *zhī gōu* Branch Ditch, TB-6
会宗 *huì zōng* Convergence and Gathering, TB-7
三阳络 *sān yáng luò* Three Yáng Connection, TB-8
四渎 *sì dú* Four Rivers, TB-9
天井 *tiān jǐng* Celestial Well, TB-10
清冷渊 *qīng lěng yuān* Clear Cold Abyss, TB-11
消泺 *xiāo luò* Dispersing Riverbed, TB-12
臑会 *nào huì* Upper Arm Convergence, TB-13
肩髎 *jiān liáo* Shoulder Bone-Hole, TB-14
天髎 *tiān liáo* Celestial Bone-Hole, TB-15
天牖 *tiān yǒu* Celestial Window, TB-16
翳风 *yì fēng* Wind Screen, TB-17
瘈脉 *qì mài* Tugging Vessel, TB-18
颅息 *lú xī* Skull Rest, TB-19
角孙 *jiǎo sūn* Angle Vertex, TB-20
耳门 *ěr mén* Ear Gate, TB-21
和髎 *hé liáo* Harmony Bone-Hole, TB-22
丝竹空 *sī zhú kōng* Silk Bamboo Hole, TB-23

胆经
Gallbladder Channel

瞳子髎 *tóng zǐ liáo* Pupil Bone-Hole, GB-1

听会 *tīng huì* Auditory Convergence, GB-2

上关 *shàng guān* Upper Gate, GB-3

颔厌 *hàn yàn* Forehead Fullness, GB-4

悬颅 *xuán lú* Suspended Skull, GB-5

悬厘 *xuán lí* Suspended Tuft, GB-6

曲鬓 *qū bìn* Temporal Hairline Curve, GB-7

率谷 *shuài gǔ* Valley Lead, GB-8

天冲 *tiān chòng* Celestial Hub, GB-9

浮白 *fú bái* Floating White, GB-10

头窍阴 *tóu qiào yīn* Head Orifice Yīn, GB-11

完骨 *wán gǔ* Completion Bone, GB-12

本神 *běn shén* Root Spirit, GB-13

阳白 *yáng bái* Yáng White, GB-14

头临泣 *tóu lín qì* Head Overlooking Tears, GB-15

目窗 *mù chuāng* Eye Window, GB-16

正营 *zhèng yíng* Upright Construction, GB-17

承灵 *chéng líng* Spirit Support, GB-18

脑空 *nǎo kōng* Brain Hollow, GB-19

风池 *fēng chí* Wind Pool, GB-20

肩井 *jiān jǐng* Shoulder Well, GB-21

渊腋 *yuān yè* Armpit Abyss, GB-22

辄筋 *zhé jīn* Sinew Seat, GB-23

日月 *rì yuè* Sun and Moon, GB-24

京门 *jīng mén* Capital Gate, GB-25

带脉 *dài mài* Girdling Vessel, GB-26

五枢 *wǔ shū* Fifth Pivot, GB-27

维道 *wéi dào* Linking Path, GB-28

居髎 *jū liáo* Squatting Bone-Hole, GB-29

环跳 *huán tiào* Jumping Round, GB-30

风市 *fēng shì* Wind Market, GB-31

中渎 *zhōng dú* Central River, GB-32

膝阳关 *xī yáng guān* Knee Yáng Joint, GB-33

阳陵泉 *yáng líng quán* Yáng Mound Spring, GB-34

阳交 *yáng jiāo* Yáng Intersection, GB-35

外丘 *wài qiū* Outer Hill, GB-36

光明 *guāng míng* Bright Light, GB-37

阳辅 *yáng fǔ* Yáng Assistance, GB-38

绝骨 *jué gǔ* Severed Bone, GB-39

悬钟 *xuán zhōng* Suspended Bell, GB-39

丘墟 *qiū xū* Hill Ruins, GB-40

足临泣 *zú lín qì* Foot Overlooking Tears, GB-41

地五会 *dì wǔ huì* Earth Fivefold Convergence, GB-42

侠溪 *xiá xī* Pinched Ravine, GB-43

足窍阴 *zú qiào yīn* Foot Orifice Yīn, GB-44

肝经
Liver Channel

商阳 *shāng yáng* Shang Yáng, LR-1

二间 *èr jiān* Second Space, LR-2

三间 *sān jiān* Third Space, LR-3

合谷 *hé gǔ* Union Valley, LR-4

阳溪 *yáng xī* Yáng Ravine, LR-5

偏历 *piān lì* Veering Passageway, LR-6

温溜 *wēn liù* Warm Dwelling, LR-7

下廉 *xià lián* Lower Ridge, LR-8

上廉 *shàng lián* Upper Ridge, LR-9

手三里 *shǒu sān lǐ* Arm Three Li, LR-10

曲池 *qū chí* Pool at the Bend, LR-11

肘髎 *zhǒu liáo* Elbow Bone-Hole, LR-12

手五里 *shǒu wǔ lǐ* Arm Five Li, LR-13

臂臑 *bì nào* Upper Arm, LR-14

肩髃 *jiān yú* Shoulder Bone, LR-15

巨骨 *jù gǔ* Great Bone, LR-16

天鼎 *tiān dǐng* Celestial Tripod, LR-17

扶突 *fú tú* Protuberance Assistant, LR-18

禾髎 *hé liáo* Grain Bone-Hole, LR-19

迎香 *yíng xiāng* Welcome Fragrance, LR-20

任脉
Controlling Vessel

会阴 *huì yīn* Meeting of Yīn, CV-1
曲骨 *qū gǔ* Curved Bone, CV-2
中极 *zhōng jí* Central Pole, CV-3
关元 *guān yuán* Pass Head, CV-4
石门 *shí mén* Stone Gate, CV-5
气海 *qì hǎi* Sea of Qì, CV-6
阴交 *yīn jiāo* Yīn Intersection, CV-7
神阙 *shén què* Spirit Gate Tower, CV-8
水分 *shuǐ fēn* Water Divide, CV-9
下脘 *xià wǎn* Lower Stomach Duct, CV-10
建里 *jiàn lǐ* Interior Strengthening, CV-11
中脘 *zhōng wǎn* Central Stomach Duct, CV-12
上脘 *shàng wǎn* Upper Stomach Duct, CV-13
巨阙 *jù què* Great Tower Gate, CV-14
鸠尾 *jiū wěi* Turtledove Tail, CV-15
中庭 *zhōng tíng* Center Palace, CV-16
膻中 *dàn zhōng* Chest Center, CV-17
玉堂 *yù táng* Jade Hall, CV-18
紫宫 *zǐ gōng* Purple Palace, CV-19
华盖 *huá gài* Florid Canopy, CV-20
璇玑 *xuán jī* Jade Swivel, CV-21
天突 *tiān tú* Celestial Chimney, CV-22
廉泉 *lián quán* Ridge Spring, CV-23
承浆 *chéng jiāng* Sauce Receptacle, CV-24

督脉
Governing Vessel

长强 *cháng qiàng* Long Strong, GV-1
腰俞 *yāo shū* Lumbar Transport, GV-2
腰阳关 *yāo yáng guān* Lumbar Yáng Pass, GV-3
命门 *mìng mén* Life Gate, GV-4
悬枢 *xuán shū* Suspended Pivot, GV-5
脊中 *jǐ zhōng* Spinal Center, GV-6
中枢 *zhōng shū* Central Pivot, GV-7
筋缩 *jīn suō* Sinew Contraction, GV-8
至阳 *zhì yáng* Extremity of Yáng, GV-9
灵台 *líng tái* Spirit Tower, GV-10
神道 *shén dào* Spirit Path, GV-11
身柱 *shēn zhù* Body Pillar, GV-12
陶道 *táo dào* Kiln Path, GV-13
大椎 *dà zhuī* Great Hammer, GV-14
哑门 *yǎ mén* Mute's Gate, GV-15
风府 *fēng fǔ* Wind House, GV-16
脑户 *nǎo hù* Brain's Door, GV-17
强间 *qiáng jiān* Unyielding Space, GV-18
后顶 *hòu dǐng* Behind the Vertex, GV-19
百会 *bǎi huì* Hundred Convergences, GV-20
前顶 *qián dǐng* Before the Vertex, GV-21
囟会 *xìn huì* Fontanel Meeting, GV-22
上星 *shàng xīng* Upper Star, GV-23
神庭 *shén tíng* Spirit Court, GV-24
素髎 *sù liáo* White Bone-Hole, GV-25
人中 *rén zhōng* Human Center, GV-26
水沟 *shuǐ gōu* Water Trough, GV-26
兑端 *duì duān* Extremity of the Mouth, GV-27
龈交 *yín jiāo* Gum Intersection, GV-28

Index

AUTHORS' BIOGRAPHIES

Nigel Wiseman was born in England on April 21, 1954. He received a Bachelor's degree in Spanish and German interpreting and translation in 1976 from Heriott-Watt University in Edinburgh. He has lived in Táiwān for the last 19 years and taught at China Medical College for many years. He now teaches Chinese medical English in the newly established Department of Traditional Chinese Medicine of Chang Gung University, Táiwān. He is author or coauthor of a number of Chinese medical works including *Fundamentals of Chinese Medicine*, *Fundamentals of Chinese Acupuncture*, *An English-Chinese Chinese-English Dictionary of Chinese Medicine*, and *Shāng Hán Lùn* (On Cold Damage): *Translation and Commentaries*. He has recently completed his doctorate in Complementary Health and Applied Linguistics at the University of Exeter, England.

Féng Yè (馮曄) was born in Táiwān on November 26, 1967. He graduated from the Chinese Medical School of China Medical College, Táiwān in 1994, and holds R.O.C. licenses in Chinese and Western medicine. He received his Master's degree from the Institute of Chinese Medical Sciences, China Medical College, in 1997. He has co-authored several Chinese medical works including *An English-Chinese Chinese-English Dictionary of Chinese Medicine* and *Shāng Hán Lùn* (On Cold Damage): *Translation and Commentaries*. He is now a resident doctor in the Chinese Internal Medicine Department of Chang Gung Memorial Hospital and lectures in diagnostics in the Department of Traditional Chinese Medicine at Chang Gung University's College of Medicine. His special fields of interest other than general internal medicine include pulse theory, *shāng hán* (cold damage), diagnostics, acupuncture, and external injury.

英文中医词汇入门
英文中醫詞彙入門

Wiseman & Féng's

Introduction to

ENGLISH TERMINOLOGY OF CHINESE MEDICINE

This book serves several basic needs. For the beginning Western student of Chinese medicine, it defines basic concepts. For the learner of Chinese, it furnishes all terms in Chinese characters, both simplified and complex, together with intoned Pīnyīn pronunciation. For Chinese practitioners learning clinical English, it provides English terms with pronunciation in KK transcription. For Táiwān students and practitioners unfamiliar with mainland China's Pīnyīn system, it provides conversion tables for Mandarin Phonetic Symbols (ㄅㄆㄇㄈ). The full index helps readers to locate all terms in the body of the text and furthermore serves as an Chinese-English English-Chinese dictionary.

Features

- Introduces 1129 basic concepts in thematic order.

- Provides both simplified and complex Chinese characters with intoned Pīnyīn for each term.

- Gives English pronunciation for non-native speakers of English.

- Sets nearly 900 questions to test progess, with answers at the end of the book.

- Provides a guide for Pīnyīn pronunciation.

- Includes a Pīnyīn Conversion Table for Mandarin Phonetic Symbols for Táiwān students and practitioners.

- Includes an appendix of 548 basic characters together with examples of terms in which they appear.

- Contains a full index including the names of medicinals and formulas that allows any Chinese term or English equivalent to be accessed.

Other books in the Chinese Medicine Language Series include *Chinese Medical Chinese: Characters* and *Chinese Medical Chinese: Grammar and Vocabulary*.

CHINESE   MEDICINE   LANGUAGE   SERIES

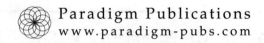

Paradigm Publications
www.paradigm-pubs.com

Wiseman & Féng's

Chinese Medical Chinese:
Grammar and Vocabulary

This is a very sophisticated and highly useful work that provides a sound basis for reading both modern and classical texts for anyone wishing to learn original Chinese medical language. The work assumes readers already have knowledge of how Chinese characters are composed, how they are written by hand, and how they are pronounced.

This book is divided into two parts. The first part describes the basic features of literary Chinese medical language and its relationship to both the classical language and to the modern vernacular of northern China, known as Mandarin. It explains many grammatical constructions commonly encountered in Chinese medical texts, and describes how Chinese medical terms are composed. The second part presents the vocabulary and terminology of Chinese medicine as its component characters.

The lessons are organized by Chinese medical categories and the characters are introduced in sets according to subject matter; for example, terms related to the five phases, terms related to inspection of the tongue, terms related to pulse-taking, or terms related to women's diseases. Each of these sets is followed by a section that presents examples of compound terms formed from characters already introduced. These examples are then followed by drills that self-test these vocabularies.

In all, this text covers basic theories, four examinations, diseases, pathomechanisms and disease patterns, principles and methods of treatment, pharmaceutics, and acupuncture. It includes etymologies of terms, gives component characters in simplified and complex form with their significs, and explains term translations for 1027 characters and 2555 compound terms. The back matter includes answers to the 910 drill questions, appendices containing the names of commonly used medicinals, formulas, and acupuncture points, and a copious index.

CHINESE   MEDICINE   LANGUAGE   SERIES

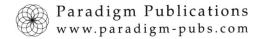

Paradigm Publications
www.paradigm-pubs.com

CHINESE MEDICAL CHINESE: CHARACTERS, VOLUME ONE

Nigel Wiseman, Zhang Yu Huan, Ken Rose

This work forms an integral part of the *Chinese Medicine Language Series* for students and practitioners who are engaged in the study of Chinese medical language. It presents the first 100 characters based upon frequency of use in medical texts, as well as an overall program designed to help the student acquire the necessary tools for building a thorough vocabulary.

This first volume presents the basics of Chinese characters along with the etymologies of the 100 most commonly seen characters. Designed as a workbook, it offers students practice in learning to read, recognize, and write the characters and provides the basic tools that students need to become familiar with the written language of Chinese medicine and thereby enrich their studies.